Hematology Laboratory Management and Practice

Hematology Laboratory Management and Practice

Edited by

S. M. Lewis BSc, MD, FRCPath, DCP
Emeritus Reader and Senior Research Fellow, Department of Haematology, Royal Postgraduate Medical School, London, UK

and

John A. Koepke BS, MS, MD, FCAP
Professor of Pathology and Associate Professor of Medicine, Duke University Medical Center, Durham, North Carolina, USA

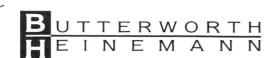

Butterworth-Heinemann Ltd
Linacre House, Jordan Hill, Oxford OX2 8DP

$\mathcal{R}$ A member of the Reed Elsevier plc group

OXFORD   LONDON   BOSTON
MUNICH   NEW DELHI   SINGAPORE   SYDNEY
TOKYO   TORONTO   WELLINGTON

First published 1995

© Butterworth-Heinemann Ltd 1995

British Library Cataloguing in Publication Data
Hematology Laboratory: Management and
Practice
 I. Lewis, S. M. II. Koepke, John A.
 616.15

ISBN 0 7506 0964 8

Library of Congress Cataloguing in Publication Data
Hematology laboratory management and practice/edited by S.M. Lewis
 and J.A. Koepke
   p.   cm.
 Includes bibliographical references and index.
 ISBN 0 7506 0964 8
 1. Hematology.   2. Pathological laboratories–Management.
 I. Lewis, S. M. II. Koepke, John A., 1929–
   [DNLM: 1. Laboratories—organization & administration.
 2. Hematologic Tests—standards.   3. Quality Control.   QY 23 H487
 1995]
 RB45.H54   1995   94–35300
 616.1′—dc20   CIP

Typeset by Datix International, Bungay and printed in Great Britain by Martins the Printers, Berwick upon Tweed.

Contents

Contributors

Paul Bachner MD
University of Kentucky Medical Center, Lexington,
Kentucky, USA

Daniel M. Baer MD
Veterans Affairs Medical Center, Portland, Oregon,
USA

Richard E. Belsey MD
Oregon Health Sciences University, Portland,
Oregon, USA

Willard E. Boyd III JD
Nyemaster and Partners, Des Moines,
Iowa, USA

B. Brozović MD PhD FRCPath
North London Blood Transfusion Centre
London, UK

M. Brozović MD FRCPath
Consultant Haematologist, Central Middlesex
Hospital, London, UK

Brian S. Bull MD
Department of Pathology and Laboratory Medicine,
Loma Linda University, Medical Center,
Loma Linda, California, USA

Lawrence W. Diamond MD
Pathology Institute, University of Cologne,
Germany

J. M. England MB PhD FRCPath
UKNEQAS(H), Watford General Hospital,
Watford, UK

Thomas M. Habermann MD
Division of Hematology and Internal Medicine,
Mayo Medical School, Rochester, Minnesota,
USA

William B. Hamlin MD
Laboratory of Pathology Inc.
Nordstrom Medical Tower, Seattle, Washington,
USA

D. A. Kennedy PhD FIBMS
Device Technology and Safety Group,
Medical Devices Agency, Department of Health,
London, UK

George G. Klee MD PhD
Department of Laboratory Medicine and Pathology,
Mayo Medical School, Rochester, Minnesota,
USA

John A. Koepke BS, MS, MD, FCAP
Duke University Medical Center, Durham, North
Carolina, USA

Mark D. Koepke JD
Health Plus – Presbyterian Hospital, Albuquerque,
New Mexico, USA

S. M. Lewis BSc MD FRCPath
Department of Haematology, Royal Postgraduate
Medical School, London, UK

Doyen T. Nguyen MD
Pathology Institute, University of Cologne,
Germany

A. Richardson-Jones
Clinical Laboratory, Coulter Corporation,
University of Miami Hospital and Clinics, Miami,
Florida, USA

R. M. Rowan FRCP MRCPath
Haematology Department, Western Infirmary,
Glasgow, UK

John A. Shively MD
Department of Pathology and Laboratory Medicine,
University of South Florida, College of Medicine,
Tampa, Florida, USA

A. Simmons PhD FIBMS
National Reference Laboratory, Nashville, Tennessee,
USA

Laurence P. Skendzel MD
Munson Medical Center, Traverse City,
Michigan, USA

Kent A. Spackman MD PhD
Department of Pathology, Oregon Health Sciences
University, Portland, Oregon, USA

John Stuart MD FRCP FRCPath
Department of Haematology, Medical School,
University of Birmingham, Birmingham, UK

O. W. van Assendelft MD PhD
National Center for Infectious Diseases,
Atlanta, Georgia, USA

R. L. Verwilghen MD PhD
Department of Haematology, University of Leuven,
Belgium

Preface

There are three essential components in good laboratory practice, namely: interlaboratory harmonization, quality assurance, organizational management. The International Council (originally Committee) for Standardization in Haematology was established in order to achieve harmonization by consensus on methods used in diagnostic tests and to define written and material standards. Its work has resulted in international recommendations on haemoglobinometry, cytometry, diagnostic tests with radionuclides, as well as various quantitative and qualitative tests on the constituents of the blood. The recommendations have appeared in selected scientific journals, and also in the ICSH published books and WHO manuals which are listed below. ICSH has organized symposia on quality assurance at the congresses of the International Society of Hematology which have been included in some of these publications.

Books previously published by ICSH

Erythrocytometric Methods and their Standardization (Ed. C. G. Boroviczeny) Karger, Basel, 1964.

Standardization, Documentation and Normal Values in Haematology (Ed. C. G. Boroviczeny) Karger, Basel, 1965.

Standardization in Haematology III (Ed. C. G. Boroviczeny) Karger, Basel, 1966.

Standardization in Hematology (Ed. G. Astaldi, C. Sirtori and G. Vanzetti) Franco Angeli Editore, Milan, 1970.

Modern Concepts in Hematology (Ed. G. Izak and S. M. Lewis) Academic Press, New York, 1972.

Abnormal Haemoglobins and Thalassaemia (Ed. R. M. Schmidt) Academic Press, New York, 1975.

Quality Control in Haematology (Ed. S. M. Lewis and J. F. Coster) Academic Press, London, 1975.

Advances in Hematological Methods: The Blood Count (Ed. O. W. van Assendelft and J. M. England) CRC Press, Boca Raton, Florida, 1982.

Quality Assurance in Haematology (Ed. S. M. Lewis and R. L. Verwilghen) Baillière Tindall, London, 1988.

WHO Manuals (World Health Organization, Geneva)

Quality Assurance in Haematology (S. M. Lewis), 1986.
Calibration and Maintenance of Semi-automated Haematology Equipment (J. M. England, S. M. Lewis, E. Lloyd and R. M. Rowan), 1992

Technical proficiency has always been the cornerstone of the laboratory, but in recent years professional expertise in the organization and management of the laboratory has assumed an important role in good laboratory practice, especially taking account of the dramatic way in which laboratory practice has changed in recent years: the advent of sophisticated instruments and automation, increasing costs of labour, equipment and reagents as well as increasing demands for diagnostic tests, and expectation of accuracy by clinicians who have become reliant on the laboratory. The laboratory is accountable to hospital management, to auditors, and to national health authorities as well as to its customers. The laboratory director has legal and ethical obligations to ensure that the tests which are carried out are appropriate for the diagnostic problems and provide reliable analytic results; he or she must also ensure the safety and welfare of those who work in the laboratory. And we are now facing a further challenge as the long-established traditions of laboratory service change to meet market forces by the use of industrial methods which are leading to increasing regulatory controls. It becomes important that the laboratory should be in the vanguard in structuring these regulations.

ICSH has accepted the challenge to provide guidance on these topics, including those concerned with the complexities of regulatory affairs. Each subject is dealt with in one or more chapters in which the opinions of internationally recognized experts are presented under the aegis of ICSH.

S. M. Lewis
J. A. Koepke

Part One

Role of the Physician in Hematology Laboratory Practice

1

Proper use of the hematology laboratory

M. Brozović and S. M. Lewis

The hematology laboratory of today is no longer simply the laboratory where blood counts are performed and blood films looked at. Although blood counts comprise a significant proportion of the work, hospital blood transfusion service, cytochemistry, cell surface markers, red cell enzyme measurement, investigation of abnormal hemoglobins, tests of hemostasis, and many other investigations form an integral part of a modern hematology laboratory. In some instances the laboratory is burdened by unnecessary demands; conversely it may be underused if the facilities provided and the clinical usefulness of the tests are not fully appreciated.

Hematological investigation is usually requested for one of the following reasons:

1. *To screen for a possible abnormality.* Preoperative blood tests, antenatal screening, screening for insurance or employment purposes, general health checks and tests on industrial workers exposed to potentially toxic substances fall into this category. The repertoire of tests used for screening is limited and they are generally performed using automated equipment. The proportion of abnormal results is low and specialist physician expertise is required in a few cases only.

2. *To diagnose or exclude blood disease or to help establish a specific medical diagnosis* characterized by unique hematological features, such as malaria, malabsorption syndromes, etc. The initial tests are usually simple and often performed using automated equipment. The definitive diagnostic tests may, however, be technologically complex and require time and expertise. Input from a specialist hematologist is essential.

3. *To monitor treatment or provide appropriate supportive care.* This is the case when providing blood and blood components for surgery; providing blood products and components for patients with hemorrhagic diathesis; providing appropriate support for chemotherapy and radiotherapy; or monitoring antithrombotic or thrombolytic treatment. This aspect of laboratory work requires specialized services and

cannot function without continuous input from a specialist hematologist.

4. *To provide hematological tests and blood transfusion services in an emergency, 24 hours a day.* The tests performed are usually simple and the total volume of work may be small, but a reliable and continuous presence of laboratory facilities and of expert advice impose important organizational constraints.

5. *To provide specialist investigations* necessary for diagnosis and/or monitoring of some blood diseases. These include the diagnosis and classification of acute leukemia, minimal residual disease, complicated tests of hemostasis or thrombosis, peripheral blood stem cell collection and related services, and investigations for hemoglobinopathy.

6. *To evaluate new methods and equipment.* This function is becoming increasingly important because of the rapid development of new technologies and aggressive marketing techniques by manufacturers.

7. *To monitor extra-laboratory or near-patient testing* whether performed within the hospital or in health centers or doctor's offices. Although there are at present relatively few hematological tests used in this way, extra-laboratory testing is likely to expand in volume and importance in the future (see Chapter 5).

8. *To provide laboratory facilities for hematological research.* The laboratory support for hematological research may be provided in two ways: The state of art technology can be used to investigate or identify new aspects of blood diseases, or, alternatively, research laboratories may provide sophisticated technology and/or large volume automated tests for drug trials or epidemiological studies.

1.1 The organization and siting of different functions

In some large units all aspects of hematological laboratory work may be represented within one department.

In other units, different aspects are separated; for example, screening, diagnostic and emergency services may be directed and run by a general clinical pathologist, whereas the specialized and monitoring services are supervised by a specialist hematologist.

In the UK, all hematological laboratory services including the hospital blood transfusion services, have traditionally been united under a specialist hematologist who is also in charge of patients with blood diseases (BCSH, 1991). The unity of specialist and generalist provision for hematology ensures high quality medical and technological expertise even in small laboratories. Most, if not all hematological disorders can be reliably diagnosed and safely treated in the local unit, thus saving time, effort and transport costs. Nevertheless, this strategy carries certain disadvantages. If every laboratory is to provide a full and reliable service regardless of the size of workload, the cost per test becomes prohibitive. If, however, agressive cost cutting is applied, new techniques and equipment cannot be acquired, and the quality of service inevitably deteriorates.

The alternative approach, common in other European countries and in the USA, is for the specialist hematologist to run his own specialist laboratory service. Screening and high volume diagnostic tests are performed by a general laboratory, usually in conjunction with blood biochemistry, urine microbiology and biochemistry, and simple microbiological techniques.

This approach ensures that the general laboratory has a rapid throughput and is cost-effective. It also encourages research and development within the general laboratory. The disadvantages are the lack of specialist expertise in the general laboratory and the consequent need to refer abnormal test results for further investigations. It is also possible that subtle but important hematological changes, e.g. those detected on the blood film such as a few blast cells, will be missed by the generalist in the high volume automated laboratory and a potentially dangerous delay in diagnosis may be incurred.

The specialist laboratory can concentrate on complex investigations and develop expertise without the burden of a large number of tests with results within the normal reference range. The majority of patients investigated are those already looked after by the specialist in charge; this ensures the continuity of care and a full understanding of the implications of the test results. The disadvantages of an isolated specialist laboratory include the increasingly high level but narrow specialization of the staff and the danger of relaxing the discipline which is imposed by the quality assurance procedures inherent in running large numbers of tests.

The supervision of extra-laboratory or near-patient testing is an important new function likely to be carried out by the general or by the British style of unified laboratory. Many biochemical investigations have been ingeniously adapted to the new technology; the hematological repertoire is at present limited but such diverse investigations as the measurement of hemoglobin concentration, coagulation tests and sickle solubility test can be performed at the bedside or in the doctor's office without laboratory space or expertise. The advantage of this approach is the immediate availability of the result to the clinician and to the patient. However, satisfactory quality assurance is difficult to achieve and the sensitivity of the technology is limited, so that some abnormalities cannot be reliably detected. Furthermore, the near-patient technology at present remains costly in comparison with the conventional approach. To ensure that this promising new approach is used in a cost-effective and clinically safe way, close supervision, quality assurance and continuing training of the user is essential; these roles are best undertaken by the local hospital laboratory.

In developing countries, the problems of hematological laboratory investigations are different. At the local level, even under favourable economic circumstances, only a few simple tests can be performed. Specialized and/or more complex tests are usually only available centrally. The World Health Organization (1987) is especially concerned with the development of laboratory services and the provision of appropriate technology. Three levels of laboratory facilities are recommended:

Primary Health Centre with a small laboratory facility, staffed by laboratory assistants, where hemoglobinometry using a comparator, erythrocyte sedimentation rate, leukocyte count in a counting chamber and microscopic examination of blood film for cell morphology and parasites are performed.

Primary Level District Hospital, where a laboratory with trained technologists can perform more sophisticated tests such as blood cell counting using non-automated simple counters, hemoglobinometry, microhematocrit, blood grouping and cross-match, simple coagulation tests and microscopy. However, in many cases even simple cell counters are not available, and counts must be carried out in hemocytometer chambers.

Regional and Central laboratories should have the facilities to perform more sophisticated blood counting techniques, all coagulation tests, enzyme assays, cytochemistry, to deal with advanced morphological problems and to carry out radio assays, immunophenotyping, and chromosome analysis, as well as investigations using DNA technology.

The proper use of any hematology laboratory thus depends on the local philosophy of the laboratory organization and usage.

1.2 The place of a unified hematology laboratory

A unified hematology laboratory, where every sample is treated as having a potentially significant blood abnormality, has many advantages and is attractive to technologists and specialist hematologists. A careful screening procedure inherent in this approach ensures that no significant abnormality is missed and that appropriate additional investigations are instituted without delay. Technologists and doctors are exposed to a spectrum of hematological problems and acquire enviable and unique expertise. This allows the most effective use of available resources and optimal care for patients with hematological problems.

One of the misuses of the unified laboratory arises as a result of potential overinvestigation of trivial problems. For example, full investigation for hemoglobinopathy may not be necessary in every patient showing red cell microcytosis and normal iron status. It is becoming increasingly clear that carefully designed protocols (practice guidelines) for laboratory investigations of common blood disorders should be applied to provide a balance between not investigating in sufficient depth and overinvestigating.

In order to remain cost-effective, unified laboratories must be subject to planned centralization of some highly specialized services, such as DNA technology, cytogenetics, complex tests of hemostasis, etc. The decision as to which services might be centralized must be made with full knowledge of local circumstances. For example, if the hospital contains a Hemophilia Centre, complex tests of hemostasis are required on site and should not be transferred to another institution.

Supportive and monitoring services are best performed by the unified laboratory: costly blood products and components are dealt with by staff familiar with clinical cases and possible problems. Continuity of care and rationalization of usage can be accomplished.

Unified laboratories are an important teaching and training resource for technologists, nurses and doctors, as well as for undergraduate and postgraduate students.

1.3 Hematology as a part of general clinical pathology laboratory

An increasing number of tests (full blood count, white cell differential, erythrocyte sedimentation rate, reticulocyte count, serum vitamin B_{12}, folate and ferritin measurements, one-stage prothrombin time, partial thromboplastin time, thrombin time, coagulation factor assays, etc.) can now be performed using fully automated equipment with large throughput. Reliable software is available for quality assurance. The new technology enables large workloads to be processed quickly and without operator fatigue. The flagging process for results outside the reference range can be finely adjusted to ensure that abnormal results are identified and acted upon.

One of the most important traditional hematological skills, that of microscopy and blood film morphology, is almost inevitably reduced and eventually lost in a general automated laboratory. The sensitivity and accuracy of automated differential counting and its concordance with careful manual differential counts was recently studied in Britain (Birch et al., 1991a). The results from two large general hospitals (Birch et al., 1991b) showed that they could safely use automated differential counting in combination with 11 parameter profile to reduce the percentage of blood films examined microscopically to just over 20%. There was less than 9% of false negatives and only 2 of them showed clinically significant missed abnormalities. By comparison, in teaching and specialized units (Lewis and Rowan, 1991), which dealt with many abnormal films, automated differential counting reduced the number of films examined by 20 to 45%. The percentage of false negatives was between 1.6 and 4.8 and none had clinically significant abnormalities. The main limitation of the algorithms used by the participating units was the generation of a relatively large number of false positives, that is films where no abnormality was detected on microscopic examination. Thus, algorithms require to be prepared specifically for the local situation. There is no doubt that careful use of an appropriate algorithm with automated differential counters can significantly reduce the need for microscopic examination of blood films. Nevertheless, the skill of microscopic morphology can never be completely compensated for by the automated instruments as these have well recognized shortcomings: for example, differential cell counters cannot reliably detect small numbers of blasts cells, or fine morphological features of the red cells, such as basophilic stippling.

The training of technologists and clinical pathologists working in general laboratories should always include traditional manual hematological skills; continuing professional education should ensure that the skills are retained and improved.

It is important that technologists and general pathologists on the one hand, and the physicians using the laboratory on the other, recognize the limitations of large-scale automated technology and adapt their practice to the changed standards. If there is a strong clinical suspicion of a hematological abnormality, a negative or normal result should be confirmed using specialized or more specific tests, and a blood film should always be examined by an experienced morphologist, even though this may present organizational difficulties and cause a significant delay.

Carefully designed and regularly reviewed and up-dated protocols are essential to ensure that general laboratories possess a safety net for most blood abnormalities.

Large general laboratories provide a quick, 24-hour per day laboratory service and are usually very cost-effective. New technology and organizational innovations are welcomed and introduced early. In contrast, a small general laboratory cannot be as cost-effective and is in danger of staff loss because the volume of work in any one discipline is insufficient to maintain interest and standards. There is thus a critical size for an efficient automated general laboratory. Small multidisciplinary laboratories must use different technology, staff training and protocols.

The role of medically qualified pathologists in general laboratories has been debated for many years (College of American Pathologists, 1993). Medical skills are not essential for the management and organization of large factory-like laboratories; this is not to say that a medically qualified clinical pathologist may not excel in and enjoy running a large automated laboratory. Nevertheless, medical input is essential for a general laboratory: the place and role of laboratory investigations in the wider context of health care can only be fully appreciated by an individual trained in both clinical medicine and laboratory sciences. Medical input should never be haphazard: a planned and systematic input provides not only the interpretation of complex laboratory investigations but also ensures that appropriate technology is used and that continuous development of the service takes place. Frequent interaction with other disciplines and awareness of the needs of individual patients, groups of patients and services (such as gastroenterology or cardiology) is a hallmark of a successful hematological section of a general laboratory and can only be provided by a medically qualified pathologist.

Hematological medical input is even more important for a small multidisciplinary laboratory where expertise and standards can easily fall: medical input becomes a combination of consultation and education.

The training of laboratory-orientated hematologists has become increasingly complex because of the need to acquire knowledge and expertise in analytical, research and clinical aspects of hematology, as well as in communication, team leadership, management and public relations (College of American Pathologists, 1993). The training programmes do not always reflect these rapidly changing goals and must be regularly and carefully scrutinized. A curriculum which has been proposed by the European Division of the International Society of Hematology is shown in the Annexe (see page 9).

1.4 Specialist hematology laboratory

A specialist laboratory may be completely separate or may complement a large general pathology laboratory. The size and scope is dictated by the local circumstances. In many academic institutions, a specialist laboratory carries out many research functions. The supportive functions (provision of blood and blood products, monitoring of chemotherapy, thrombolytic therapy or bleeding problems) are usually supervised by a specialist hematologist and may be a part of the specialist laboratory. Some specialist laboratories have evolved into supra-specialist referral centres for specific and complex situations, and they fulfil an important and often unique function.

It may be difficult to obtain specialist opinion for the common hematological problems such as anemia of chronic disorder or mild neutropenia, when the specialist laboratory is small and entirely dedicated to one aspect of hematology, e.g. leukemia or hypercoagulable states. In such a situation, provisions for diagnosis, and treatment of common hematological conditions must be established and if necessary, tests 'farmed out' to a central general laboratory or to an appropriate specialist service.

The need to adhere to the quality assessment and laboratory accreditation schemes must always be kept in mind, however small, narrowly specialized or eminent the laboratory may be. The training and professional development of the technologists and doctors staffing specialist laboratories deserves particular attention. Continuing education should always retain some basic general hematological tecniques appropriate to the laboratory in question. Specialist laboratory is in itself an important educational resource for the generalist and should be freely available for teaching and training of the technologists and doctors working in other specialities.

Decision on which tests are performed by the general as opposed to the specialist laboratory often causes problems. A valuable research investigation frequently evolves into a widely used test, which is eventually adapted for a fully automated method capable of large throughput. The decision whether such a test joins the battery of tests performed by the general laboratory or not, should always be made formally, on the basis of available expertise, workload and cost. If large throughput tests are indiscriminately left to the specialist laboratory, the flexibility and the specialist character of the laboratory may eventually be lost.

Another important issue for the specialist laboratory is whether or not to accept all referred investigations. Some investigations may be clinically unjustified, some may be sent with insufficient patient information and some may be so costly as to be justifiable only after full standard investigation has been completed. The criteria for accepting a specialist investigation must be firmly established and implemented.

The dichotomy between the specialist and the generalist may be a positive force inducive of research and development, but may also cause serious professional problems and lead to less than optimal care with costly duplication of effort and equipment on the same site. A formal and regular review of services offered by all laboratories within an institution should be carried out by the management and professions to minimize the risk of this happening.

1.5 Near-patient testing in hematology

Erythrocyte sedimentation rate, hemoglobin measurement and sickle solubility tests have been performed as side-room tests for many years (see also Chapter 5). Many new card or cartridge tests, sometimes using a hand-held electronic or optical reader, are now available; they arc becoming increasingly attractive to doctors and patients. The repertoire of such tests is widening. At present, the technology is relatively primitive and the tests are unable to detect some important abnormalities reliably. Nevertheless, it is only a question of time before the dry chemistry technology is applied to hematology, and the reliability and accuracy of various tests reaches a satisfactory level.

One of the main roles of near-patient testing is likely to be an immediate triage of abnormal results for further referral. On one hand, early exclusion (identification) of abnormality has important cost, convenience and, above all, clinical implications. On the other hand, if rapid proliferation of near-patient testing occurs in the primary care without appropriate controls or education of the user, it may paradoxically result in missed diagnostic opportunities, delays in treatment and increased costs for the health service. The long-term effect of such proliferation of near-patient testing on conventional laboratories must also be kept in mind.

To ensure that near-patient technology is used to the patient's best advantage, each test must be validated and its use and usefulness closely monitored. The user must be trained how to collect samples, use the equipment or kit, record and interpret the results. The users should participate in an external quality assessment scheme. A procedure for dealing with abnormal results must be set. It will also be necessary to register and accredit each user of near-patient technology. The most effective way forward is to place all users of near-patient facilities under the jurisdiction of the local hospital laboratory; the trained personnel from the hospital will then monitor the equipment and the use of kits, check quality assurance performance and provide necessary training. Accreditation can also be obtained through the parent laboratory. This approach will also ensure that near-patient testing is not perceived as competition against the conventional laboratory, but rather as a complementing and enhancing development.

Interpretation of results of near-patient testing requires particular care. The limitations of the definition of 'normality' in near-patient testing must be made abundantly clear to the user, for example, hemoglobin concentration within the reference range does not exclude macrocytosis due to megaloblastic anemia with all its subsequent clinical symptoms.

Near-patient coagulation tests are, in theory, ideally suited for monitoring anticoagulant therapy in a large number of geographically dispersed patients on life-long treatment. This can be achieved if the methodology is reliable, subject to stringent quality control and sufficiently simple to guarantee operator compliance. A systematic field check of the safety and reliability of such a system, as well as the participation in quality assurance, must be an intrinsic part of near-patient control of anticoagulation.

Appropriate legislation is necessary to make near-patient testing a safe and reliable option.

1.6 Emergency hematology

Laboratories with large workloads often work extended hours or a shift system, and many tests are available 24 hours per day without the need for special arrangements. In contrast, small laboratories usually function during the day only, and special arrangements must be made to provide a limited repertoire of tests and blood transfusion facilities should an emergency arise outside the working hours. Ideally, the technology used during the day and the technologist who normally performs the tests should be employed. The number of staff may be too small to allow internal cover for the emergency service and outside staff may be employed. In this case, their skills and reliability must be regularly checked.

In some circumstances, where the emergency workload is small, the technology used is different from that normally used. Kits and near-patient technology are some of the options. Careful monitoring of performance, as well as the use of external quality assurance schemes which include exercises specifically designed for checking emergency and after-hour services is required in this case. If the workload is very small, alternative arrangements, such as the use of an outside laboratory, should be considered.

1.7 Selection of tests for different organizational models

Simple tests are suitable for the primary care environment, but the simplicity of execution does not necessarily mean that the test can be interpreted as a simple yes–no or normal–abnormal. Some simple tests, such as ESR or one-stage prothrombin time, may be required at specialized facilities because of their universal screening value. Sophisticated tests may be adapted for simple technology requiring little technical skill, but such tests may only be indicated after a detailed preliminary investigation. A laboratory with a small throughput may decide to use a manual and labour intensive technique for an infrequently used test; the same test may be performed using simple automated technology or kits in a central laboratory with a large throughput. The definition of simple and sophisticated is only meaningful in the context of a single laboratory; the test and technology selection are dictated by the clinical need, size of workload, financial and staffing constraints and by many other factors.

1.8 On the misuse of hematology laboratory facilities

Hematological laboratory facilities can be misused in the following general ways:

1. Inappropriate or unnecessary tests may be offered to the user.
2. Inappropriate or unnecessary tests may be requested by the clinician.
3. Appropriate investigations may be misinterpreted or ignored.
4. Tests essential for diagnosis or monitoring of treatment may be omitted or are unavailable.

1.8.1 Inappropriate choice of tests by the laboratory

The choice of tests is dictated by the availability of technology, local needs, tradition and personal preferences of the hematologist-in-charge. In many laboratories there is an inherent inertia which may prevent timely change; manufacturers have a tendency to avoid costly and risky enterprise technology, and to concentrate their efforts on improving the well-established tests. This favours obsolete approaches and concepts.

In contrast, laboratories may be tempted to try new techniques or equipment because of commercial pressures; tests of limited value may be offered free of charge or at reduced cost under the guise of trial, often to laboratories with little or no expertise. Regular audit of new technology may help identify such a situation and discourage further similar occurrences. A careful balance between obsolete, and new but unknown must be established and maintained at all times.

1.8.2 Overuse

The best weapon against overuse of any laboratory facility is education; in-service, undergraduate, postgraduate and continuing education have an often overlooked role in ensuring appropriate use. The use of laboratory facilities is an important but costly diagnostic tool and should be taught like any other skill to doctors, nurses, technologists and other health professions. Battery testing and indiscriminate screening for any abnormality have no place in today's cost-conscious society. Hematologists must take a leading role in educating the user on what, when and how of laboratory hematology.

Good and professionally knowledgeable management is an equally effective tool for ensuring that the laboratory is used properly. Hematology is part of the health care offered to the community. It must be subject to the same planning and management rules as all other aspects of the care offered and must meet the needs of the community it serves. For example, laboratory facilities for investigation of hemoglobinopathies are essential if there are many thalassemia or sickle-cell disease sufferers within the community. A large group of hemophiliacs needs access to a reliable hemostasis laboratory and blood transfusion facility. A laboratory service built in response to a perceived local need is likely to be used appropriately because there is already a wealth of local expertise and understanding of the problem.

Protocols and professional guidelines, such as the recently published Standard Haematology Practice, prepared by the British Committee for Standards in Haematology, refered to above, provide standards that can be applied to all laboratories regardless of their size and type and may help ensure appropriate use. Such guidelines should always be kept simple and user friendly.

1.8.3 Misinterpretation

Test results may be misinterpreted or ignored for a variety of reasons: from a simple mechanical failure to send or receive reports, to a failure to appreciate the true significance of an 'abnormal' or a 'normal' result. The expectation of the user is for an immediate, absolute and correct result; this expectation is fostered by continuing improvements in information technology. The user often fails to realize that there is an unavoidable and possibly irreducible margin of error in a multi-stage complex process of laboratory investigation. The limitations of the test and technique are forgotten and simple yes–no philosophy is applied. It is essential that information technology is used to ensure that the user is aware of the true significance of any one result of any one test. Tables, algorithms and graphical presentation of results are preferable to a simple reference range.

Increasing devolvement of tests for use in primary

care must be accompanied by information technology which will allow a knowledgeable and appropriate interpretation of results.

1.8.4 Underuse

When limited resources do not allow all required investigations to be offered to the patient and his doctors, the limitations of the service must be made clear to the users and whenever possible arrangements made for essential investigations to be carried out elsewhere. The legal liability for the laboratory services not provided because of the shortage of funds rests with the hospital management or the health authority who ultimately hold the responsibility for the allocation of funds at the local level.

A strict demarcation between service on one hand, and research and development on the other, becomes necessary in a situation where resource is scarce. In ideal circumstances service follows research and development closely and is poised to use the latest developments to the best advantage of the patient as soon as possible. This usually results in improved clinical service at an increased cost, so that an objective assessment of cost-effectiveness should be made.

1.9 The future

With advancing technology, the hematology laboratory of the future will be able to provide not only a virtually immediate test result for common tests such as full blood count, coagulation tests, serum concentration of various hematinics, etc., but also a wide variety of complex investigations such as investigation of disorders of hemostasis, hemoglobin abnormalities, cell surface markers and many others.

Many tests will inevitably be carried out in primary care using dry chemistry or simple miniaturized equipment. They will be subject to the same stringent monitoring, quality assurance and interpretation as the tests performed in the laboratory. Samples for further investigation from the primary care and samples collected within the hospital will initially be analysed using rapid turn-over, automated tests. All flagged specimens will be referred to an appropriate specialist facility. Whether the screening and the specialized facility remain under one roof will probably be determined by tradition, geographic and economic factors.

The repertoire of sophisticated tests will continue to expand and pressure to move such tests from a specialist to a screening facility will increase because of the commercial implications of large-scale usage of reagents and equipment. How are the hematologists to determine whether or not a new test can justifiably be used on a large scale?

It is no longer feasible to wait for the results of large trials or for many reports on vast numbers of controls and patients; peer opinion and acceptance are notoriously slow in the milieu of consumer and market pressures. The significance of a test may also depend on local factors, for example, a simple test to exclude the presence of malaria parasites in blood without microscopy is of little interest in a laboratory in Northern Europe, but is a major advance to be widely used in tropical countries.

It will become necessary to establish a mechanism for introducing new tests and technology. This mechanism must balance cost containment and improvements in patient care against salesmanship and sometimes conflicting professional advice. In order to avoid fragmentation of effort and ensure that all hematologists share their experiences and expertise, a regular review of technology, both new and old, should be conducted and the information made available to each laboratory. This can be achieved through a central government or profession-run organization, possibly using designated units to assess new technology. With increasing specialization, such an approach may become essential in maintaining contact with complex investigative techniques and new ideas in hematology.

Another possible scenario must be considered for the post-industrial society: that of diminishing resources imposing general reduction rather than expansion in the future. If such a reduction becomes reality, essential services should be safeguarded. The decision as to what are the essential and what are the luxury services, must be made by the profession in consultation with authorities, users and patient representatives. It is unlikely that a completely satisfactory and safe solution can be achieved, but the profession must attempt to safeguard the best essential services as perceived at the time, while still keeping a potential for research and development. Let us hope that the future is not bleak and that the hematology will continue to strive for improvement, new knowledge and the ultimate goal of perfection.

Annexe

Model training programme in hematology
(Keith Shinton. Formerly Chairman Education and Training Committee of the European and African Division of the International Society of Hematology.)

The Education and Training Committee of the European and African Division of the International Society of Hematology decided in 1988 that a harmonized training programme in Hematology was required for Europe. To achieve this the current arrangements for training in Hematology were collected by the chairman of the training committee following circulation of a questionnaire and where necessary interview with an appropriate national hematologist concerned in training. The results of this survey were given as a communication to the Training Committee and subsequently published (Shinton, 1993). By consensus discussion the Training Committee developed a Model Training Programme which combined clinical and laboratory hematology training and was compatible with other medical training programmes of the European Union of Medical Specialties (UEMS). This Model Training Programme is reproduced below.

Specialist/postgraduate training in general hematology. Model Curriculum recommended by the International Society of Hematology (European and African Division)

1. Postgraduate training leading to a recognized specialist qualification in general hematology should be entered after successful completion of at least 6 years undergraduate medical training which includes a period as intern or pre-registration clinical training. This should be followed by a period of 2–3 years clinical vocational training in internal medicine, including pediatrics.
2. Hematology is recognized as both a clinical and laboratory based discipline including the subspecialities of hemostasis and hospital blood transfusion. This general hematology training curriculum is the minimum required for a general hematologist practising at a general hospital.
3. Postgraduate training foreseen in this model curriculum should extend over at least 3 years fulltime education, or its equivalent if training is undertaken on a part-time basis.
4. Training must be undertaken in departments of hematology in hospitals where all aspects of the speciality are practised and where instruction and experience provided will enable the trainee to take full responsibility for the investigation and management of patients with primary hematological disorders.
5. Training must consist of an appropriate and planned balance between clinical and laboratory teaching.
6. The training should be subject to some form of structured evaluation. Successful completion of training should be confirmed by the award of a diploma, certificate or other evidence of formal qualification.
7. Hematology is a rapidly changing subject and the total content of the training programme will need to be reviewed at regular intervals. At the present time minimum range of training should include:

a. CLINICAL HEMATOLOGY

Bone marrow failure and role of bone marrow transplantation.

Anemias.

Disorders of hemoglobin structure.

Hematological malignancies including leukemias, lymphoma, myeloma, myelodysplastic syndromes and chronic myeloproliferative disorders.

Congenital and acquired bleeding disorders.

Thrombo-embolic disorders.

Hospital Blood Transfusion including collection and storage of blood and cell separation.

Hematological problems associated with antenatal, delivery and postnatal care; intensive care; renal medicine, organ transplantation, orthopedic and cardiovascular surgery.

Consultations regarding patients with secondary hematological disorders in other departments.

b. LABORATORY HEMATOLOGY

Collection of blood samples, their transport and storage.

Morphology of blood cells and marrow aspirates including cytochemistry, cytogenetic and immunological techniques.

Hemoglobin estimation in whole blood and plasma with its catabolic products.

Hemoglobin electrophoresis with measurement of Hb F, A_2 and detection of abnormal hemoglobins.

Blood cell counting and sizing by both visual and automated methods.

Erythrocyte sedimentation rate and plasma viscosity.

Erythrocyte osmotic fragility, autohemolysis and detection of PNH.

Erythrocyte enzyme determinations.

Hemostatic measurement: bleeding time, platelet function.

Coagulation factor studies by prothrombin time, partial thromboplastin time, thrombin time and individual factor assays.

Control of anticoagulant and thrombolytic therapy.

Basic immunological methods.

Basic molecular techniques applied to inherited and acquired hematological disorders.

Use of radionuclides for blood volume, red cell mass, erythrokinetics, ferrokinetics, vitamin B_{12} folate and ferritin measurement.

Identification of blood group antigens and antibodies.

Compatibility testing of blood transfusion.

Investigation of blood transfusion reactions.

Auto-immune antibody testing.

Emergency procedures.

Principles of laboratory practice, organization and management training, particularly in resource allocation, budget control, audit, quality assurance and personnel supervision.

Standardization and statistical methods as applied to analytic data.

Epidemiology and geographic pathology.
Laboratory safety of staff.
Medical ethics.

c. COMPLETION OF A SMALL RESEARCH PROJECT.

References

Birch, A. J., Brozovic, M., Lewis, S. M. *et al.* (1991a) Role of blood film with automated blood counting systems. In: Roberts B. (ed.), *Standard Haematology Practice*. Oxford: Blackwell Scientific Publications, pp. 19–22.

Birch, A. J., Brozovic, M., Lewis, S. M. *et al.* (1991b) Assessment of the need for blood film examination with blood counts by second generation light scatter counters. In: Roberts B. (ed.), *Standard Haematology Practice*. Oxford: Blackwell Scientific Publications, pp. 23–33.

British Committee for Standards in Haematology (BCSH) – General Haematology Task Force (1991) Code for good laboratory practice in Haematology Laboratories (including hospital blood banks): In Roberts B. (ed.), *Standard Haematology Practice*. Oxford: Blackwell Scientific Publications, pp. 1–18.

College of American Pathologists (1993) Issues in pathology residency training. Pathology patterns. *Am. J. Clin. Pathol.*, **100** (supplement), 1–47.

Lewis, S. M. and Rowan, R. M. (1991) Assessment of the need for blood film examination with blood counts by aperture – impedence systems. In: Roberts, B. (ed.), *Standard Haematology Practice*. Oxford: Blackwell Scientific Publications, pp. 34–42.

Shinton, K. (1993) Postgraduate Education, Training and Specialization in Haematology. *Haematologia*, **25**, 1553–1640.

World Health Organization (1987) Laboratory Services at the Primary Health Care Level. World Health Organization Publication, WHO/LAB/87.2.

2

Interpretive aspects of hematology tests with a focus on the blood film

John A. Shively

'I have a turn both for observation and for deduction.'
Sherlock Holmes in '*A Study in Scarlet*'

2.1 Introduction

The interpretation of hematology test data in diagnosis is dependent on a number of considerations by a physician. Not only are the results important and useful in the diagnosis of primary hematological disorders of the bone marrow and hematopoiesis, but changes in hematological data may also be seen in diseases affecting other organs and tissues. These manifestations are initially or even chiefly alterations of hematology values and in reality are only a secondary expression of systemic disturbances or disorders (Zuelzer, 1957). Secondary hematological changes may be manifest as anemias of infection, renal failure, malignant disease or as leukemoid reactions associated with bacterial, viral or parasitic infections, as well as the thrombocytopenia secondary to portal hypertension and the associated splenomegaly. These inter-relationships with systemic diseases is perhaps best exemplified by the definition of hematology, proposed by some wag, who stated that hematology was 'all of the diseases of the blood and all of the organs through which it flows!'

An initial and important consideration in the interpretation of hematological data is the accuracy and validity of numerical values, i.e. blood counts, hemoglobin concentration, and hematocrit. With the use of automated blood cell counters and instruments that also perform leukocyte differential counts, the accuracy of data from the hematology laboratory has improved in recent years so that the precision as well as accuracy of these tests are quite acceptable. However, standardization of the procedures and the validity of test data are dependent on a disciplined program of quality control with the use of accurate standards and quality control specimens which are needed to maintain both accuracy and precision. Also needed is a program of quality assurance that ensures proper identification of specimens, correct ratio of anticoagulant to blood specimen, prompt transmission of data in order that the clinician can make a timely decision for patient care, all of these being important. The sensitivity and specificity for the individual test values are significant benchmarks for the interpretation of hematological test data as is the predictive value for the suspected disease in the patient population being tested.

In the automated counting systems, the presence of qualitative flags or quantitatively abnormal results indicate the need to review the blood film and/or perform a manual differential count. Using a 'three-part' automated differential count, review rates (screen or manual differential) have varied from 5% on a population of ambulatory patients (Kalish, Goldberg and Roberts, 1987) to 42% in hospitalized patients (Ross *et al.*, 1985). In one series with slightly more sophisticated instrumentation, approximately 50% of the automated differential counts in a hospital population had to be manually counted or screened (Krause, 1990) (see also pages 5 and 191).

The interpretation and use of hematological test data varies as to whether the tests are being used as a screening procedure for the presence or absence of disease, i.e. problem sensing, or whether the tests are providing essential criteria to be met for the diagnosis of a specific disease. The data may also be used in the monitoring or maintenance of an optimal level of a hematological component during therapy of a disease process. While accuracy is always a laudable goal, precision is essential in this setting and significant changes will influence dosage of drugs and management decisions. This stage in the interpretation of hematological data should be considered as information processing with determination of normal versus abnormal values for the red cell, leukocyte and platelet counts as well as distinguishing between normal and abnormal hemoglobin and hematocrit values. Equally important is an assessment of the red cell indices, and examination of the histograms of red cell and platelet sizes, in addition to an evaluation of the values and the scattergrams of the leukocyte differential count.

Table 2.1 Average normal blood values in infancy and childhood (from Miller, Bachner and McMillian, 1984)

Age	Hemoglobin (g/dl)	RBC (× 10¹²/l)	Hematocrit	MCV (fl)	MCV (pg)	MCHC (%)	Reticulocytes (%)
Cord blood	16.8	5.25	63	120	34	31.7	3.2
1 day	19	5.14	61	119	36.9	31.6	3.2
3 days	18.7	5.11	62	116	36.5	31.1	3.8
7 days	17.9	4.86	56	118	36.2	32	0.5
2 weeks	17.3	4.8	54	112	36.8	32.1	0.5
3 weeks	15.6	4.2	46	111	37.1	33.9	0.8
4 weeks	14.2	4	43	105	35.5	33.5	0.6
2 months	10.7	3.4	31	93	31.5	34.1	1.8
3 months	11.3	3.7	33	88	30.5	34.8	0.7
6 months	12.3	4.6	36	78	27	34	1.4
8 months	12.1	4.6	36	77	26	34	1.1
10 months	11.9	4.6	36	77	26	34	1
1 year	11.6	4.6	35	77	25	33	0.9
2 years	11.7	4.7	35	78	25	33	1
4 years	12.6	4.7	37	80	27	34	1
6 years	12.7	4.7	38	80	27	33	1
8 years	12.9	4.7	39	80	27	33	1
10 12 years	13	4.8	39	80	27	33	1
Adult men	16	5.4	47	87	29	34	1
Adult women	14	4.8	42	87	29	34	1

2.2 Reference ranges and physiological variations

The theory of reference values is described in chapter 15. In this context 'What is normal?' is an important question that needs to be considered for each component of hematological test data. The age of the patient influences the normal reference range of values, especially during the newborn period and subsequent childhood, as shown in Tables 2.1 and 2.2, with a stabilization and consistency of the values in later adult life showing only male/female differences in the red cell count, hematocrit and hemoglobin levels (Table 2.3). The age-related changes in the leukocyte and differential count are depicted in graphic format as average values in Figure 2.1 with the leukocyte count in the first 24 hours postnatal period and the predominance of lymphocytes in the differential count during early childhood being potential interpretive issues for the patient's physician. There is little or no variation in the normal older individual from the middle-aged adult, but the black population has been found to have a slightly lower hemoglobin level than caucasians (Van Assendelft, 1991). Also, black persons have consistently lower mean leukocyte counts than white persons as well as a lower segmented neutrophil mean count (Van Assendelft *et al.*, 1977).

The concentration of red blood cells per unit volume is influenced by blood volume alterations, the most consistently predictable example being seen in normal pregnancy as demonstrated in Table 2.4 (Hytten, 1985). The units in which the results are reported are important. Le système international

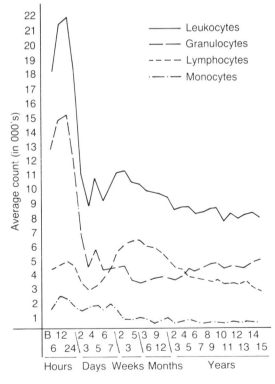

Figure 2.1 Graphic presentation of average leukocyte counts from birth to 15 years of age. (From Kato, 1935)

d'unités (SI units) is used extensively in Europe and has been recommended by World Health

Table 2.2 Normal leukocyte counts (from Dallman, 1977)

Age	Total leukocytes		Neutrophils			Lymphocytes			Monocytes		Eosinophils	
	Mean*	(Range)*	Mean*	(Range)*	(%)	Mean* (Range)*		(%)	Mean*	(%)	Mean*	(%)
Birth	18.1	(9.0–30.0)	11	(6.0–26.0)	61	5.5	(2.0–11.0)	31	1.1	6	0.4	2
12 hours	22.8	(13.0–38.0)	15.5	(6.0–28.0)	68	5.5	(2.0–11.0)	24	1.2	5	0.5	2
24 hours	18.9	(9.4–34.0)	11.5	(5.0–21.0)	61	5.8	(2.0–11.5)	31	1.1	6	0.5	2
1 week	12.2	(5.0–21.0)	5.5	(1.5–10.0)	45	5	(2.0–17.0)	41	1.1	9	0.5	4
2 weeks	11.4	(5.0–20.0)	4.5	(1.0–9.5)	40	5.5	(2.0–17.0)	48	1	9	0.4	3
1 month	10.8	(5.0–19.5)	3.8	(1.0–9.0)	35	6	(2.5–16.5)	56	0.7	7	0.3	3
6 months	11.9	(6.0–17.5)	3.8	(1.0–8.5)	32	7.3	(4.0–13.5)	61	0.6	5	0.3	3
1 year	11.4	(6.0–17.5)	3.5	(1.5–8.5)	31	7	(4.0–10.5)	61	0.6	5	0.3	3
2 years	10.6	(6.0–17.0)	3.5	(1.5–8.5)	33	6.3	(3.0–9.5)	59	0.5	5	0.3	3
4 years	9.1	(5.5–15.5)	3.8	(1.5–8.5)	42	4.5	(2.0–8.0)	50	0.5	5	0.3	3
6 years	8.5	(5.0–14.5)	4.3	(1.5–8.0)	51	3.5	(1.5–7.0)	42	0.4	5	0.2	3
8 years	8.3	(4.5–13.5)	4.4	(1.5–8.0)	53	3.3	(1.5–6.8)	39	0.4	4	0.2	2
10 years	8.1	(4.5–13.5)	4.4	(1.8–8.0)	54	3.1	(1.5–6.5)	38	0.4	4	0.2	2
16 years	7.8	(4.5–13.0)	4.4	(1.8–8.0)	57	2.8	(1.2–5.2)	35	0.4	5	0.2	3
21 years	7.4	(4.5–11.0)	4.4	(1.8–7.7)	59	2.5	(1.0–4.8)	34	0.3	4	0.2	3

*10^9/l

Table 2.3 Blood cell values in a normal adult population (from Williams et al., 1990)*

	Men	Men and women	Women
White cell count, ($\times 10^9$/l)		7.8 (4.4–11.3)	
Red cell count, ($\times 10^{12}$/l)	5.21 (4.52–5.90)		4.60 (4.10–5.10)
Hemoglobin (g/dl)	15.7 (14.0–17.5)		13.8 (12.3–15.3)
Hematocrit, ratio	0.46 (0.42–0.50)		0.40 (0.36–0.45)
Mean corpuscular volume (fl/red cell)		88.0 (80.0–96.1)	
Mean corpuscular hemoglobin (pg/red cell)		30.4 (27.5–33.2)	
Mean corpuscular hemoglobin concentration (g/dl RBC)		34.4 (33.4–35.5)	
Red cell distribution width (CV (%))		13.1 (11.5–14.5)	
Platelet count ($\times 10^9$/l)		311 (172–450)	

*Mean and range

Organization for use worldwide. But in spite of considerable efforts to use the system, for the past several decades in the United States, the traditional conventional units of measurement are being maintained as the method of choice in reporting hematological and biochemical values in practice with many medical journals continuing to use both systems. An interest in obtaining laboratory reference values information by testing a large group of unselected subjects has been revived recently. This was first proposed approximately thirty years ago by Hoffmann who derived reference limits from data of tests performed on routine patient specimens sent to the clinical laboratory (Hoffmann, 1963). Using this method or a variant thereof, it has been found that the reference limits derived in this manner are 'tighter' than those obtained by more conventional methods and while there is a theoretical increase in test **sensitivity**, there is a concomitant decrease in test **specificity** which is not likely to be of clinical benefit (Millward and Dix, 1992).

The diurnal variation as well as the longer day-to-day biological variation of values in a single individual must be considered in addition to the analytical precision in the laboratory. Equally important are the clinician's criteria for medically significant changes in laboratory data that will be used in the diagnosis, treatment and management of the patient; results of a survey using coefficient of variation (CV) as the benchmark are compared to the analytical

Table 2.4 Blood volume changes in normal pregnancy (from Hytten, 1985)

	Non-pregnant	Weeks of pregnancy		
		20	30	40
Plasma volume (ml)	2600	3150	3750	3850
Red cell mass (ml)	1400	1450	1550	1650
Total blood volume (ml)	4000	4600	5300	5500
Body hematocrit (%)	35	32	29	30
Venous hematocrit (%)	39.8	36.4	33	34.1

Table 2.5 Comparison of medically-derived versus analytical performance requirements (adapted from Skendzel, Barnett and Platt, 1985)

Test	Medically Useful (CV%)	Laboratory (Precision CV%)
Hemoglobin	3.6	1.1
Hematocrit	5.4	1.6
Leukocytes	16.4	3.3
MCV	3.2	
Prothrombin Time	15.2	3.3

Table 2.6 Average intra-individual biologic variation and derived objective analytical goal (from Fraser, 1987)

Test	Biologic Variation (CV%)	Goal (CV%)
Hemoglobin	2.4	1.2
Hematocrit	2.5	1.3
Platelets	6.6	3.3
Leukocytes	15.6	7.8
Neutrophils	24.6	12.3
Lymphocytes	11	5.5
Monocytes	16.2	8.1
Eosinophils	21.1	10.6
Basophils	13.2	6.6

precision in the laboratory in Table 2.5 (Skendzel, Barnett and Platt, 1985). The within-subject biological variability of hematology test data has been studied, utilizing the approach that also has been used for chemical tests (see also Chapter 11). This has been found to be consistent in several studies, and it is the basis for the consideration that the between-day variability of each test in an individual is half of the average of the within-subject biological variability, as depicted in Table 2.6 (Statland *et al.*, 1978; Fraser, 1987; Fraser *et al.*, 1989; Dot, Miro and Fuentes-Arderiu, 1992). The biological variability does not vary with age although there is some cyclic variation of the leukocyte concentration which has been related to the menstrual cycle in women.

2.3 Characteristic blood cell responses

Abnormalities in the blood cell lines, i.e. granulocytes, erythrocytes, platelets, monocytes and lymphocytes indicate whether there is a stem cell disorder present or only changes in one or more of the differentiated cell lines due to neoplasia, deficiencies, toxins, infectious agents or autoimmunity.

2.3.1 Red cell correlations

Hypochromic, microcytic red cells usually indicate iron deficiency, ovoid macrocytes with hypersegmented granulocytes are found in folate and/or vitamin B_{12} deficiency, and leptocytes indicate liver disease or hemoglobinopathies. Anisocytosis is seen in impaired red cell maturation, poikilocytes are associated with ineffective erythropoiesis, schistocytes with angiopathic hemolytic disease and spherocytes with red cell membrane disorders or injury. All of these pathophysiological correlations can be projected into diagnostic considerations.

2.3.2 White cell correlations

The presence of increased numbers of band neutrophils (left shift), toxic granulation, vacuolization of segmented neutrophil and Döhle bodies are indicative of inflammatory states, but are also seen in pregnancy (Bain, 1989). Eosinophilia suggests parasitic disease, skin disorders or atopic allergy, or a rarer variant of a myeloproliferative disease. Increased numbers of basophils in the adult frequently are indicative of a more specific chronic granulocytic leukemia. Large abnormal granules in the neutrophils may be seen in the rarer anomalies of Chediak–Higashi syndrome or the Adler–Reilly anomaly. Hypogranulation and dysplasia may be seen in both mature and immature neutrophilic granulocytes as a reflection of drug toxicity or a myelodysplasic process. The presence of an Auer rod in a blast cell or immature granulocyte is indicative of leukemia or myelodysplasia.

The presence of variant (atypical) lymphocytes is usually a reflection of a viral infection (hence the occasional designation as virocytes) with plasmacytoid lymphocytes frequently indicating an immune response by the host. Monocytosis is generally an indication of a chronic infectious process although in the elderly patient with a refractory anemia, with or without thrombocytopenia, myelodysplasia must also be considered. The presence of increased numbers of smudge cells in a middle-aged or older adult with a marginal or modest elevation of the lymphocyte count is almost always indicative of a variant of chronic lymphocytic leukemia.

2.3.3 Platelet correlations

The presence of a thrombocytopenia immediately raises the issue of whether it is due to underproduction or increased destruction as one searches for other morphological changes in the blood film that would indicate the cause. Thrombocytosis in the presence of hypochromic microcytic cells in a child is frequently only a reflection of iron deficiency. Larger platelets (increased MPV) are indicative of younger platelets which are produced as a response to a variety of stimuli.

2.4 The blood film review

After the information processing stage in the interpretation of hematological data, there is information utilization for pattern recognition and clinical correlation which focuses on the examination of a well-prepared, well-stained peripheral blood film linked to the information from a complete blood count. All blood specimens collected for complete blood counts by automated instruments should have blood films prepared for examination and potential reference. This utilizes the ability and skill of the clinical pathologist or laboratory physician in making subjective observations and adds qualitative information in the interpretive and diagnostic process rather than relying only on objective or quantitative data. Confirmation of red cell, white cell, and platelet concentrations as reflected by the blood film can be carried out, as well as the review of morphology of each of these cell series. An estimate of the red cell and white cell count can be made from a well-prepared blood film under the low power objective, the red cells being placed closely to each other at the end of the feather edge of the film in polycythemia as contrasted to the wide separation of cells that extends back into the butt end of the film in a patient with severe anemia. In an area of the film where the red cells have an even distribution, neither overlapping each other or being widely separated, a rough estimate of the leukocyte count can be made with approximately fifteen white cells per low power field equivalent to 5.0×10^9 leukocytes/l.

The presence of a bluish background in the Romanowsky stained film is an anomaly due to either the use of a heparinized blood specimen or a dysproteinemia associated with multiple myeloma. Rouleaux formation of the red cells near the 'feather' edge of the blood film may be seen with myeloma, pregnancy and inflammatory states in which there is elevation of fibrinogen concentration as well as other large molecular weight proteins. Rouleaux formation is also associated with an increased sedimentation rate.

2.4.1 Platelet review

The next step in this process is to confirm the validity of the platelet count by estimating the number of platelets in an appropriate oil immersion field of the film, generally five platelets in a well prepared film being equivalent to approximately 20×10^9 platelets/l. An artefactual thrombocytopenia due to platelet clumping or satellitism, often associated with a fallacious neutropenia, may be detected in the blood count produced by an automated instrument by the examination of the blood film (Dale and Schumacher, 1982). Large platelets can be identified, these being frequently an index of platelet regeneration or if they are especially large, as evidence of dysplasia.

2.4.2 Red cell review

The red cell morphology is then correlated with the indices, which with automated counting devices, are very accurate because of the sample size of cells which are measured for their calculation. Minor populations of abnormal red cells must be searched for since these may not be detected in alterations of the indices because of an average normal cell size with a concealed minor population of cells such as spherocytes; also, two populations of cells may be secondary to blood transfusion or indicative of more than one clone of erythrocyte precursors in the bone marrow. Careful examination of the cell histograms may reveal a so-called dimorphic red cell population and the red cell volume distribution width (RDW) may also detect dual populations of erythrocyte. Anisocytosis and hypochromia can be confirmed on the film and these can be correlated with the values. Proponents of the RDW indicate that it is increased with a heterogeneous variation in the cell volume of erythrocytes, as for example in the hypochromic cells in the usual iron deficiency anemia, and that there are narrower values with more homogeneous changes of erythrocytes in a patient with thalassemia minor. However, the RDW, as the coefficient of variation of the volume distribution, has limitations that must be recognized, i.e., RDW values are increased in some cases of α- and β-thalassemia trait and normal in a subgroup of blood donors with iron deficiency (Brittenham and Koepke, 1987). Hence, the RDW, while often diagnostically helpful, should be checked by correlation with the examination of the blood film.

2.4.3 White and nucleated red blood cell review

Examination of the white blood cells will reveal the presence or the absence of hypersegmented or band forms, as well as evidence of immaturity, reactive changes and dysplasia of the granulocytes, lymphocytes or monocytes. The presence or absence of nucleated red cells is determined; frequently if present in small numbers they will be seen only by examination with the low power objective, but their detection will usually have diagnostic or prognostic significance in the patient.

2.5 Bone marrow and lymph node examination

The same analytical process can be applied to examination of the bone marrow preparations and histological sections of both marrow and lymph nodes to which are added the additional hematological parameters of histochemists or immunochemistry, cytogenetic abnormalities, flow cytometry and surface markers, gene rearrangement studies, as well as the polymerase chain reaction (PCR), any or all of which are invaluable in developing a definitive diagnosis.

A comprehensive discussion of the bone marrow examination including the various special studies has been published (Shively, 1991). It includes reference values for marrow cell populations, including those for children, as well as a discussion of the evaluation of bone marrow tissue sections.

2.6 Clinical correlations

Given only the additional information of the patient's age, and with the presence or absence of drumsticks in the segmented neutrophils indicating the sex, the systematic and orderly examination of the peripheral blood film is the foundation of making deductions and inferences from the changes present by the application of the method of Zadig. This form of observation and deduction was used by Sir William Osler as a teaching exercise for students in medical education and by the physician author Arthur Conan Doyle in his mystery novels with the fictional detective Sherlock Holmes (Belkin and Neelon, 1992). What has been called the 'capacity for noticing or for raising questions', the power of informed observation is a useful diagnostic tool as well as being an effective educational process. Each item in the observation of the blood film is correlated with the pathophysiology of the variation found and is a useful exercise as a pattern of changes develop and the generation of diagnostic possibilities and considerations for further investigation. Frequently a definitive diagnosis can be made from this type of disciplined examination; the entire process may be considered to be an extension of the physical examination.

A variant of this mechanism was used by the pioneer Austrian pathologist, Karl von Rokitansky, who started his analysis of postmortem studies by extrapolating backwards from the autopsy findings and only at the end of this exercise were his results compared with the report of his clinical colleagues on the history and physical finding as well as the clinical course of the patient's illness (Ludwig, 1993). The reverse clinical pathological conference in medical education is another example of the same process.

2.7 Cases correlating observation and deductive reasoning

In the previous section the more common and straightforward correlations of morphological abnormalities with clinical conditions were outlined. In this section more complex cases, many with diagnostic implications, are presented. Previous experience with clinical medicine is coupled with morphological expertise to arrive at a possible diagnosis (or at least a differential diagnosis) which will explain the array of laboratory findings, including the blood film review, in a rational manner. Whilst the variety of cases may be enormous, for illustration a number of such correlations will be given.

As an example, the presence of Howell-Jolly bodies can indicate a previous splenectomy, congenital asplenia or a functional asplenia as seen in sickle-cell disease or after bone marrow transplantation. A leuko-erythroblastic blood picture, i.e. nucleated red blood cells and immature granulocytes (metamyelocyte or myelocytes), is usually indicative of myelophthisis with the disruption of normal hematopoiesis by the delivery of moderately differentiated cells into the peripheral blood; extramedullary hematopoiesis or major stress on the bone marrow by massive hemorrhage and sepsis are also possible causes. Myelofibrosis as a form of a myeloproliferative process involving megakaryocyte proliferation usually demonstrates leukoerythroblastosis and is frequently associated with ineffective erythropoiesis and the presence of tear drop shaped poikilocytes in the peripheral blood.

An indication of prognosis may also be projected from examination of the peripheral blood film. Nucleated red blood cells are normally found only in the peripheral blood of the fetus and newborn infant with some being found in marrow stress during childhood. However, if these cells are found in the peripheral blood of adults, it usually is a poor prognostic sign, regardless of etiology, with a mortality rate of almost 50% being reported in one study of the presence of circulating nucleated red cells in hospitalized patients (Schwartz and Stansbury, 1954). Leukoerythroblastosis is frequently found in patients with myelophthisis due to carcinomatosis or malignant hematological disorders, re-affirming it as an unfavorable prognostic feature.

In the post-mastectomy patient, the appearance of myelocytes and/or a rare nucleated red blood cell in the peripheral blood film frequently is an early indicator of metastatic disease in the bone marrow. Another poor prognostic sign in patients with non-Hodgkin's lymphoma is the biochemical finding of elevated serum lactic acid dehydrogenase and serum β_2 microglobulin levels (Amlot and Adinolti, 1979; Ferraris, Giuntini and Gaetani, 1979). This demonstrates the inter-relationships of morphological benchmarks and biochemical values in the interpretive process, i.e. vitamin B_{12}, folate, or ferritin. In cases of autoimmune hemolytic anemia, a rapid or accelerated drop in the hemoglobin level associated with reticulocytopenia as reflected by the absence of polychromatophilic red cells indicates a fulminant and potentially fatal course that usually requires transfusion of type-specific red cells in spite of an unsatisfactory cross-match.

The final step in the interpretation of hematological test data is the process of information application which is aided by the inter-relationship and the ability of the clinical pathologist or hematologist to communicate with the patient's clinician. As the diagnostic possibilities are considered, the age of a patient is important clinical information. Since pediatric hematological responses are frequently different from that of an adult and reference ranges vary for different age groups, these variables influence the working hypothesis in the process of pattern recognition.

2.8 Illustrations of the utility of blood film reviews

The usefulness as well as the validity of these correlations are demonstrated by several vignettes:

A 24-year-old male medical technologist, on a routine health examination, was found to have a normal complete blood count and normal red blood cell indices with a total serum bilirubin of 2.2 mg/dl (38 μmol/l) but other liver function tests were normal. Examination of the peripheral blood film revealed an occasional microspherocyte. There was a history of the patient's mother having a cholecystectomy at the age of 26 years. Further investigation revealed compensated hemolytic disease due to congenital spherocytosis with the instrument-generated red cell indices being unaffected by a minor population of abnormal cells.

A 35-year-old male with a hemoglobin level of 22.5 g/dl (225 g/l) had normal erythrocyte morphology as well as normal platelet, leukocyte, and differential leukocyce counts. A preliminary diagnosis of secondary polycythemia was made on the basis of the age of the patient, the normal leukocyte and platelet values and the absence of a hepatosplenomegaly. This was subsequently confirmed by the discovery of pulmonary stenosis.

2.9 The special case of malaria and other infections

The diagnosis of malaria infections is made from the examination of the blood film and the identification of the specific species of the Plasmodium organism influences treatment of the patient as well as the prognosis of the disease process. *P. vivax* and *P. ovale* infections are generally mild as are those due to *P. malariae*. However, *P. malariae* has a greater propensity for asymptomatic lifetime dormancy that may be a hazard for transfusion-induced malaria from a blood donor who acquired the infection much earlier in life.

P. falciparum is the most pathogenic and life threatening of the malarias; it can be recognized by the intra-erythrocyte, delicate ring forms or trophozoites which frequently are multiple and maybe in an applique position on the surface of the red cell which is not enlarged. However, occasionally a seriously ill patient may have only an occasional parasite or even no detectable organism on the initial blood examination. Conversely, up to 40–50% of the erythrocytes may be infected and the degree of parasitemia is used to guide exchange transfusions along with the use of intravenous quinine or quinidine in the management of cerebral malaria which is the most serious form of *P. falciparum* infection. The goal is to reduce the parasitemia to less than 1%, which is monitored by examination of blood films and the return of a normal mental status (Muller, Greenberg and Campbell, 1989). If there are large numbers of crescent/banana-shaped gametocytes with only an occasional trophozoite or ring form, the clinical severity of the infection is generally less serious since gametocytes are seen approximately ten days after the appearance of the asexual ring forms. These are short lived and die if there is no further mosquito transmission (Finch, 1987).

Babesia microti must be distinguished from *P. falciparum* organisms with the former being characterized by ring forms which may be up to 12 per RBC in contrast to 3–4 for *P. falciparum*; the Babesia rings tend to be clustered in groups of four, are larger than those of *P. falciparum* and may also be seen in extra-erythrocytic locations.

Fungi (histoplasma) or Leishmania organisms may be present in the cytoplasm of monocytes or granulocytes. Bacteria may be seen in the cytoplasm of granulocytes and this rare finding is an indication of sepsis that requires immediate attention and treatment. Trypanosomes and microfilariae may be a startling discovery when the film is scanned under low power magnification.

2.10 The future for blood film reviews

With increasingly sophisticated hematology analysers being used in many clinical hematology laboratories, there is a temptation to ask if microscopes are becoming extinct. Despite those concerns, there still remains a need and a role for individuals experienced in blood film examination and interpretation. The present-day instruments, by and large, identify or flag blood specimens for further evaluation and this requires the examination of a properly made and stained blood film. There is a concern that the skills as well as the number of such individuals may be diminishing since lesser numbers of blood films are being examined. Although these skills are still present in more experienced clinical pathologists and hematologists, there is an impression that trainees are no longer acquiring the necessary experience to interpret a blood film correctly.

In the blood film review process, the production of accurate and precise information and the ability of the clinical pathologist/hematologist to recognize patterns of changes in hematological test data, will initiate other diagnostic tests and gives material assistance in making a definitive clinical diagnosis. This orderly and well-disciplined process of observation and deduction utilizes morphological and quantitative changes that are associated with pathophysiological mechanisms of disease in the clinical patient. It maximizes the benefits obtained from the interpretation of the hematology test data and exploits the usefulness of the examination of a well-prepared, well-stained blood film. This may be the most informative single procedure performed in the clinical laboratory.

References

Amlot, P. L. and Adinolfi, M. (1979) Serum B₂-microglobulin and its prognostic value in lymphomas. *Eur. J. Cancer*, **15**, 791–796.

Bain, B. J. (1989) *Blood Cells – A Practical Guide*. Philadelphia: Lippincott, pp. 42–46.

Belkin, B. M. and Neelon, F. A. (1982) The art of observation: William Osler and the method of Zadig. *Ann. Intern. Med.*, **116**, 863–866.

Brittenham, G. M. and Koepke, J. A. (1987) Red blood cell volume distributions and the diagnosis of anemia. *Arch. Pathol. Lab. Med.*, **111**, 1146–1148.

Dale, N. L. and Schumacher, H. R. (1982) Platelet Satellitism-new spurious results with automated instruments. *Lab. Med.*, **13**, 300–304.

Dallman, P. R. (1977) In: Rudolph, A. M. (ed.), *Pediatrics*, 16th edn. Appleton-Century-Crofts, New York, p. 1178.

Dot, D., Miro, J. and Fuentes-Arderiu, X. (1992) Within-subject biological variation of hematological quantities and analytical goals. *Arch. Pathol. Lab. Med.*, **116**, 825–826.

Ferraris, A. M., Giuntini, P. and Gaetani, G. F. (1979) Serum lactic dehydrogenase as a prognostic tool for non-Hodgkin lymphomas. *Blood*, **54**, 928–932.

Finch, C. D. (1987) Malaria. In: Feigin, R. D. and Cherry, J. D. (eds), *Textbook of Pediatric Infectious Disease*. Philadelphia: Saunders, pp. 2050–2066.

Fraser, C. G. (1987) Desirable standards for hematology tests: a proposal. *Am. J. Clin. Pathol.*, **88**, 667–669.

Fraser, C. G. *et al.* (1989) Biologic variation of common hematology laboratory quantities in the elderly. *Am. J. Clin. Pathol.*, **92**, 465–470.

Hoffmann, R. G. (1963) Statistics in the practice of medicine. *JAMA*, **185**, 864–874.

Hytten, F. (1985) Blood volume changes in normal pregnancy. *Clin. Hematol.*, **14**, 601–612.

Kalish, R. J., Goldberg, G. and Roberts, K. (1987) Automated three part leukocyte differential counts in the preoperative evaluation of ambulatory surgery patients. *Arch. Pathol. Lab. Med.*, **111**, 1155–1157.

Kato, K. (1935) Leucocytes in infancy and childhood. *J. Pediatr.*, **7**, 11.

Krause, J. R. (1990) Automated differentials in the hematology laboratory. *Am. J. Clin. Pathol.*, **93**, Suppl. 1, 511–516.

Ludwig, F. C. (1993) Pathology in historical perspective. *Pharos*, Spring, 5–11.

Miller, D. R., Bachuer, R. L. and McMillian, C. W. (1984) *Blood Diseases of Infancy and Childhood*. St Louis: Mosby, p. 28.

Millward, M. and Dix, D. (1992) Determining reference ranges by linear analysis. *Lab. Med.*, **23**, 815–818.

Muller, K. D., Greenberg, A. E. and Campbell, C. C. (1989) Treatment of severe malaria in the United States with continuous infusion of quinidine gluconate and exchange transfusion. *N. Eng. J. Med.*, **321**, 65–70.

Ross, D. W., Watson, J. S., Davis, P. H. *et al.* (1985) Evaluation of the Coulter three part differential. *Am. J. Clin. Pathol.*, **84**, 481–484.

Schwartz, S. O. and Stansbury, F. (1954) Significance of nucleated red blood cells in peripheral blood. *JAMA*, **154**, 1339–1340.

Shively, J. A. (1991) Examination of the bone marrow. In: Koepke, J. A. (ed.), *Practical Laboratory Hematology*. New York: Churchill Livingstone, pp. 173–192.

Skendzel, L. P., Barnett, R. N. and Platt, R. (1985) Medically useful criteria for analytic performance of laboratory tests. *Am. J. Clin. Pathol.*, **83**, 200–205.

Statland, B. E. *et al.* (1978) Evaluations of biologic sources of leukocyte counts and other hematologic quantities using very precise automated analyzes. *Am. J. Clin. Pathol.*, **69**, 48–54.

Van Assendelft, O. W. (1991) Interpretation of the quantitative blood cell count. In: Koepke, J. A. (ed.), *Practical Laboratory Hematology*. New York: Churchill Livingstone, pp. 61–98.

Van Assendelft, O. W., Mcgrath, C., Murphy, R. S. *et al.* (1977) The differential distribution of leukocytes. In: Koepke, J. A. (ed.) *Differential Leukocyte Counting*. Chicago: College of American Pathologists, pp. 11–22.

Williams, W. J. *et al.* (ed.) (1990) *Hematology*, 4th edn. New York: Mc Graw-Hill, p. 10.

Zuelzer, W. W. (1957) Diagnostic principles in pediatric hematology. *Pediatr. Clin. North Am.*, May, 347–356.

3

Role of the physician in the coagulation laboratory

John A. Koepke

3.1 Introduction

The relationship between laboratory results and clinical care is probably nowhere closer than in the evaluation and treatment of patients with problems in hemostasis and/or thrombosis. Take, for example, Factor VIII assays and the transfusion of Factor VIII concentrates to hemophiliacs undergoing surgery or recovering from trauma. Another example would be the periodic monitoring of the prothrombin time in patients receiving long-term oral anticoagulation therapy. Congenital coagulation abnormalities require very sophisticated and accurate testing in order to diagnose accurately these disorders. In the recent past platelet disorders have been divided and subdivided into a number of functional disorders largely on the basis of platelet aggregometry done with a variety of agonists. All of these clinical conditions require the availability of good coagulation testing for accurate and specific diagnosis as well as appropriate monitoring of therapy.

The hemostatic system has been one of the most intensely researched aspects of human biochemistry. The synthesis of the numerous systems and subsystems has confirmed the great complexity of the hemostatic system with no end yet in sight. This discipline has been a fertile field for both the practical application of these studies to large numbers of patients most often with acquired defects. But also it has a great appeal to the investigator who has a penchant for Sherlock Holmes mysteries.

3.2 Training and experience of the laboratory physician

The unravelling of the normal process of hemostasis and in particular the biochemistry of blood coagulation has been a fairly recent development in laboratory medicine. Depending upon the orientation of the basic science faculty of the medical school, medical students may have a varying exposure to this fascinating process. A 'bare bones' curriculum will include a description of the several named factors and also their inter-relationship in the so-called coagulation cascade. The contribution of platelets to the initiation of the coagulation process was subsequently elucidated. The relationship of platelets to microaggregates which may trigger transient ischemic attacks as well as the development of atherosclerosis have been a fertile field of investigation. More recently, an exploration of the role of fibrinolysis has received an increased amount of study. A variety of agents are being used to lyse thrombi. The best way to monitor this type of therapy is still being debated and the physician in the coagulation laboratory can play a pivotal role in the development of this new mode of therapy.

Although the biochemistry of coagulation may be taught in some medical schools, the usual time at which physicians learn about this topic is during their residency and/or fellowship experience. In pathology training programmes this would primarily include technical matters while in internal medicine/hematology training programmes they would concentrate on the clinical aspects of hemostasis and its investigation.

The medical director of the coagulation laboratory must be conversant with the complexities of hemostasis. In addition, however, the director must be able to inter-relate the laboratory tests which seek to measure the various steps in this process either directly or more often in indirect ways. The methodology used in the laboratory must be understood in some detail in order to interpret the results of the testing properly. It is beyond the scope of this discussion to give a treatise of the biochemical aspects of hemostasis, nor can the laboratory aspects of testing including interpretation be covered here. Rather, the interested reader is referred to several useful books listed in the References at the end of this chapter. These or comparable reference texts should be included in the laboratory library.

Probably most important for the director is experience in the diagnosis and treatment of problems of hemostasis as well as thrombosis. This is usually acquired by long practice in this field. Training in a large laboratory where there is direct ongoing communication with clinicians as well as patients is most valuable. For instance, daily working coagulation 'rounds' where the clinical history is correlated with the results of testing is probably the most efficient way of acquiring the appropriate knowledge. At these rounds further testing is determined which then is discussed at the following session. Since the clinicians are regular participants, the clinical history as well as follow-up reports are especially useful. In a university hospital where I formerly practised these sessions were held each morning. After the clinical resident presented the patient's pertinent history and physical findings, the coagulation test results were shown on a transparency using an overhead projector. Figure 3.1 is given as an example of a case as presented over several days. At the conference the laboratory results are discussed and a diagnosis and treatment plan may be proposed. But if the diagnosis was not certain, various options are debated and follow-up laboratory studies decided on. Subsequent cases are presented in a similar way. Occasionally some of the group might visit the patient, remembering that the patient's history might provide invaluable clues to the diagnosis. For instance, was the patient taking aspirin unbeknown to the physician? Or, not infrequently, the patient might have an indwelling catheter which the house officer was keeping patent with an occasional bolus of heparin from a vial of this potent anticoagulant kept in his jacket pocket.

Finally, continuing education is especially important in this rapidly changing field. This includes national and international meetings, either of societies concentrating on hemostasis (e.g. the International Society on Thrombosis and Hemostasis and its Scientific and Standardization Committees) or those in which there are major sessions on hemostasis (e.g. International Society of Hematology). The American Society of Hematology as well as the American Society of Clinical Pathologists offer continuing education workshops on coagulation topics of significance. Regional as well as local seminars and workshops sometimes sponsored by manufacturers are also opportunities to keep up with coagulation testing.

A type of in-service education of special value to laboratory workers is the evaluation of new coagulation instruments. These may be evaluations contracted with the manufacturer to generate clinical and laboratory correlations (so-called beta sites) as they seek approval of the US Food and Drug Administration (FDA) to market a new or improved instrument system and/or reagent; or it may involve a new instrument being evaluated by the laboratory as they consider it for purchase. In both cases the dynamic limits of testing should be evaluated and a variety of clinical specimens should be studied.

3.3 Testing strategies – screening, panel and definitive tests

To provide coagulation testing appropriate for the institution an analysis of the patient population to be served is in order. Most general hospitals would undoubtedly have a more or less standard panel of tests appropriate for the clinical needs of the institution. A basic panel would include the prothrombin time (PT), partial thromboplastin time (PTT), fibrinogen and platelet count. Also, screening tests for disseminated intravascular coagulation (DIC) would most likely be included since this syndrome can arise in so many different common clinical situations. While in the past a screening test for fibrin degradation products has been widely used for DIC screening, newer more specific tests are now available. Beyond this basic panel either more definitive procedures or the availability of a good coagulation referral laboratory must be provided. Table 3.1 gives examples of basic as well as specialized or focused coagulation panels.

Partly in an effort to supplant the skin bleeding time as a screen for platelet disorders, platelet aggregation studies have become more popular in the past several years. A variety of instruments are available, some requiring the preparation of platelet-rich plasma while others can use whole blood as a sample. By using a variety of different platelet agonists, or activators, a number of congenital as well as acquired platelet defects have been delineated using platelet aggregometry. Undoubtedly these studies will become more popular in the future.

The medical director must be well acquainted with the methods as well as the interpretation of the basic tests. The conditions and/or medications which may cause artefactual changes in the tests must be known and considered. For example, in some hospitals the most common cause for an unexpected elevation of the partial thromboplastin time was the periodic injection of heparin into indwelling catheters by house officers in order to prevent thrombus formation. As a general rule of thumb, an unexpectedly prolonged partial thromboplastin time is due to heparin until proven otherwise. Similarly, the patient's use of aspirin may invalidate platelet aggregation studies.

The concept of panels of tests appropriate to certain clinical conditions is well developed in the coagulation. The wide variety of panels are available in the laboratory (see Table 3.1). The panels are set up both as an aid to the clinician who may not be well acquainted with the intricacies of the coagulation

Patient Name   Hospital Number

Clinical History: Excessive bruising and occasional hemarthroses, since childhood. Bleeding following dental extractions.

TEST	Date 3–25	3–26	3–27	Reference Range
Prothrombin Time(s)	11.6			**9–10**
PTT (s)	54	50	49	**22–35**
Fibrinogen (mg/dl)	225			**152–344**
Platelet count ($\times 10^9$/l)	315			**150–450**
Thrombin time (s)				**within 3s**
Reptilase time (s)				**within 3s**
Frag D-dimer (μg/ml)				**< 2**
FDP (μg/ml)				**< 10**
Other tests				
Factor VIII (%)		34		**50–200**
Bleeding Time (m)		17		**3–10**
vWF: Ag (%)			27	**50–150**

Final diagnosis: von Willebrand's Disease

Figure 3.1 Coagulation case review

Table 3.1 Coagulation test panels*

Basic panel includes:
  Prothrombin time (PT)
  Partial thromboplastin time (PTT)
  Fibrinogen, and
  Platelet count

Special panels include the basic panel (above) plus the indicated tests:
Disseminated intravascular coagulation – Fragment D-dimer
von Willebrand disease (vWD) – Factor VIII assay, vWD factor antigen, vWD factor activity, ristocetin cofactor
Thrombosis – Antithrombin III activity, plasminogen activity, protein C activity, protein S antigen, and Reptilase time
Lupus anticoagulant – Incubated mix, thrombin clotting time and dilute Russell's viper venom time (DRVVT)
Fibrinolysis – Euglobulin lysis time, fragment D-dimer, plasminogen antigen and activity, 2–plasmin inhibitor level

*From *Coagulation Manual* (1993). Panels may vary among laboratories.

laboratory and also as a method for the laboratory to do a creditable evaluation in a particular case.

With a panel of tests the sensitivity and the specificity of the testing is maximized and a valid diagnosis is determined or excluded as quickly and efficiently as possible. Panels will vary from one institution to another but they should be delineated in such a fashion so as to take advantage of their evident merits. Incidentally, panel tests provide the backbone of the clinical coagulation conference discussed previously.

3.4 Reference Ranges

A significant amount of time and effort should be given to the establishment and/or confirmation of reference ranges for these tests. It is not always appreciated that even the common tests such as the prothrombin time and in particular the partial thromboplastin time may have significantly different reference ranges depending upon the test system (instrument plus reagent). One only has to examine the participant result summaries of interlaboratory surveys to confirm this fact. Table 3.2 presents character-

Table 3.2 Prothrombin time system biases*

Thromboplastin	Instrument			
	MLA Electra	Ortho Koagulab	OTC Coag-a-Mate	IL ACL
Dade Thromb-C Plus	1.06			
Dade Thromb-C	.96			
Ortho Brain		1.08		
OTC Auto			.85	
OTC Excel			1.11	
IL PT FIB				1.06

*Expressed as ratio of mean PT for group to the overall mean PT of 17.1 s for survey specimens CG2–03 and CG2–05 done by 853 laboratories.

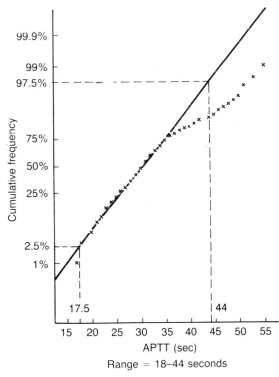

Range = 18–44 seconds

Figure 3.2 Normal probability plot of PTT results from outpatients

istic data from a recent College of American Pathologists (CAP) Survey (CAP, 1993). It has only recently been appreciated by many that coagulation systems are quite unique and dependent upon the method of end-point detection as well as reagent and activator differences. A system is defined as the combination of an instrument or method with the reagent.

Published methods for reference range studies often outline very extensive and laborious procedures which few laboratories can carry out without a very significant expenditure of technical time and statistical effort (NCCLS, 1992a). But it is not easy to recruit the required large group of normal individuals. Gender and age variations are not well studied. This problem is particularly difficult when one seeks to develop reference ranges for infants and children (Hathaway, 1987).

When pressed for a practical method to develop reference ranges (as now required by federal regulation in the USA) the method of log normal distribution of test results from 100 consecutive patients seen in the outpatient or emergency department would be appropriate. While undoubtedly there is a group of abnormal results in this population, when the cumulative results are plotted on normal probability paper, the Gaussian distribution of the normal individuals can be identified. Table 3.3 and Figure 3.2 summarize a study done for the partial thromboplastin time (Stewart and Koepke, 1987). When such specimens are collected and identified, several common coagulation tests can be run and the data added to the normal value study.

For the less common tests, the manufacturer's suggested reference ranges can be used initially but these ranges should be confirmed with at least 20 normal individuals.

The determination of the International Normalized Ratio (INR) requires the individual laboratory to determine the Mean Normal Prothrombin Time (MNPT), *not* the control prothrombin time as many laboratories continue to do. The MNPT is used with the patient's prothrombin time to determine the INR (ICTH/ICSH, 1979). Unfortunately clinicians continue to look for the 'control prothrombin time' and are sometimes even supported in this practice by the warfarin manufacturers in their package inserts (Koepke, 1993b).

3.5 Reporting conventions

While historically many coagulation tests have been reported in functional terms (i.e. seconds or other time intervals) newer tests are being measured increasingly in milligram, microgram or even picogram concentrations of a procoagulant. This evolution was led by quantitative fibrinogen measurements after many years of being estimated by performing a bedside thrombin time. Now only the prothrombin time, partial thromboplastin time and the bleeding time continue to be reported in terms of time intervals.

Functional testing will most likely continue to be the preferred method to screen for isolated factor deficiencies or DIC. However, for monitoring oral anticoagulant therapy the implementation of the

Table 3.3 PTT results from one hundred consecutive emergency department patients

Value	Freq.	Cum. Freq.	Value	Freq.	Cum. Freq.	Value	Freq.	Cum Freq.
17	1	1	31	7	55	45	1	89
18	2	3	32	6	61	46	2	91
20	2	5	33	4	65	47	1	92
21	3	8	34	4	69	48	1	93
22	2	10	35	5	74	49	1	94
23	4	14	36	3	77	50	1	95
24	4	18	37	2	79	51	2	97
25	3	21	38	2	81	53	1	98
26	5	26	39	1	82	55	1	99
27	3	29	40	1	83	56	1	100
28	6	35	41	2	85			
29	6	41	42	2	87			
30	7	48	44	1	88			

International Normalized Ratio (INR) is recommended. In the late 1970s the International Committee for Thrombosis and Hemostasis in collaboration with the International Council for Standardization in Hematology developed a method for the standardization of prothrombin time reporting (ICTH/ICSH, 1979). This method allows for the interlaboratory correlation of anticoagulation intensity so that patients can be anticoagulated at a level comparable to that used in large trials which have determined optimal levels of oral anticoagulation. While this system has been widely adopted in the Netherlands and the UK as well as other countries, the implementation in the USA has been relatively tardy (Triplett and Brandt, 1993).

In order to hasten the move toward INR reporting, the director of the coagulation laboratory should be well acquainted with the method for the assignment of the International Sensitivity Index (ISI) for the particular prothrombin time system (thromboplastin and instrument) being used in the laboratory and should make the reporting of the INR available to the patients receiving oral anticoagulants. While clinicians may be reluctant to change to a different reporting method, they should be made aware of the significant advantages of this method for their patients. For example, a recent review of several clinical studies concluded that patient care would be improved if clinical laboratories uniformly report the intensity of anticoagulation as the INR (Eckman, Levine and Pauker, 1993).

The use of microchemical and immunologic methods to measure the concentration of coagulation components will undoubtedly increase in the future. These methods are especially useful in the diagnosis of complex coagulopathies, the subclassification of some factor deficiencies and the identification of carriers of coagulation disorders. Finally, they also appear to be useful for the investigation of prethrombotic states (Bertina, 1986).

3.6 Testing methods

There continues to be an attachment to past methods used for prothrombin time and partial thromboplastin time testing. Many laboratories still do duplicate testing because that is the way these tests were done in the past when manual methods were used. But with significant improvements in coagulation instrumentation and reagents duplicate testing is probably not necessary, although this practice continues in many laboratories. A statistically and clinically valid system to evaluate if duplicate testing is necessary has been devised. In this method 32 specimens equally distributed over four quartiles of prothrombin times and/or partial thromboplastin times, i.e. normal, mildly, moderately and markedly elevated, are analysed in duplicate. A statistical analysis is done and any duplicates beyond the determined limits are reviewed (Koepke *et al.*, 1994). The final judgment is made on a clinical basis – would either of the 'disparate' values result in a difference in diagnosis or treatment? If the answer is 'no', duplicate testing is no longer necessary. Before a new instrument or reagent (or lot) is placed in service, the evaluation of the validity of single testing is repeated.

The collection and storage of coagulation specimens have in the past been beset with rather rigid requirements which has resulted in a considerable amount of needless work for the laboratory. For years, immediate icing of the coagulation specimen after collection was required. But only later was it appreciated that, in fact, this was deleterious to the specimen (apparently Factor VII is activated). Similarly, specimens were collected in 3.8% (129 mmol/l) citrate anticoagulant even though a lower concentration of citrate (e.g., 3.2% or 109 mmol/l) is probably preferable since it would decrease the incidence of artefactual prolongations of coagulation tests in patients with higher hematocrits (Koepke *et al.*, 1975).

Finally, it has been difficult, at times, to comply with the requirement to 'immediately' test coagulation specimens. However, several studies have shown conclusively that the prothrombin time and the partial thromboplastin time are quite stable over many hours (Simmons, 1993). The latest guidelines for coagulation specimen collection and storage are appropriately making these requirements less rigid (NCCLS, 1991). Nevertheless, by repeating the test 6–8 hours after the initial testing and using the same program as was used for duplicate testing evaluation to evaluate the results, a laboratory can easily show its own personnel as well as laboratory inspectors that longer holding times prior to testing are acceptable.

The current guidelines include factor assays in the battery of tests which might be deleteriously affected by delays in testing (NCCLS, 1991). While this may be so, certainly one does not need to apply such rigid standards to the more common tests. But keep in mind, if 'add on' testing is done in the laboratory, that the routinely collected specimen may not be adequate for some tests.

3.7 On-site or bedside coagulation testing

The utility of on-site coagulation testing has been evident for many years. For example, the activated coagulation time (ACT) has provided immediate turnaround times for the monitoring of heparin therapy in cardiac surgery and renal dialysis (Hattersley, 1984). More recently, several bedside coagulation instruments which are used to perform prothrombin times and partial thromboplastin time have become available and results, at least for the prothrombin time, appear to be quite acceptable. These instruments automatically determine the INR making them convenient for cardiac outpatient anticoagulation clinics. It is important to ensure that the bedside and laboratory methods are comparable – if both report the INR this should not be a problem since the INR system is 'blind' to coagulation system. However, if the INR system is not used, comparability studies between the central laboratory results and those generated by the device should be done (Rose *et al.*, 1993).

One bedside test, the skin bleeding time, has been a bone of contention between clinicians and laboratories for many years. Many clinicians have the mistaken belief that the bleeding time can accurately predict operative bleeding problems. But a number of studies refute this (Barber *et al.*, 1985; Burns and Lawrence, 1989). In some situations, a pre-operative

bleeding time may be considered 'standard practice' and abandoning it may pose a problem. The medical director of the coagulation laboratory should take a leadership role in the hospital to teach the clinicians the appropriate use of the test as well as common abuses. Also, he should guarantee that, if appropriately ordered, the laboratory will do the test properly, quickly and without complaint.

3.8 The special role of the laboratory physician

As medical director of a laboratory offering coagulation testing the physician has several different but interrelated functions. First, he functions as a teacher both to the laboratory staff but also more importantly to the clinicians served by the laboratory. He also serves as a consultant in the evaluation of coagulation tests results but also any other laboratory studies which may be pertinent to the case. And finally he may, particularly if he also has responsibilities for the transfusion service, be expected to advise on therapy particularly with blood products. Let us examine these requirements.

It is commonly appreciated that the process of hemostasis (platelet aggregation, plasma coagulation and fibrinolysis) is complex and sometimes poorly understood. Therefore the medical director should realize the existence of this problem and work to improve the level of expertise of both laboratory staff and clinicians. It has already been stated that clinical coagulation rounds are an excellent way to educate both students and practitioners. Attendance at departmental and hospital staff meetings and presentations at such sessions, particularly when changes are being made in the laboratory service, are very helpful. Conversations and meetings with the residents and the clinicians are helpful. The laboratory director can let the clinicians know about new laboratory developments and also respond to questions about problems with laboratory service. This is especially useful since small problems can be resolved before they grow into larger ones.

Tertiary care medical centres are large and complex. Each year there may be literally hundreds of incoming house staff as well as attending physicians who may often come from a variety of backgrounds. While it has been the custom to present various facets of the operation to a captive house staff in the first few days of their appointments this is not an efficient way to present the myriad of facts that these house officers need to know. So, for a number of years our coagulation laboratory attending staff has published a small pocket-sized coagulation manual, now in its fourth edition, which covers a large number of topics pertinent to the most efficient use of the coagulation laboratory (Table 3.4). Each

Table 3.4 Coagulation Manual – Table of Contents

individual section outlines the problem and offers advice on the steps to be followed. Each section also includes two or three pertinent references.

While the coagulation manual answers a great many questions, some still arise which require the special expertise and experience of the medical director. For instance, how low should the prothrombin time be in order to perform a percutaneous liver biopsy safely? Can a patient with von Willebrand's disease safely undergo surgery with a Factor VIII level of 55%? These would, of course, be in addition to the interpretation of inhibitor assays, plasma mixing studies and lupus inhibitor assays.

A common problem in the past has been the interpretation of the DIC panel especially in mild or chronic cases. And if there is evidence of this syndrome what is the appropriate therapy? Should the patient be heparinized? Is there a need for platelet and/or cryoprecipitate transfusions? Is there a treatable cause for the DIC such as infection?

While it unusual for laboratory physicians in hematology or clinical chemistry to be directly involved with therapeutic consultation, it is much more common for physicians in the coagulation laboratory to be asked for such advice particularly if they have a clinical appointment. Indeed, in many laboratories the director of the laboratory may be a clinician. The important point is that this individual bridges the gap between the patient and the laboratory. With an appropriate fund of clinical as well as technical

information, advice can be given for monitoring heparin or oral anticoagulant therapy. Fibrinolytic therapy regimens are still under development and the final role of the laboratory in this important field is yet to be determined.

The inter-relationship between hemostatic abnormalities and transfusion is well illustrated by the bleeding problems in a wide variety of patients (Simpson, 1991). Such cases might include patients who have suffered extensive trauma, obstetrical patients with DIC or those receiving massive transfusions. Sometimes thrombocytopenic patients require surgery and the director of the coagulation laboratory will be asked to advise on blood transfusion therapy while the patient undergoes surgery. If the patient's platelet count is below $50 \times 10^9/l$ an adult dose of platelets, defined as an apheresis platelet preparation or a pool of 6–8 platelet concentrates from single units of blood, is usually required. In more major surgical procedures, e.g. intracranial operations, higher levels of platelet counts may be necessary. The platelets should be given an hour or two before the patient goes to the operating room. It is wise to repeat the platelet count after the transfusion to confirm that the count is at a satisfactory level. Platelet and/or cryoprecipitate transfusions may also be indicated for the occasional patient undergoing surgery who has acute disseminated intravascular coagulation associated with infection or following surgery (Koepke, 1993a).

Fibrinogen levels less than 100 mg/dl are frequently associated with increased bleeding. In such cases fibrinogen replacement with fibrinogen-rich cryoprecipitate is indicated. An appropriate dose can be calculated with the knowledge of the patient's estimated plasma volume and the fact that each bag of cryoprecipitate contains at least 100 mg of fibrinogen. Our standard dose is a pool of ten bags of cryoprecipitate, or about 1000 mg of fibrinogen. Again, the response to transfusion should be monitored by repeating the plasma fibrinogen level.

In patients with multiple coagulation factor deficiencies fresh frozen plasma (FFP) transfusions are useful. Recently, larger pools of FFP from donors who have been plasmapheresed have been prepared by blood donor centres in order to decrease the recipient's exposure to multiple donor transfusions.

A number of consensus conferences to develop guidelines for transfusion have been held under the auspices of the American National Institutes of Health (NIH, 1985, 1987). Other transfusion guidelines have been developed locally (e.g. the Duke University Medical Center Coagulation Manual, 1993), or by various professional groups (College of American Pathologists, 1993). When one examines these guidelines in detail it is apparent that the objective results from the hematology or coagulation laboratory are quite important particularly in the case of active bleeding in association with trauma or surgery. If the key laboratory data indicate that

Table 3.5 In-Vivo Quality Control of Blood Components

Deficiency	Therapy	Dosage	Expected Level	Half-Life (hours)
Factor VIII	F VIII concentrate	60 U/Kg	100% F VIII	12–15
vWF	Cryoprecipitate	2 bags/10 Kg	> 50% F VIII	12–15
	DDAVP	0.3–0.4 ug/Kg	> 50% F VIII	12–15
Factor IX	F XI concentrate	60 U/Kg	> 50% F IX	18–24
Fibrinogen	Cryoprecipitate	10 bag pool	50–100 mg/dl	90–144
Platelets	Platelet concentrate	One apheresis unit	$> 50 \times 10^9/L/M^2$	72–96

From Koepke, 1993a

there are reasonably hemostatic levels of platelets and procoagulants, the presumption is that there may be a mechanical cause for the continuing hemorrhage, e.g. an unligated blood vessel. If the vessel is not tied off, no amount of platelets, cryoprecipitate and/or fresh frozen plasma will staunch the flow of blood. These debates may become confrontational at times but we must remember to keep the patient foremost in our deliberations. The surgeon may make the decision at the time of the crisis but this may become an opportunity for continuing education in the coming days.

One useful quality assurance practice that crosses interdepartmental boundaries is the *in vivo* evaluation of transfusion products or coagulation factor concentrates. While perhaps most useful in the evaluation of patients who may have developed coagulation factor inhibitors, the same rationale is applicable to patients who are receiving platelet transfusions and who may have developed platelet antibodies. Both the blood product and the patient's blood are measured for the factor or component in question before and after transfusion. By appropriate calculation, knowing the expected space into which the component or factor is diluted, one can determine if the expected effect has been achieved (Table 3.5). If, for example, the hemophiliac patient does not achieve the expected level of Factor VIII after infusion of a known amount of Factor VIII (the product is assayed for total Factor VIII), there is the possibility of a Factor VIII inhibitor which can then be measured and appropriate measures taken. In the case of platelet transfusions the calculation of the corrected count increment (CCI) is useful in the identification of the refractory state. Better yet, of course, is the provision of so-called HLA matched platelets which have been rendered free of contaminating leukocytes which apparently promote the development of platelet antibodies and subsequent suboptimal responses to platelet transfusion.

Cryoprecipitate was one of the early Factor VIII concentrates used in hemophilia and therefore blood centres have assayed these products for acceptable Factor VIII concentration. Over the years, commercially prepared Factor VIII materials have replaced cryoprecipitate in the care of hemophiliacs. However cryoprecipitate has significant amounts of fibrinogen

and therefore has been used increasingly in the treatment of hypofibrinogenemia. But fibrinogen levels are not usually measured on cryoprecipitate. Depending upon the method of manufacture as well as thawing and pooling the hoped-for amounts of fibrinogen may not be found. Attention is thus drawn to improving the production and use of fibrinogen-rich cryoprecipitate, and patient care is significantly improved (Hoffman, Koepke and Widmann, 1987).

3.9 Summary

The physician director plays an important leadership role in the development and management of a clinical coagulation laboratory. The diagnosis and treatment of problems of hemostasis require both an understanding of the technical aspects of testing and a knowledge of the clinical aspects of thrombosis, hemostasis and fibrinolysis. In addition, there is a close association with the appropriate provision of blood products to patients. Thus, this field combines several different aspects of medical care in an interesting as well as important fashion, leading to the best care possible for our patients.

References

Barber, A., Green, D., Galluzzo, T. *et al.* (1985) The bleeding time as a preoperative screening test. *Am. J. Med.*, **78**, 761–764.

Bertina, R. M. (1986) Coagulation testing: Activity versus concentration. *LabMedica*, **3**. (Aug/Sept), 23–26.

Burns, E. R. and Lawrence, C. (1989) Bleeding time – a guide to its diagnostic and clinical utility. *Arch. Pathol. Lab. Med.*, **113**, 1219–1224.

Comprehensive Coagulation Survey Participant Summary – Set CG2-A (1993) Northfield, ILL. College of American Pathologists.

College of American Pathologists (1993) *Practice Parameter for the Use of Fresh Frozen Plasma, Cryoprecipitate and Platelets.* Northfield, ILL. pp. 1–12.

Duke University, Medical Center (1993). *Coagulation Laboratory Manual.* Durham, NC.

Eckman, M. H., Levine, H. J., Pauker, S. G. (1993) Effect of laboratory variation in the prothrombin time ratio on the results of oral anticoagulant therapy. *N. Engl. J. Med.*, 329, 696-702.

Hathaway, W.E. (1987) Hemostatic disorders in the newborn. In: Bloom, A. L. and Thomas, D. P. (eds), *Haemostasis and Thrombosis*, 2nd edn. Edinburgh; Churchill Livingstone, pp. 554–569.

Hattersley, P. G. (1984) Heparin anticoagulation. In Koepke, J. A. (ed.), *Laboratory Hematology*, New York; Churchill Livingstone, pp. 789–818.

Hoffman, M., Koepke, J. A. and Widmann, F. K. (1987) Fibrinogen content of low volume cryoprecipitate. *Transfusion*, 27, 356–358.

ICTH/ICSH (1979) Prothrombin time standardization: Report of the expert panel on oral anticoagulant control. *Thromb. Haemostasis*, 42, 1073–1114

Koepke, J. A. (1993a) Diagnosis and management of perioperative bleeding. Glenside, PA: Toltzis Medical Communications, 4, No. 5.

Koepke, J. A. (1993b) Reporting prothrombin time for patients taking anticoagulants (letter). *Am. J. Clin. Pathol.*, 99, 762.

Koepke, J. A., Gilmer, P. R., Filip, J. D. *et al.* (1975) Studies of fibrinogen measurement in the CAP survey program. *Am. J. Clin. Pathol.*, 63, 984–989.

Koepke, J. A., McLaren, C. E., Wijetunga, A. *et al.* (1994) A method to examine the need for duplicate testing of common coagulation tests. *Am. J. Clin. Pathol.*, 102, 242–247.

Koepke, J. A., Rodgers, J. L. and Ollivier, M. J. (1975) Pre-instrumental variables in coagulation testing. *Am. J. Clin. Pathol.*, 64, 591–596.

National Committee for Clinical Laboratory Standards (1992a) How to define, determine and utilize reference intervals in the clinical laboratory; proposed guideline. NCCLS Document C28-P (ISBN 1–56238–143–1). Villanova, PA: NCCLS.

National Committee for Clinical Laboratory Standards (1992b) One-stage prothrombin time test (PT); tentative guideline. NCCLS document H28-T (ISBN 1–56238–167–9) Villanova, PA: NCCLS.

National Committee for Clinical Laboratory Standards (1991) Collection, transport and processing of blood specimens for coagulation testing and performance of coagulation assays – second edition. Approved Guideline.

NCCLS document H21-A2 (ISBN 1–56238–129–6). Villanova, PA: NCCLS.

National Institutes of Health (1985) Fresh frozen plasma: indications and risks. *JAMA*, 253, 551–553.

National Institutes of Health (1987) Platelet transfusion therapy. *JAMA*, 257, 1777–1780.

Rose, V. L., Dermott, S. C., Murray, B. F. *et al.* (1993) Decentralized testing for prothrombin time and activated partial thromboplastin time using a dry chemistry portable analyzer. *Arch. Pathol. Lab., Med.* 117, 611–617.

Simmons, A. and Paulo, M. A. (1993) Prothrombin time stability and precision using buffered sodium citrate. *LabMedica*, 10(b), 22–24.

Simpson, M. B. (1991) Transfusion therapy for hematologic diseases. In: Koepke, J. A. (ed.), *Practical Laboratory Hematology*. New York, Churchill Livingstone, p. 1141–1173.

Stewart, C. E. and Koepke, J. A. (1987) Reference intervals. In: *Basic Quality Assurance Practices for Clinical Laboratories*. Philadelphia: Lippincott, pp. 61–73.

Triplett, D. A. and Brandt, J. (1993) International Normalized Ratios – has their time come? *Arch. Pathol. Lab. Med.*, 117, 590–592.

General References

Bloom, A. L. and Thomas, D. P. (eds) (1987) *Haemostasis and Thrombosis*, 2nd edn. Edinburgh: Churchill Livingstone.

Koepke, J. A. (ed.) (1991) *Practical Laboratory Hematology*. New York: Churchill Livingstone.

Ruggeri, Z. M. (ed.) (1985) Coagulation Disorders. *Clinics in Hematology* 14:2, London: Saunders.

Thomson, J. M. (ed.) (1980) *Blood Coagulation and Haemostasis, – A Practical Guide*, 2nd edn. Edinburgh: Churchill Livingstone.

Triplett, D. A. (ed.) (1984) Coagulation. *Clinics in Laboratory Medicine* 4:2, Philadelphia: Saunders.

Triplett, D. A. (ed.) (1986) *Advances in Coagulation Testing: Interpretation and Application*. Skokie, ILL. College of American Pathologists.

4

Blood transfusion service

B. Brozović

4.1 Introduction

Blood transfusion service is the hematology subspecialty with the widest range of activities. Although structure and organization of the blood transfusion service vary considerably in different countries the main aim of the service is to provide a safe supply of blood and blood components to the patients in need of transfusion support. In some countries the transfusion service is nationwide and under centralized management, for example the National Blood Authority in the UK. In other countries it may be wholly operated by the National Red Cross Society, as for example the Canadian Red Cross. The American National Red Cross Blood Services provides about half of the blood transfused, the remaining blood being provided by other suppliers in the USA. In other countries the transfusion service is provided by a number of independent non-profit and for-profit organizations, operating side by side, often in open competition, as for example in Germany.

The fundamental principles of ethics of blood transfusion are based on voluntary non-remunerated donations of blood by donors (André, 1980; Moore, 1993).

The voluntary non-remunerated blood donor, whether donating whole blood or plasma for fractionation, is less likely to conceal an event(s) in his medical and social history which would preclude the donation of blood. Such events may indicate that he belongs to the category of individuals at high risk of transmitting an infection to the recipient, and should lead to his rejection as a donor. The donor who benefits from the donation by receiving either money or inducements in kind (e.g. goods, tickets for sports events or theatre, etc.) should also be avoided. That is the reason why many countries strive to achieve self-sufficiency through voluntary unremunerated blood donation not only by promoting blood donation using the public relations campaigns but also by providing an appropriate legal framework (as for example the Recommendation No. R(88)4 of the

Committee of Ministers of Council of Europe, 7 March 1988).

However, a substantial proportion of plasma products marketed by several multinational manufacturers has been processed from plasma drawn from paid donors. While this trade receives criticism from ethical purists and objecting scientists, it satisfies the demand for these products which exists in the countries unable to achieve self-sufficiency. It is certain that current methods of viral inactivation should render these products free from the risk of transmitting most of the known viruses and in particular HIV. However, many experts in blood transfusion share the view that the safety of plasma products will be further increased when plasma is collected only from volunteer unpaid donors (Huestis and Taswell, 1994; Strauss et al., 1994).

The chain of procedures which take place from the moment of blood collection from the donor to its administration to the patient is complex and it is served by numerous professionals with diverse qualifications and training (Table 4.1). The procedures can be conveniently grouped into those related to the collection of blood and testing of blood donors, usually carried out at blood centres, those related to the provision of compatible blood and appropriate blood components for the patient, traditionally performed in the hospital transfusion service*, and those accompanying the administration of blood to the patient, almost invariably carried out on the ward or operating theatre. It is, therefore, convenient to use three models to describe different types of provision of services (Table 4.2). In Model 1, blood centres in the UK serve a geographic area with a population of half a million to 5 million, collect blood from blood donors who represent between 5 and 10% of population, and provide 10–100 hospitals with blood and services. Hospital blood banks carry out immuno-

---

* The British Transfusion Services equate with Blood Banks in the USA; to avoid confusion in this chapter these are termed Blood Centres. The term Transfusion Service is used to refer to a hospital unit or department.

Table 4.1 The chain of events that link the blood donor and the patient receiving transfusion and the health care professionals who participate in the chain

Events	Health care professionals
Blood donor	
Recruitment	Public Relations staff
Selection	Medical Officer
Blood collection	Donor Attendant
Blood processing	MLA*
Donor testing	
Immunohematological testing	MLSO† or Clinical Scientist
Microbiological testing	MLSO or Clinical Scientist
Blood stock maintenance	Clerical Officer
Reconciliation of documentation	IT‡ staff
Blood issue	Clerical Officer
Blood delivery	Driver
Blood reception	MLSO or Clinical Scientist
Blood stock maintenance	MLSO or Clinical Scientist
Compatibility testing	MLSO or Clinical Scientist
Blood processing (where required)	MLSO or Clinical Scientist
Reconciliation of documentation	MLSO or Clinical Scientist
Blood issue	MLSO or Clinical Scientist
Patient	
Reconciliation of documentation	RGN§
Administration	Physician or Surgeon
Follow-up	Physician or Surgeon

*MLA, Medical Laboratory Assistant. †MLSO, Medical Laboratory Scientific Officer. ‡IT, Information Technology staff. §RGN, Registered General Nurse.

hematological investigations and ensure that compatible blood and appropriate blood components are issued to the wards for transfusion to the patient. Some blood centres, in proximity to a hospital, provide not only the supply of blood but also all the services traditionally undertaken by a hospital transfusion service (Model 2). In Model 3 the transfusion service of a hospital carries out the collection and processing of blood, and testing of donors in addition to its conventional tasks. In all three models the functions of the blood centre, hospital transfusion service and staff on the wards remain the same (see also Hollan *et al.*, 1990 and Gibbs and Britten, 1992).

The relationships which exist between the blood centre, hospital transfusion service and hospital ward and the lines of demand and supply of blood, from the donor to the patient, are illustrated in Figure 4.1. The activities required to maintain that line and the role of the hematologist in support and supervision of these activities are described below.

4.2 Blood centres

Blood centres provide services on a district or regional basis serving a community of up to 5 million people. They have similar aims and objectives (Table 4.3) although their size, annual rate of blood collection, organization and range of services may vary enormously (Table 4.4). The main features of blood centers which make them unique among the health care providers are as follows.

4.2.1 The public dimension

Blood centers recruit donors from the general public. Recruiting campaigns, donor selection procedures, retention of established donors and similar activities must be carried out with sensitivity to current political, social and local issues, for example when targeting ethnic minorities, as blood transfusion exists on the goodwill of voluntary non-remunerated donors (in most countries).

Many advances, and occasionally a disaster, which have happened in the field attract the interest of the public in general and the mass media in particular. Press releases, photo-opportunities and interviews are frequent occurrences for the staff of blood centers.

The medical screening of donors may discover the presence of an abnormal condition or a disease of which the donor is unaware. Medical staff have then to decide which one of several of the following actions to follow: refer the donor to his general practitioner or to a specialist, investigate further, counsel where appropriate, follow-up and/or advise him not to donate in the future.

4.2.2 High volume testing

It is standard practice that a sample of blood taken from each donor at the time of donation is tested using hematological and immunological methods. Blood centers may test between 100 and 2000 samples a day with a number of mandatory and optional tests (Table 4.5). The high volume testing has driven the blood centres towards an increasing use of automation and computerization (Barbara, 1989, 1992). In particular, demands for error-free processing, testing and reporting of mandatory immunological tests have led to the development of modular add-on systems as well as to complete units for processing (e.g. the Abbott 'Prism', the Behring BEP-III, the Hamilton 'FAME', the Organon MPP system, etc.). These demands have also made it necessary to develop fully integrated computerized systems for the management of the donor panels on the one hand and the collection, processing, testing and release of the blood units on the other hand. These systems have been developed as recommended by official documents such as the Guidelines for Preparing Standard Operat-

Table 4.2 Models for provision of transfusion services

A. Collection and processing of blood, testing of donors, stock maintenance and issue of blood and blood components

B. Patient testing, compatibility testing, stock maintenance and issue of compatible blood and appropriate blood components

C. Assessment of the patient's transfusion needs, generation or request, administration of transfusion, follow-up

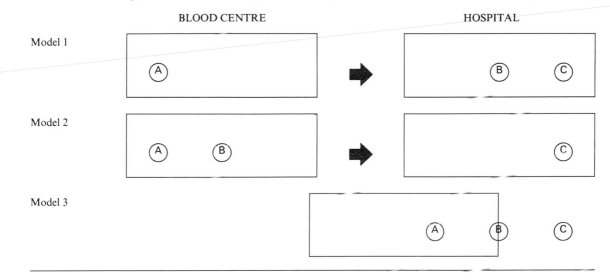

ing Procedures for Blood Bank Computer Systems by the American Association of Blood Banks.

4.2.3 Reference laboratory

Blood centres provide reference services for immuno-hematological problems on a 24 hour basis. The reference laboratory is not only a diagnostic laboratory for investigation of patients with antibodies against red cells, but also a focal point which provides advice on the management of patients and their follow-up, on the investigation and management of women attending prenatal clinics, and provides phenotyped and/or compatible units of blood

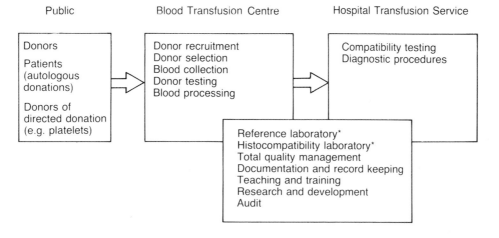

* May be located in blood transfusion centre and/or hospital transfusion service

Figure 4.1 Blood transfusion service links the donor, the member of the public, and the patient in a hospital, through a wide range of activities carried out in the blood centre and the hospital transfusion service

Table 4.3 Aims and objectives which are applicable to a typical blood centre

Aims
- To produce and supply blood, and blood components for clinical use and plasma for fractionation in an appropriate, timely and cost-effective fashion
- To provide the relevant specialist clinical, technical and scientific services
- To ensure that the needs of customers (both donors and users) are fully met
- To provide training and advice on all aspects relating to blood transfusion for internal and external medical, technical and scientific staff
- To improve the quality and safety of the blood supply through research and development
- To raise public awareness of blood transfusion service

Objectives
- To achieve the target set for whole blood donations
- To meet the demand for blood and blood components and respond to the users' requirements
- To update working practices and extend the range of components where required
- To promote good transfusion practices at hospitals
- To implement total quality management
- To implement a programme of internal audit, and at a request by customers carry out external audit
- To provide useful management information
- To achieve a balanced budget

for transfusion. Although a reference laboratory is a unit with low-volume/high-cost activity it provides an indispensable service to the hospitals.

4.2.4 Preparation of blood components

Blood centres in developed countries process almost all of the units of blood collected. Red cells, platelet concentrates and fresh frozen plasma are three main components prepared by processing of blood. The facility to connect packs using sterile docking devices (SDD) has enabled the practice of dividing individual components into several small volume units for transfusion to neonates, or, alternatively, in pooling several units into one pack, as for example pooling platelet concentrates. Large transfusion centres may have on their list of components 20–30 different components and prepare over 500 000 units in a year. The processing has to be carried out according to the current good manufacturing practice (cGMP) embodied in the Rules Governing Medicinal Products in the European Community (1992) and within the framework of the Guidelines for the Blood Transfusion Service (1993).

4.2.5 Statutory requirements

In the UK, blood centres operate under manufacturer's 'specials' licence issued by the Medicines Control Agency and are regularly inspected at two-year inter-

vals. The licence covers all activities related to collection, processing, testing, storage and issue of blood and blood components. The Agency's inspector has to be satisfied that all the statutory requirements, directives, regulations, guidelines, etc. are implemented before the manufacturing licence is renewed. Similar statutory requirements are in operation in other countries, so, for example, the Food and Drug Administration (FDA) in the USA where blood is regulated as a 'drug'.

4.2.6 Teaching and education

There are many difficulties in defining the requirements for teaching and education in a subspecialty of hematology (in some countries a specialty in its own right) which requires broad general medical knowledge and interfaces with many clinical disciplines and specialties (Table 4.6). In the UK the Royal College of Pathologists is responsible for designing the curriculum and examination in blood transfusion as part of the MRCPath Part I and Part II examinations. This issue has also been raised by the International Society of Blood Transfusion on several occasions in the recent past with the aim to formulate the minimum curriculum for specialist training in transfusion medicine within the European Union (Rossi and Cash, 1991, 1992). In view of the complexity of the issue it is unlikely that a training program which would satisfy training requirements in all countries will be designed in the foreseeable future.

4.3 Hospital transfusion services

Main functions of a hospital transfusion service are the provision of diagnostic immunohematological services and the provision of compatible blood and/ or blood component(s). Other functions of the hospital blood bank are listed in Table 4.7.

The hospital transfusion service requires sufficient resources, i.e. staff, equipment and revenue budget, to meet the demand for testing and for purchasing blood and to provide professional advice. Organization in the transfusion service should enable a continuous 24 hours service with clear lines of communication with laboratories in the hospital and to the regional transfusion centre. Useful information about establishing and maintaining a transfusion service in a developing country can be found in the publication Laboratory Services at the Primary Care Level (WHO, 1987).

The hospital transfusion service is in a unique position among other hospital laboratories and departments (with the exception of hospital pharmacy) as it receive supplies of blood and blood components directly from the blood centre. It is responsible for

Table 4.4 Organization and range of services of a blood center

Department	Services
Donor services	
Public relations	Donor recruitment, donor call-up, donor awards, publicity, press and TV visibility
Donor records	Maintenance of the donor records
Mobile collection teams	Selection of donors, collection of blood, transport
Static clinics	Collection of blood, plasmapheresis, plateletpheresis, collection of peripheral blood stem cells
Components laboratory	Processing of blood and preparation of components. Cryopreservation of red cells and platelets
Testing laboratories	
Immunohematology	Donor testing, phenotyping, preparation and testing of reagents, supply of reagents to customers
Microbiology	Donor screening with mandatory tests, additional testing, confirmatory testing of repeatedly reactive samples, collection of epidemiological data, investigation of transfusion transmitted infections
Diagnostic laboratories	
Reference laboratory	Investigation of patients, provision of compatible blood, prenatal investigation, anti-Rh(D) quantitation
Histocompatibility laboratory	HLA typing, investigation of patients with suspected antibodies against leukocyte and platelet antigens
Biochemistry laboratory	Determination of serum proteins and enzymes, detection of hemoglobinopathies
Medical department	
Donor services	Preparing and monitoring selection procedures, monitoring welfare of donors, counselling and follow-up of donors, communication with clinicians, epidemiological studies
Patient services	Advice on patient management, dealing with the hospital clinician
Audit	Internal audits, external (hospital) audits
Teaching and training	Organization of lectures, courses, meetings and symposia for medical, technical, scientific and nursing staff, management training, continuous medical education, continuous professional development, supervision of students studying for academic degrees
Research and development	Conducting a programme of applied research and development
Support services	
Quality department	Implementation of total quality management
Information technology department	Integrated computerization of the centre
Support departments	Finance, human resources, supplies and stores, transport, estates, etc. perform their specific tasks

Table 4.5 Immunohematological and microbiological testing of donors

Immunohematological tests	Microbiological tests
	Generally mandatory tests
Blood grouping: ABO	Hepatitis B surface Antigen (HBsAg);
Rh(D)	Anti-Human Immunodeficiency Virus 1 and 2 (HIV 1 and 2)
Antibody screening	Anti-Hepatitis C Virus (anti-HCV)
	(TPHA)*
	Mandatory tests in some countries
	Anti-Hepatitis B core (HBc)
	Alanine aminotransferase (ALT)
	Human T-cell lymphotrophic virus (HTLV) I and II
	Anti-*Trypanosoma cruzi*
	Optional tests
Extended Rh phenotype	Anti-cytomegalovirus (CMV)
Full red cell phenotype	Neopterin†
Anti-HLA screening	Human Immunodeficiency Virus (HIV) antigen
	Anti-*Plasmodium falciparum*
	Anti-*Toxoplasma gondii*

* *Treponema pallidum* hemagglutination assay.

† A lymphocyte activation marker.

Table 4.6 Relationships between blood transfusion specialty and its activities and other medical specialties and institutions

Blood transfusion specialty, activities	Related specialty or institution

Core activities
  Donor management
  Collection and processing of blood
  Donor testing	

Provision of components, support and advice for treatment	Hematology Oncology Neonatology/ Perinatology Surgery Obstetrics
Transfusion microbiology	Microbiology
Immunology of red cells, platelets and leukocytes	Immunology
Histocompatibility testing	Immunology
Teaching and training	Royal Colleges Universities Medical Specialty Boards (USA)
Research and development	Medical Research Council National Heart Lung and Blood Institute of the National Institutes of Health (USA) Charities Industry

Table 4.7 Activities and procedures in a hospital transfusion service

Activities	Procedures
Pretransfusion testing	Blood grouping, phenotyping Antibody screening, antibody identification Compatibility testing
Stock control (red cells, platelet concentrates, FFP, cryoprecipitate, volume expanders, albumin solutions, coagulation factor concentrates)	Stock maintenance Contract monitoring
Support for special units (cardiac surgery, oncology, hematology, nephrology, neonatal medicine, ICU)	Provision of appropriate blood components
Processing of blood and platelet concentrates	Filtration, pooling
Investigation of autoimmune hemolytic anemias	Immunohematological testing
Quality control, validation and testing of reagents and equipment	
Provision of care to hemophiliac patients	Investigation and treatment
Hemapheresis	Collection of platelets, PBSC*, lymphocytes, etc. Therapeutic hemapheresis
Autologous blood collection	Collection, testing and storage of autologous units of blood
Formulation of the hospital blood transfusion policies	Implementation of policies; participation in Hospital Transfusion Review Committee
Record keeping and documentation Teaching and training of medical and scientific staff Audit, internal and external	

* PBSC, peripheral blood stem cells.

the inventory and operates stock control and issue of products. In addition, further processing of blood, as for example leukofiltration, may be carried out. These activities should be carried out within the framework of the Consumer Protection Act (1987) Part I in the UK and under similar regulations in other countries of the European Union.

The medical director in charge of the blood bank has several roles. First, he is ultimately responsible for the organization and function of the transfusion service in accordance with the Code for Good Laboratory Practice in Haematology Laboratories (1991) and recommendation of the Blood Transfusion Task Force (1991) on documentation and procedures. Secondly, his responsibilities are extended to the interpretation of all immunohematological results and to the provision of advice on matters of transfusion medicine to the medical staff in the hospital. Finally, he is responsible for development and implementation of policies on the appropriate use of blood and blood components as well as for an appropriate use of transfusion services in the hospital. One of the recent changes promulgated by the medical staff is the practice of autologous blood donation (Kruskall, 1989, 1992). The medical director has the central role in organizing of and participating in the hospital transfusion review committee. In a large hospital the medical director is expected to spend full time on matters of transfusion medicine.

4.4 Wards and operating theatres

Many health care professionals directly involved in patient care have to deal with some if not all aspects of administration of blood and blood components to the patient. It is, therefore, essential that they receive appropriate education and training in blood transfusion. It is also essential that they are aware of the hospital policies on blood transfusion embodied into the hospital transfusion manual and incorporated in the hospital nursing manual.

4.5 Hospital transfusion review committee

Hospital transfusion review committee is the body with an executive power to change practices of blood transfusion and implement new ones within the hospital. Its members are representatives of major users of hospital transfusion services. The terms of reference of the committee may vary depending on the local circumstances, but are invariably directed towards promoting better blood transfusion practices. One of the main tasks of the committee is to monitor the practice of blood transfusion by audit.

4.6 Hospital transfusion audit

Audit of different aspects of hospital transfusion service is instigated at the request of the hospital transfusion review committee. The gathering of information, whether retrospectively or prospectively carried out, and the analysis of the results are carried out by designated personnel, and the report is presented to the committee for deliberation. The decision to introduce changes, where required, is then made by the committee. Audit has become a powerful tool to improve the blood transfusion practice on the one hand and to reduce costs of service on the other hand. It is an inseparable part of quality assurance in hospital transfusion practice (Nicholls, 1993).

4.7 The future

At present transfusion services in many countries are undergoing reorganization. In the West that has been brought about by the drive for cost-efficiency at the time of an increasing demand for safe supply of blood made by the public and enacted by legislation. In developing countries the reorganization has been the result of the desire to establish a national transfusion service and achieve self-sufficiency. Some factors affecting planning of blood transfusion service in the future are listed in Table 4.8.

One way to reduce the cost of the service and at the same time to increase efficiency, standardize procedures and improve quality, is to centralize the testing of donors in a few laboratories only. In this model, to be implemented in the future by the American National Red Cross Blood Services, the collection of blood will be undertaken by 52 blood centres but testing of donors will be carried out in only 14 centres. The economies of scale will be achieved by using fully automated testing equipment and an integrated computer system, which will enable each of the testing centres to test up to 500 000 samples a year.

Advances in the development of oxygen-carrying substances, such as polymerized hemoglobins and perfluorocarbons, have been slow, and none is currently available on the market. Human recombinant FVIII has been licensed by FDA in the USA and it is possible that recombinant albumin will become available on the market in the not too distant future. There is no doubt that availability of blood substitutes will have a profound effect on the organization of blood transfusion services. It is at present difficult to design a scenario of their effects without knowledge of a reasonably reliable timetable.

It is certain, however, that the demand for platelet concentrates used for supporting thrombocytopenic patients receiving cytotoxic therapy will increase despite the use of cell growth factors, as the number of patients treated will increase. In response to that demand blood centres will expand the use of cell separators and diversify services, e.g. collection and preservation of peripheral blood stem cells. Other procedures such as collection of lymphocytes for *ex vivo* expansion in adoptive immunotherapy or gene transfer as well as extracorporeal photochemotherapy will become commonplace.

While the blood centres are likely to offer a variety of different services, the hospital transfusion services may get smaller in size and closer to the

Table 4.8 Some factors affecting planning of blood transfusion service for the future

Population changes
Numerical changes – population shifts
Changes in age distribution of the population (ageing population)
Changes in ethnic mix of the population
Changes in clinical practice
Reduction in numbers of acute beds
Increasing use of outpatient services, e.g. same day surgery
Expansion of existing modalities of treatment and introduction of new ones
– bone marrow transplantation
– use of cell growth factors
– dose intensification regimens for chemotherapy
– increased intensive care of premature neonates
– increased use of autologous transfusion
– availability of recombinant coagulation factors concentrates
Changes in disease pattern
Hip replacement revisions
Coronary bypass repeats
Organ transplantation repeats
Changes in staff structure
Medical staff – decreased numbers of trainees
Scientific staff – increased requirements for in-service training and day-release courses
Automation and information technology
Drive for centralization of services (establishment of consortia) to maximize benefits of automation and information technology
Emerging technologies
Use of gel techiniques for blood grouping, antibody screening and compatibility testing may enable near patient testing

patient. We can expect that the techniques for blood grouping, antibody screening and compatibility testing in gel solutions may improve to the extent which will make these acceptable for near-patient testing. However, all the concerns for near-patient testing, discussed in Chapter 1, will also have to be resolved before immunohematological testing in that format becomes standard practice. In addition, instant access to available stocks of blood and blood components will have to be secured to enable the transfusion service operating the near-patient testing policy to respond quickly in an emergency.

References

American Association of Blood Banks: (1991). Guidelines for Preparing Standard Operating Procedures for Blood Bank Computer Systems. Arlington.

André, A. (1981) Montreal 1980: A code of ethics for blood transfusion. *Vox Sang.*, **40**, 303–305.

Barbara, J. A. J. (1989) Defining the information flow in the transfusion-microbiology laboratory. In: Smit Sibinga C.Th, Das P. C., Högman C. F. (eds): *Automation in blood transfusion*. London: Kluwer. pp. 91–96.

Barbara, J. A. J. (1992) Automation in transfusion microbiology. *Buletin*, **14**, 187–189.

Blood Transfusion Task Force (1991) Hospital blood bank documentation and procedures. In: Roberts, B. (ed.); *Standard Haematology Practice*, Oxford: Blackwell Scientific Publications. pp. 128–138.

Code for Good Laboratory Practice in Haematology Laboratories (including hospital blood banks), (1991) In: Roberts, B. (ed.), *Standard Haematology Practice*, Oxford: Blackwell Scientific Publications. pp. 1–18.

Consumer Protection Act 1987, Chapter 43, Part I.

Gibbs, W. N. and Britten, A. F. H. (eds) (1992) Guidelines for the Organisation of a Blood Transfusion Service. Geneva: WHO.

Guidelines for the Blood Transfusion Service (1993) 2nd edn. London: HMSO.

Hollan, S. R., Wagstaff, W., Leikola, J. and Lothe, F. (eds) (1990) *Management of Blood Transfusion Services*. Geneva: WHO.

Huestis, D. W. and Taswell, H. F. (1994) Editorial: Donors and Dollars. *Transfusion*, **34**, 96–97.

Kruskall, M. S. (ed) (1989) The changing face of transfusion practices: autologous blood and other alternatives to routine transfusion. *Transfusion Science*, **10**, 77–145.

Kruskall, M. S. (1992) Autologous transfusions – past, present, and future. *Mayo Clinic Proceedings*, **67**, 392–393.

Moore, B. P. L. (1993) A guide to ethical conduct in transfusion medicine. *Haematologia*, **25**, 293–299.

Nicholls, M. (1993) Quality assurance of hospital transfusion practice. *Med. J. Aust.* **159**, 295–296.

Rossi, U. and Cash, J. D. (1991) *Teaching and Education in Transfusion Medicine*. Council of Europe and Commission of the European Communities.

Rossi, U. and Cash, J. D. (1992) *Teaching and Education in Transfusion Medicine*. Council of Europe and Commission of the European Communities.

Rules Governing Medicinal Products in the European Community (1992) Volume IV, Good manufacturing practice for medicinal products. Commission of the European Communities, Luxembourg.

Strauss, N. G., Ludwig, G. A., Smith, M. V. *et al.* (1994) 'Concurrent comparison of the safety of paid cytapheresis and volunteer whole-blood donors.' *Transfusion*, **34**, 116–121.

WHO (1987) *Laboratory Services at the Primary Health Care Level*. World Health Organisation Publication, WHO, Lab 87.2.

5

Physician's office testing

Daniel M. Baer and Richard E. Belsey

5.1 Rationale for laboratory testing in the physician's office

Laboratory testing takes place in many locations outside the conventional clinical laboratory. Within hospitals, glucose testing at patients' bedsides, operating room blood gas measurement, dialysis unit activated clotting times, and emergency room hematocrits are some of the more common non-laboratory testing sites. Outside hospitals, testing occurs in physicians' offices and clinics and in health care centres without physicians such as family planning clinics. In most cases, this testing is performed by nurses, medical assistants or individuals without either laboratory or medical care training such as office receptionists. This chapter will focus on laboratory testing within physicians' offices and clinics.

In the USA primary care physicians commonly have an office laboratory. It has been estimated that 90% of family practitioners and general physicians (internists) have some tests analysed in their offices and that hematological or chemical analyses are performed in as many as 90 000 medical offices, most of them single or dual practices.

For many practitioners the reasons for office test analysis are patient convenience, more rapid diagnoses and medical management, avoidance of repeat visits, and streamlining of patient care and office administration. For the majority of practitioners profit motive is a minor factor for instituting office testing. Many practitioners wish to perform tests in the office laboratory and take action on the test results before the patient leaves the medical office. Patients, especially those who live a long distance from the physician as well as elderly patients, may find it difficult to make repeated visits to the physician. For these patients it is a great convenience to include testing with the medical visit so that a diagnosis can be made or therapy can be initiated or evaluated in a single trip to the physician. For the physician and office staff, performing, evaluating and acting on a laboratory test result while the patient is still in the office, prevents multiple filings and retrievals of the patient's chart, and obviates the need for phone calls to the patient and pharmacy. Avoiding these added steps undoubtedly saves a significant amount of staff time for each patient whose test results are available before leaving the office, as long as 14 minutes per patient has been suggested by some observers.

Hematological tests commonly performed in the physician's office include quantitative and morphological examination of blood cells, erythrocyte sedimentation rate, either as an indication of inflammatory disease or for monitoring of rheumatic diseases, and prothrombin time for management of oral anticoagulant therapy. In our practice, for example, home health nurses perform prothrombin time tests in the patients' homes, using a small portable test system. This allows them to adjust anticoagulant therapy on single visit to the patient, thus providing better patient care while achieving greater productivity.

5.2 Characteristics of people doing point of care testing

Two studies (Brock *et al.*, 1977; Gwyther and Kirkman-Liff, 1982) suggested that approximately one-third of the technical staff in physician office laboratories had some laboratory technical training while the remainder who were not technically trained included nurses, medical assistants and clerical staff. Approximately one-third of the individuals doing the testing had no health care training of any kind. Registration and licensing of laboratories in the USA required by the Clinical Laboratory Improvement Amendments of 1988 (CLIA '88) will eventually provide an accurate picture of the training and experience of individuals performing point of care testing in US office laboratories.

Most individuals who have no laboratory technical training have little appreciation of the limitations of testing technology, analytic variability associated with testing, and the quality management techniques required for consistent production of precise and accurate results. Because of the high quality of test results from professionally directed and staffed laboratories, many have a false reliance on quality being built 'into the testing box'. These individuals are unaware of the steps that must be taken to ensure a high standard of quality. Such common laboratory quality management practices as procedure manuals, use and documentation of quality control samples, external proficiency testing, regularly scheduled instrument maintenance, and technical staff in-service education are not part of the culture of individuals without technical training.

In a study performed in the state of Idaho in 1986 (Crawley *et al.*, 1986) we found that 20% of the individuals responsible for point of care testing in physicians' offices were no longer employed in the same office six months later and 50% had changed jobs in a one-year period. This turnover of personnel presents significant problems in providing appropriate training for individuals who perform tests and indicates that there is a high probability that the laboratory staff has not been adequately trained for the procedures they perform.

The physician's office laboratory director is usually the physician himself, but he or she generally has had no preparation for the management and supervision of laboratory testing in the office and has no basis for selection of equipment and methods other than the recommendation of the salesperson. The Clinical Laboratory Improvement Amendments of 1988 recognizes this by requiring that each laboratory that is not directed by a laboratory professional has a qualified medical technologist or other laboratory professional who is responsible for selection of test methods. This technical consultant has broad responsibility for the quality of testing, training and evaluation of the testing personnel (see Chapter 21).

5.2.1 Test selection

The tests performed in the office laboratory should be selected on the basis of the clinical needs of the physician but they frequently also reflect the test menu of the analytic system. For instance, the family practitioner or general internist may require only a total leukocyte count to help differentiate a bacterial from viral respiratory illness. However, if the cell counter is a multiparameter one, a full set of test results would be produced by the analytic system.

Other factors influencing the selection of tests to be performed include the availability of simple technology appropriate to the technical capabilities of the laboratory staff; the degree of automation to allow laboratory staff with multiple office duties to start a test then leave it unattended while performing other duties; and cost of test performance versus reimbursement (Baer and Belsey, 1986).

5.2.2 Test systems

Blood cell counters

The current models of blood cell counters marketed to physicians' office laboratories are generally multiparameter systems providing RBC count, hemoglobin/hematocrit, red cell indices including MCH, MCV, MCHC, and perhaps RDW, WBC count and a three-part differential leukocyte count, platelet count, and possibly the PDW. Most of the systems provide graphic cell distribution histograms or scattergrams on a computer screen and/or in printed form. These tests systems, which usually employ an impedance counting principle, have automated pipetting and some even use closed vacuum tube sampling, using a cap puncturing device. These systems generally retail in the range of $20 000–25 000. Simpler, less expensive systems performing RBC count, hemoglobin/hematocrit and WBC counts are becoming outmoded in the USA. One estimate indicates that only 15% of instruments sold in 1992 were of this simpler, less expensive variety. Major manufacturers of cell counters include the Coulter Corporation, Abbott Laboratories (Celldyne), Roche Diagnostic Systems, Danam, Serono–Baker and Sysmex.

Becton-Dickinson's QBC (Wardlaw and Levine, 1983) has been aggressively marketed to the physician's office laboratory market. This instrument measures the relative volume of red cells (i.e. microhematocrit), two classes of leukocytes (granulocytes and mononuclears) and platelets which are selectively separated during centrifugation in a capillary tube with a specially designed plastic float. A fluorescent stain within the tube allows for the identification of the different cell populations. The instrument is available either as a manual configuration or as an auto-reader model. In the manual instrument the operator observes the centrifuged capillary through a magnifier and moves a pointer to the interfaces between cell populations to obtain the readings. The auto-reader model automatically performs this task taking multiple readings of each interface. This latter model is said to be more accurate and objective in its readings. An interesting feature of the auto-reader model is the optional incorporation of interpretative reports based on excerpts from Wintrobe's hematology text although users are warned that these are only suggestions based on a limited examination of a part of a patient's hematological status, and should not be accepted as a complete clinical diagnosis. Some users of this system have commented on a potential hazard from broken capillary tubes (FDA, 1993). These can expose the operator to puncture wounds and infection from blood-borne pathogens such as hepatitis viruses and HIV. The substitution of plastic capillary tubes might remedy this problem.

Microhematocrit measurements are commonly performed in physicians' office laboratories as well as in out-of-laboratory testing sites within hospitals. This technology suffers from the same potential hazard of exposure to blood-borne pathogens as the QBC. Because of its simplicity and freedom from operator-induced errors, it has been classified as a waived test under US federal laboratory licensing rules, and is not subject to regulation by CLIA '88.

Hemoglobin measurements are included in the test menus of a variety of common physician's office chemical analysers such as Kodak Ektachem DT-60, Abbott Vision, Boehringer–Mannheim Reflotron, and Miles Serolyzer and Clinistat. The Mallinckrodt HemoCue is a single purpose hemoglobinometer that accurately analyses hemoglobin with a disposable reagent cuvette. It measures hemoglobin very accurately as hemiglobinazide (Bridges, Parvin and Van Assendelft, 1987). This method is also classified as a waived test under CLIA '88.

Sedimentation Rate

The erythrocyte sedimentation rate (ESR) is performed in some physicians' office laboratories but is not as popular in the United States as in Europe. Several test systems using disposable 300 millimetre Westergren tubes with self-adjusting zeroing features, collection tubes containing appropriate amounts of citrate diluent and tube racks are available for physicians' office laboratories. Systems using the shorter Wintrobe tube are less commonly sold to physician's offices. Some companies market 'micro sedimentation rate' systems. The Zeta sedimentation rate system formerly sold by Coulter, is no longer marketed.

Infectious hazards from the manipulation of blood during the dilution and filling steps of this test is a potential hazard to the operator. There are now several closed test systems which use integrated diluting tubes and self-adjusting disposable measuring tubes. Automated systems are also available, e.g. the Ves-matic system (Diesse Diagnostica Senese, Monteriggioni, Italy) which uses a special plastic blood collection tube containing the proper volume of diluent. This tube is placed directly into the instrument, which measures the sedimentation rate over a 30-min interval (Koepke, Caracappa and Johnson, 1990).

Coagulation systems

The packaging of thromboplastin in 5-ml vials, the need to reconstitute these lyophilized reagents accurately and the short shelf life of reconstituted thromboplastin limits the selection of test systems for laboratories performing a low volume of prothrombin time tests. Systems that do not depend on the formation of a traditional thrombin clot are therefore attractive in the physician's office laboratory setting. Several manufacturers provide chromogenic assays for their chemical analysers. The Abbott Vision instrument is one such method. The Ciba–Corning Biotrak 512 (also marketed by DuPont as the Coumatrak) is a prothrombin time instrument that utilizes a disposable reagent card (Belsey, Fischer and Baer, 1991). The Biotrak 512 is also capable of performing a PTT test. This hand-held portable instrument first warms the card to 37°C then instructs the user to apply a large drop of finger tip whole blood into the orifice on the card. Blood is drawn by capillary action into a channel coated with thromboplastin. End-point of the reaction is detected by the instrument as the cessation of Brownian movement by red cells as the fibrin clot forms. Results are given in seconds as well as the INR system. Whole blood normal and abnormal control specimens are provided by the manufacturer. Other portable analysers for coagulation testing are becoming available (Rose et al., 1993).

A recent paper compared the incidence of hemorrhagic and thrombotic events in ambulatory patients receiving warfarin who had prothrombin time tests performed in physicians' office laboratories. Patients from laboratories that performed few prothrombin time tests had significantly more adverse events than those whose tests were performed in higher volume laboratories (Mennemeyer and Winkelman, 1993). A survey of physicians' office laboratories suggests one reason for this: only 15% of the office laboratories performing prothrombin time tests tested quality control samples.

In hospitals and free-standing dialysis centres, heparin anticoagulation and protamine neutralization are controlled using the activated clotting time (ACT) test. Test systems are Hemochron (International Technidyne Corporation) and HemoTec (Medtronic HemoTec, Inc.). In our hospital, this test is performed by the cardiopulmonary perfusionists in the operating room, the cardiac catheterization laboratory and the dialysis unit. Although quality control materials are now available for the ACT test, quality control testing is not commonly performed.

5.3 Quality management and regulatory issues in the USA

The regulations for maintaining quality standards in clinical laboratories in the USA (CLIA '88) are described in Chapter 21. Although the Clinical Laboratory Improvement Act of 1967 and the Conditions for Medicare Reimbursement, implemented at about the same time, required quality management and personnel qualification for laboratories engaging in interstate commerce or accepting Medicare or Medicaid payment, physician office laboratories and other point of care testing sites were exempt. The 1988 amendments extended federal regulation to all sites

Table 5.1 Waived tests

The following tests are not subject to the provision of CLIA '88. Laboratories performing these tests must register with HCFA and follow the manufacturers' directions for running the tests.

Dipstick or tablet reagent urinalysis (non-automated) for the following:
  Bilirubin
  Glucose
  Hemoglobin
  Ketone
  Leukocytes
  Nitrite
  pH
  Protein
  Specific gravity
  Urobilinogen
Ovulation test – visual colour comparison tests for human luteinizing hormone;
Urine pregnancy tests – visual colour comparison tests;
Erythrocyte sedimentation rate – non-automated;
Hemoglobin – copper sulphate, non-automated;
Hemoglobin by single analyte instrument (HemoCue),
Fecal occult blood;
Spun hematocrit;
Blood glucose by glucose monitoring devices cleared by FDA specifically for home use;
Whole blood cholesterol measurement using device cleared by FDA specifically for home use.

Table 5.2 Exempt physician-performed tests

The following physician-performed microscopic tests are not subject to the provisions of CLIA '88. If performed by individuals other than a physician, personally for his/her own patients, these tests are classified as moderately complex, and are subject to CLIA '88 rules.

Urine sediment examinations
Postcoital examinations
Wet mounts for parasites and fungus
Wet mounts of prostatic secretions
KOH preparations for fungus
Pinworm examinations
Fern tests for estrogen effect

---

performing laboratory tests for patient care or health screening.

Under the rules of CLIA '88, tests are regulated according to their complexity. A very small number of tests are placed in a waived category which are exempt from regulation (Table 5.1). The most commonly performed tests, including most which would be conducted in a physician's office, are classified as moderately complex. These tests may be performed by individuals, frequently without technical training, currently performing tests of this kind. Certain tests involving microscopic examination are also exempt from the regulations if examined by a licensed physician for his or her own patients (Table 5.2). If, however, these test are performed by someone other than the physician they are subject to the full regulatory burden required for moderately complex testing. Examination of peripheral blood film, bone marrow or body fluids is not exempt from the rules. Identification of blood cells is of particular interest because, when the blood cells are normal, the test is categorized as a moderately complex test. However, identification of abnormal blood cells categorizes the test as highly complex, requiring a higher level of personnel and supervision. This requires many physicians' office laboratories encountering an abnormal blood film to send it to a fully qualified laboratory for further examination.

In addition to CLIA '88 seventeen states and territories of the United States have laws regulating laboratories including point of care testing such as physicians' offices.

5.4 The role of professional laboratorians in quality management

Partly as a result of the implementation of CLIA '88, professional laboratorians will need to interact with point of care testing sites including physician's office and ancillary testing sites in hospitals and nursing homes. Many physicians are either not qualified to serve as directors of their office laboratories or may not wish to undertake the extensive duties required of the director. All regulated laboratories, regardless of their complexity level, must have either a qualified technical consultant or a qualified supervisor. As defined by CLIA '88, the technical consultant is a qualified medical laboratory technologist or doctoral level laboratory professional. A clinical hematologist is qualified to serve in this role, but only for hematological tests. This individual must ensure that quality management activities of the laboratory are carried out, that only qualified individuals perform testing, and that there is a programme of continuing education for laboratory staff members. The technical consultant or supervisor is responsible for selection of test methods and validation of their performance prior to being put in to use.

To be effective, professional laboratorians, including laboratory physicians, who interact with physicians' office laboratories must become familiar with their mode of operation and their needs, which are different from those of larger laboratory. Equipment methods and procedures and even language which is appropriate for the professionally directed and staff laboratory are frequently inappropriate in a small laboratory staffed by individuals who are not technically trained. Technical consultation to point of care laboratories will emerge as an opportunity for career enhancement for qualified laboratory technologists. Other laboratory professionals will also find new and interesting opportunities in developing consultation, education and product development ventures.

References

Baer, D. M. and Belsey, R. E. (1986) Assessing an office chemistry instrument. *Primary Care*, **13**, 699–711.

Belsey, R. E., Fischer, P. M. and Baer, D. M. (1991) An evaluation of a whole blood prothrombin analyzer designed for use by individuals without formal laboratory training. *J. Family Practice*, **33**, 266–271.

Bridges, N., Parvin, R. M. and Van Assendelft, O. W. (1987) Evaluation of a new system for hemoglobin measurement. *Am. Clin. Prod. Rev.*, **6**, (April) 22–25.

Brock, D. W., Crawley, R., Anderson, G. *et al.* (1977) An analysis of Idaho private physician office laboratory facilities and testing activities through on-site inspection. Center for Disease Control, Contract 200–77–0716, 1977.

Crawley, R., Belsey, R., Brock, D. and Baer, D. M. (1986) Regulation of Physicians' Office Laboratories: The Idaho Experience. *JAMA*, **255**, 374–382.

FDA (1993) *Med. Bull.*, **23**, No. 2 (June), p. 6.

Gwyther, R. E. and Kirkman-Liff, B. L. (1982) Laboratory testing in the offices of family physicians. *Am. J. Med. Technol.*, **48**, 697–702

Koepke, J. A., Caracappa, P. and Johnson, L. (1990) The evolution of erythrocyte sedimentation rate methodology. *Labmedica*, February–March, pp. 46–48.

Mennemeyer, S. T. and Winkelman, J. W. (1993) Searching for inaccuracy in clinical laboratory testing using medicare data: Evidence for prothrombin time. *JAMA* **269**, 1030–1033.

Rose, V. L., Dermott, S. C., Murray, B. F. *et al.* (1993) Decentralized testing for prothrombin time and activated partial thromboplastin time using a dry chemistry portable analyzer. *Arch. Pothol. Lab. Med.*, **117**, 611–617.

Wardlaw, S. C. and Levine, R. A. (1983) Quantitative buffy coat analysis: A new laboratory tool functioning as a screening complete blood cell count. *JAMA*, **249**, 617–620.

Editor's Note

An excellent monograph on alternate-site testing has recently been published; it includes all aspects of laboratory testing not done in the central laboratory and contains a wealth of information on this new field:

Handorf C. R. (ed.) (1994) Alternate-site testing. *Clin. Lab. Med.* **14**, 451–676.

6

Expert systems in laboratory hematology

Lawrence W. Diamond and Doyen T. Nguyen

Improvements in automated instrumentation and the availability of new reagents and techniques for characterizing hematopoietic and lymphoid cells have led to a dramatic increase in the amount of data generated by the modern, full-service hematology laboratory. Physicians and laboratory personnel need efficient ways to collect, organize and communicate this information so that it can be effectively applied to patient management.

There have been equally dramatic improvements in microcomputer hardware and software development tools in the last decade. These advances are making it possible to use computers in the challenging task of providing decision support in laboratory hematology diagnosis. In this chapter, we will focus on the application of expert system technology to the practice of laboratory hematology including the current role of knowledge-based systems for efficient and effective interpretive reporting.

A variety of problem-solving strategies including probabilistic reasoning, statistical pattern recognition, multivariate statistical analysis, discriminant functions, and cluster analysis have been tested in the construction of computer databases and decision support systems for the hematology laboratory (Bates and Bessman, 1987; Blomberg et al., 1987; Sultan, Imbert and Priolet, 1988; Paterakis, Terzoglou and Vasilioy, 1989). These approaches, although popular, have limitations which make them unattractive for the task of interpretive reporting. The mathematical and probabilistic models of clinical reasoning (in particular, Bayes' theorem and decision analysis) have been criticized because they do not resemble the way a physician reasons in actual practice (Feinstein, 1977). For example, an effective laboratory physician or consultant hematologist does not estimate probabilities to answer the question of whether an adult patient with an absolute lymphocytosis and anemia has chronic lymphocytic leukemia. A decision is reached by getting more data, such as lymphocyte immunophenotyping or bone marrow studies. In addition, it is difficult to provide explanations for diagnostic reasoning when using mathematical models. The lack of an explanation facility is thought to be a serious deficiency in a medical decision support system because users who do not understand the system's reasoning will not readily accept it (Smith, Speicher and Chandrasekaran, 1984). For these reasons, many researchers in the field of medical informatics have turned to so-called artificial intelligence techniques ('expert system technology') in the design of computer systems for use in the hematology laboratory.

Medical expert systems attempt to simulate the reasoning process a physician uses to solve complex problems. The traditional building blocks of such a system include a knowledge base, inference engine, user interface, and explanation facility. The knowledge base of a laboratory hematology system represents the storehouse of facts, rules and practical shortcuts that can be applied to all problems within the domain. How this knowledge is represented is crucial to the design of the system. This aspect of the project is usually under the control of a team member known as the knowledge engineer. Rule-based expert systems code the knowledge into a series of statements of the basic type: IF ⟨Observation⟩ THEN ⟨Conclusion⟩. Several observations can be logically joined together using AND or OR, for example, IF ⟨Observation 1⟩ OR ⟨Observation 2⟩ THEN ⟨Conclusion⟩.

The inference engine combines the patient data with the knowledge to reach conclusions and make recommendations. A number of so-called expert system shells exist which provide a pre-programmed mechanism for reasoning using IF-THEN rules (Healy, Spackman and Beck, 1989). Many shells provide a method for assigning numerical representations of uncertainty to the diagnostic rules (Shortliffe and Buchanan, 1975). Although an expert system shell may allow a sophisticated program to be built relatively easily, its use as a programming tool leads to a definite loss of flexibility in both knowledge representation and the inference process. Logical diagnostic reasoning requires a step-wise strategy for evaluating evidence, formulating intermediate conclusions by recognizing patterns, and ordering appropriate adjunctive tests before arriving at a diagnosis (Feinstein, 1973). A reasonable plan in the design of a computerized expert system is to follow this approach to whatever extent possible.

The latest microcomputer operating systems and programming languages provide the ability for up-to-date systems to have a 'friendly' graphical user interface so that a complex series of commands need not be memorized. Explanations can be provided by a function which lists the diagnostic rules invoked, or by an on-line electronic textbook with access to photomicrographs.

A high-performance computer system should be capable of reaching intelligent conclusions about all cases coming through the hematology laboratory, including follow-up studies and cases that require supplementary information for interpretation. A database (to store clinical findings, laboratory data and the system's analysis) is a critical component of such a system.

6.1 Historical perspective

An early study on the efficient classification and correlation of clinical and laboratory findings in the differential diagnosis of hematological diseases was not a computer program but rather a system for mechanical data correlation utilizing marginal punched cards (Lipkin and Hardy, 1958). This study, published in early 1958, is quite interesting when viewed from the perspective of computer systems being developed in the 1990s and will therefore be presented in some detail. The punched cards were constructed by dividing the periphery of each card into 138 numbered spaces. A hole was punched in each space. In this way, each space represented a single piece of information, e.g. space 25 represented megaloblasts present on bone marrow examination. The four sides of the cards were assigned to case history, physical examination, peripheral blood examination, and bone marrow data (together with other laboratory work), respectively. Twenty-six diseases were selected from standard hematology textbooks, each represented by a single card. A master code was made for all data from the 26 diseases. The information about a disease was transferred to the appropriate card in the following way: when a positive finding was associated with a particular disease, a triangular wedge was punched in that space (eliminating the hole for that feature from that card). In addition, an arrow was drawn on the card next to the wedge for findings which constituted the most definitive diagnostic criteria for each disease.

This set of cards could then be used to sort on the basis of a single item of data. For example, if one wished to find all of the diseases characterized by splenomegaly, one would arrange the cards front to back and place a metal or plastic rod into the hole that had been assigned to splenomegaly. When the rod was raised, cards representing diseases with splenomegaly would fall because the triangular wedge had been punched into that space. Cards without the wedge would be raised by the rod.

To test the effectiveness of this approach in differential diagnosis, the hospital records of 80 patients with hematological diseases were consulted and each positive finding was listed in a table according to the code numbers which had been assigned to the disease cards. The 26 disease cards were again assembled front to back. The side containing clinical history was placed upright and, for each positive item of historical data in a patient, a rod was placed through the stack. If a case had more than one positive item, several rods would be inserted. When the rods where raised, cards which contained wedged out areas for all of the inserted findings fell, while cards with one or more negative findings were raised and eliminated. This procedure was repeated three more times for the physical examination data, the peripheral blood findings, and the bone marrow examination and other laboratory work. The card or cards remaining after the final elimination represented disease(s) in which all positive patient findings corresponded to features of a particular disease.

With this approach, a correct diagnosis was made in 73 of 80 cases (91.25%). In 50 cases, all data were characteristic of only one disease. The single card which remained after sorting not only contained the correct diagnosis, but each item which constituted the definitive diagnostic criteria for that disease was present in that patient. In 23 cases, two or more cards remained. When the user examined those cards for the definitive diagnostic criteria, it was seen that the data from these patients satisfied only one of the diseases whose cards remained. Several cards had appeared because items which were definitive diagnostic criteria for the incorrect diseases were not positive findings in the hospital case, and therefore had not entered into the sorting procedure. If the punched cards had contained enough spaces to code negative findings initially, the incorrect disease cards would not have appeared. The authors concluded that although punched card analysis of some cases might result in no remaining card, an incorrect diagnosis could not result from this procedure if the patient's data were correct. Furthermore, when the sorting process resulted in more than one remaining card, i.e. several diseases in the differential diagnosis, examination of those items marked as definitive diagnostic criteria would indicate which further tests were required. A diagnostic accuracy for marginal punched cards of greater than 90% along with the ability to identify any important additional information needed to make a diagnosis represent quite an auspicious milepost prior to the start of the odyssey

Table 6.1 Computer programs emphasizing routine peripheral blood and/or bone marrow findings published between 1961 and 1990

Year	Author	Subject
1961	Lipkin *et al.*	Hematology differential diagnosis
1976	Engle *et al.*	Hematology differential diagnosis
1986, 1987	Blomberg *et al.*	Classification of anemia
1986, 1988	Quaglini *et al.*	Diagnosis of anemia
1987	Bates and Bessman; Bessman, McClure and Bates	Analysis of CBC/MD
1987	Shiina, Kamei and Murakami	Peripheral blood analysis
1988	Sultan, Imbert and Priolet; Imbert *et al.*	Diagnosis of anemia
1989	Paterakis, Terzoglou and Vasilioy	Microcytic anemia
1989	Houwen	Microcytic anemia
1990	O'Connor and McKinney	Microcytic anemia
1990	Ironi, Stefanelli and Lanzola; Lanzola *et al.*	Diagnosis of anemia

CBC/MD: Complete Blood Counts and WBC manual differentials

to develop computer programs designed for decision support in laboratory hematology.

Table 6.1 lists computer programs emphasizing analysis of routine hemogram results, peripheral blood film data, and/or bone marrow findings (with or without clinical history) published between 1961 and 1990.

Lipkin, the senior author on the punched card study, designed a computer program as an aid to differential diagnosis in hematological diseases (Lipkin *et al.*, 1961). The basic procedure used by the program was similar to but not identical with the mechanical system which preceded it. The computer used a matching algorithm divided into two phases. First, 20 diseases were grouped into nine classes based on common characteristics. For each disease, the textbook characteristics pertinent to hematologic disease were included and ranked (from 1 to 10, with 10 being pathognomonic) according to their significance. Only items considered to be highly diagnostic (ranks 8, 9 and 10) were considered by the program. Forty-nine patients were studied. If the patient data corresponded to any significant disease feature, that class of diseases was chosen by the program for further analysis. If all findings needed for a diagnosis were present, the diagnosis was considered to be positively established. If one critical item was tested and found to be absent, the disease was retained in the differential diagnosis and the computer requested that this item be rechecked. If two or more significant

items were tested and found to be absent, the disease was discarded from the differential diagnosis. If one or more of the critical findings had not been tested, and the disease was not discarded because of the rule cited above, the computer printed a suggestion to test for the missing item(s). The hospital diagnosis, arrived at after consultation with staff members experienced in hematology, was considered to be the 'gold standard' with which to compare the computer's performance. In 28 of the 49 cases, the hospital diagnosis was listed as a 'positive diagnosis' by the computer program. In 12 cases, the hospital diagnosis was listed as 'possible diagnosis' because one item was untested and, in one case, two critical items were untested. In six patients, the computer included the correct diagnosis in the differential and asked for one item of data to be re-examined. In two cases, the hospital diagnosis was not one of the 20 conditions known to the program.

It was again noted that the method could not result in an incorrect diagnosis being listed as a positive diagnosis. The authors concluded that for a computer program to be of value, the system should recognize the relationship between a given pattern of patient data and the disease criteria stored in the system. Furthermore, the system should organize and report the findings in a form which is useful to the physician in making a differential diagnosis. Their program performed this task admirably by listing the critical information which needed to be tested for or 'rechecked'. Alas, the investigators noted that a potential problem with this approach 'may be the vagueness in disease classification'. Later, in a summary of this work, Lipkin noted that 'indefinite criteria for defining disease entities' was a problem area of differential diagnosis which carried over to any computer system (Lipkin, 1962). The dragon of 'quantifying and managing uncertainty in diagnostic reasoning' had reared its ugly head, ready to knock off course those who tried to forge the road towards successful hematology expert systems.

The lure of Bayes' theorem as a means of representing uncertainty (Hughes, 1989) was strong, and the program HEME (Engle *et al.*, 1976), the next attempt at computerization of hematology diagnosis, was firmly based in probability theory. As is usually the case when knowledge is represented using Bayes' theorem, the investigators asked clinicians to estimate the conditional probabilities which were to be used in the calculations. An interesting feature of HEME was the ability to 'automatically improve its diagnostic accuracy as clinical data accumulate'. In this scheme, if a physician guessed that the frequency of finding 'F' in disease 'D' was one in 10, and he was quite confident in that guess, it would be expressed in the program as $1000/10000$. If, on the other hand, the physician was uncertain about the estimate, it would be expressed as $1/10$. As new cases of disease 'D' were diagnosed, the program would automatically change the numerator and denominator of this fraction depending on whether or not the case exhibited feature 'F'. For those features where the denominator started out as a small number, actual case data (rather than a physician's guess) would eventually have a profound effect on the probabilities being used in the calculations. In a preliminary test of 44 cases, HEME listed the correct diagnosis as its first choice in 25 cases (56.8%). The correct diagnosis was ranked second or third by the program in an additional 9 cases.

Over the years, various investigators continued to design systems based on mathematical and probabilistic models (Blomberg *et al.*, 1986; Bates and Bessman, 1987; Blomberg *et al.*, 1987; Sultan, Imbert and Priolet, 1988; Bessman, McClure and Bates; 1989; Imbert *et al.*, 1989; Paterakis, Terzoglou and Vasilioy, 1989). These programs were tested primarily on cases of anemia, with particular reference in some studies to the differential diagnosis of microcytic anemia (Bessman, McClure and Bates, 1989; Houwen, 1989; Paterakis, Terzoglou and Vasilioy, 1989). Professor Claude Sultan's group in France found that, in their hands, a Bayesian approach performed better than their first attempts at a rule-based system (Imbert *et al.*, 1989). The overall diagnostic performance of the systems based on statistical theories was similar to each other and showed a slight improvement over that recorded for HEME. The programs would usually rank the correct diagnosis first in 60–70% of cases and would exhibit 'satisfactory' performance (i.e. the correct diagnosis was listed in the program's top three choices) 80–90% of the time. Bates and Bessman (1987, 1989) showed that on a small number of selected cases, their program, BCDE©, could outperform a panel of physicians.

In the mid to late 1980s, rule-based expert systems for laboratory hematology began to enter the scene. Laboratory physicians (and members of the medical informatics community) began to use the existing expert system shells to develop simple systems for the differential diagnosis of anemia (O'Connor and McKinney, 1989).

In Italy, Quaglini *et al.* (1980) used EXPERT, an artificial intelligence programming shell developed at Rutgers University, for their program ANEMIA which ran on a minicomputer. ANEMIA was developed to provide assistance in the diagnosis and management of 65 diseases. ANEMIA's performance was validated in an interesting study which compared the computer program to six hematologist's evaluation of 30 cases Quaglini *et al.* (1988). With this study design, the agreement rate between the hematologists could be tested at the same time. ANEMIA's performance was judged acceptable (by a majority vote of the evaluators) in 87% of the cases (26/30), while the hematologists agreed with their colleagues in 90% of the cases (27/30).

Table 6.2 Knowledge-based hematology systems designed for laboratory use for peripheral blood, bone marrow and flow cytometry (FCM).

Year	Author	Subject
1987b	Alvey *et al.*	Leukemia diagnosis by FCM
1991	Tolmie *et al.*	Peripheral blood analysis
1992a	Smith and Gyde	Classification of leukemias
1992b	Smith and Gyde	Bone marrow reporting
1992	Nguyen *et al.*; Diamond and Nguyen	Peripheral blood interpretive reporting
1993	Diamond *et al.*	FCM interpretive reporting
1993	Nguyen *et al.*; Nguyen and Diamond	Bone marrow interpretive reporting

Some computer scientists have tried their hand at the development of new models to capture more of the available medical knowledge. The Italian group cited above, undertook this task in their next program, NEOANEMIA (Ironi, Stefanelli and Lanzola, 1990; Lanzola *et al.*, 1990). Their idea was to expand the reasoning capabilities (and hopefully, the performance) of a system by including dynamic qualitative pathophysiological models of iron metabolism, erythropoietin metabolism, and red cell production and destruction. Their prototype ran on a sophisticated workstation computer with a high-resolution screen and had a graphical user interface. An evaluation of the performance of this approach was not provided in the publications concerning this work, however.

6.2 Systems designed with the user in mind

Many of the prototype hematology systems mentioned above were clearly designed as research projects rather than for actual day-to-day use in the laboratory. Table 6.2 lists the more recent projects which appear to break away from this mold. These projects have been designed from the start as practical aids to differential diagnosis and efficient methods for computerized interpretive reporting. They encompass routine peripheral blood evaluation, leukocyte immunophenotyping for the subclassification of malignant lymphomas and leukemias, and bone marrow reporting. In most of these projects, the developers have managed to avoid the problems of quantifying uncertainty. There are several important innovations in these projects, including: (1) a structured method of dividing the problem into more manageable sub-parts; and (2) in some cases, the use of physician with considerable experience in hematology as the knowledge engineer.

Smith and Gyde (1992, a,b) have developed two systems in this category: one with the goal of providing diagnostic advice for hematologists who manage leukemia patients and one for bone marrow reporting. The leukemia project, a rule-based system utilizing an expert system shell, has three important technical features: (1) it is interfaced to a relational database; (2) there are hypertext help facilities available; and (3) an atlas of leukemic cells stored on laser disk may be linked to the system. All knowledge engineering was performed by a research hematologist. An important point in this system is the recognition that modern leukemia diagnosis draws information from many domains including clinical, general laboratory, immunologic, morphologic and cytogenetic data. There are separate knowledge bases for each of these areas within the system and the intermediate conclusions of each sub-module are brought together in the final interpretation. In a preliminary study of 43 retrospective cases, the system diagnosis was judged to be correct in 35 cases (82%). In five cases (11%), the system could not reach a certain diagnosis but in three of these it was able to provide helpful suggestions. In two cases (4%) the system was not able to reach any diagnosis, and in one case (3%) the diagnosis reached was incorrect.

The rule-based bone marrow reporting program of Smith and Gyde (1992b) prompts the user with a series of questions which can be answered from menus using single key strokes. A laser disk atlas of blood cells can be accessed directly from the program. To encourage use of the system, the authors have allowed the menu lists and report layouts to be customized by the user. The system is reported to be in operation in several centres in Europe. The comments indicate that it is both a useful training tool and an efficient way for the experienced user to generate bone marrow reports.

Alvey, Myers and Greaves (1987) have developed a rule-based computer program for interpreting immunophenotyping data as an aid to leukemia diagnosis and have described the process necessary for converting their demonstrator class system to a high-performance system (Alvey, Preston and Greaves, 1987). In their original rule-based system, each rule contained a numerical factor for dealing with uncertainty. They tested a copy of their system with the numerical certainty factors removed and found that the modified system produced exactly the same results as the original (Alvey, Myers and Greaves, 1987). We quote their conclusion from this experiment: 'Thus the cumbersome and useless numerical uncertainty mechanism was banished from the leukemia project and it has never subsequently been missed.' Their system, which has been redesigned in Prolog, provides a thorough but somewhat unwieldy explanation facility and has achieved essentially 100% accuracy on a test series of 400 cases (Alvey, Preston and Greaves, 1987).

Tolmie, du Plessis and Badenhorst (1991) have described HEMATEX, a rule-based expert system for the interpretation of full blood counts and blood film data. The hemogram data are received from an interface with a Technicon H-1 hematology analyser. The expert system supports the technologist's interpretation by either generating a report (for normal samples and samples where the hemogram data alone are sufficient) or prompting the technologist for blood film information before making an interpretation. This system has been modified and incorporated into the laboratory information system of a private laboratory in South Africa (Tolmie, personal communication). The modified system does not have the capability of reasoning based on the peripheral blood film data that its predecessor had. Instead, it acts as an 'intelligent sieve' by identifying blood samples within its capabilities and generating an interpretive report by adding coded comments. When review of a peripheral blood film is necessary, the system will attach preliminary comments to the case before passing the specimen to a technologist for interpretation. The system has been enthusiastically received by the private laboratory which feels that it at least doubles the daily capacity for performing complete blood counts.

The programs known as *Professor Petrushka* (Peripheral blood analysis), *Professor Fidelio* (interpretation of Flow cytometry (FCM) immunophenotyping and DNA content results), and *Professor Belmonte* (Bone marrow morphology) are the first three modules in a comprehensive system for interpretive reporting in laboratory hematology (Nguyen *et al.*, 1992; Diamond and Nguyen, 1993; Diamond *et al.*, 1993; Nguyen *et al.*, 1993). These programs, for IBM-compatible computers running Windows™ 3.1, share a relational database (using Paradox® Engine), an easy-to-use graphical user interface, and a powerful model of diagnostic reasoning based on defined diagnostic patterns. All three programs are designed to be used together on a 'hematology workstation' (Nguyen and Diamond, 1993). The knowledge engineer for these projects is a trained hematopathologist.

The peripheral blood system (*Professor Petrushka*) is designed to be interfaced to state-of-the-art Coulter hematology analysers which generate automated leukocyte differentials and provide flags for suspected morphologic abnormalities within the sample. The system has been designed so that it fits into the normal work flow for a hematology laboratory.

Eighteen patterns (normal, 16 specific patterns, and one non-specific pattern) have been defined from hemogram and peripheral blood film data. Each of the patterns suggests a differential diagnosis based on common features. Since more than one pattern can coexist in the same case (e.g. in acute leukemia, the thrombocytopenic pattern and a normochromic, normocytic anemia pattern may be present in addition to the abnormal mononuclear cell pattern) the knowledge base contains a hierarchy of the patterns. The specially designed inference engine interprets the findings to establish one dominant preliminary pattern. Based on the pattern and the individual findings of the hemogram, the system recommends a specific approach to the review of the peripheral blood film from a list including scanning at low-power magnification (20 × –25 × objective), review of red blood cell, leukocyte and/or platelet morphology with a medium power (40 × –63 × oil) microscope objective, and a manual leukocyte differential count. At each stage of the peripheral blood film examination, the technologist can override the system recommendations by simple point and click operations, if desired. After the peripheral blood film review is completed, the system re-interprets the data in light of the blood film findings and calculates the final dominant pattern. The system then writes an interpretive report (Figure 6.1) which lists a differential diagnosis and recommendations as to which complementary tests should be performed to establish the diagnosis. The morphological findings entered by the technologist, the system's conclusions, and the hemogram data are saved in the database along with the patient's unique identification number. The program has been evaluated in our laboratory on over 4000 cases with excellent results. Extensive testing in other hematology laboratories is being carried out in the US, Canada and the UK.

Professor Petrushka is designed to be useful for all peripheral blood specimens, not just the first specimen from an untreated patient. Before making a final interpretation, the program checks the database for any pertinent patient information (such as a history of a myeloproliferative disorder) and checks the specimen database for any previous peripheral blood data on the patient. The system's final interpretation and recommendations take into account any information found in the database (Diamond and Nguyen, 1993).

In order to provide detailed explanations of *Professor Petrushka*'s reasoning process, an on-line electronic textbook and a series of case studies with hypertext capabilities are under development using Guide™ 3.1. Digitized photomicrographs of peripheral blood and bone marrow morphology can be accessed immediately from within the textbook and case studies. In order to make the reference material particularly useful in the day-to-day practice of hematology, *Petrushka*'s electronic textbook is organized by patterns and not individual diseases or disease categories (as is commonly the case in an ordinary textbook of hematology).

Professor Fidelio is an expert system for the analysis of flow cytometric immunophenotyping (and DNA content) data in hematology. The immunologic marker data, including fluorescence intensity, is stored in the database. The results of a cytochemical test for myeloperoxidase can also be entered when subtyping

cases of acute leukemia. The system takes into account other FCM results such as cell size by light scatter, the DNA index (i.e. whether a tumor has a diploid DNA content or an aneuploid DNA content), and the percentage of cells with S-phase DNA content (a factor which is highly correlated with grading in non-Hodgkin's lymphomas (Diamond, Nathwani and Rappaport, 1982).

We strongly believe that the modern practice of neoplastic hematology is a multiparameter discipline. The immunology results in a peripheral blood specimen must be correlated with the hemogram findings, the manual differential, and the types of abnormal cells seen on the blood film. Since all of our programs work in concert, our workstation concept makes it easy to follow this approach. *Professor Fidelio* automatically looks for the corresponding peripheral blood data saved in *Professor Petrushka*'s database and correlates the findings with the FCM results before generating an interpretive report on the specimen. In the first evaluation, the system's interpretation was correct in 98.2% of 337 cases (Diamond *et al.*, 1993). The problems encountered have been corrected and the system has now been tested with accurate results on over 800 cases. *Professor Fidelio* can also be used to generate interpretive reports (taking into account any previous results) for T-cell subset analysis in patients who are being followed for acquired immunodeficiency states.

The third module of our hematology workstation is *Professor Belmonte*, for computer-assisted bone marrow interpretation (Nguyen *et al.*, 1993). In our opinion, consideration of the approach to a bone marrow specimen should always begin with a review of the peripheral blood. For this reason, when the user enters the patient identification number at the start of a bone marrow consultation, the system automatically retrieves the corresponding peripheral blood data from *Professor Petrushka*'s database and displays it along with reminders for any special studies (e.g cytochemistries, FCM immunophenotyping, or cytogenetics) which may be indicated by the peripheral blood findings. If the system is consulted at the time the bone marrow is ordered (i.e. before it is actually performed) this feature will be effective in greatly reducing the number of repeat bone marrow procedures that are currently performed because the individual doing the procedure was not familiar with the case (or someone forgot to save unfixed material for special studies).

A physician can enter the bone marrow findings into the system by simple point and click operations with the mouse. The computer keyboard can serve as a bone marrow differential counter, if desired. *Professor Belmonte* generates an interpretive report which includes all of the available information. For example, in a case of acute leukemia from our laboratory, the report contains: (1) a summary of the peripheral blood findings; (2) the bone marrow morphologic features including the differential and the qualitative

Professor Petrushka's Interpretation and Recommendations

In this 87-year-old female the hemogram findings are characteristic of a MACROCYTIC PATTERN with
Moderate Normochromic Macrocytic Anemia
Marked Anisocytosis
Mild Thrombocytosis

Differential diagnosis: B12/Folate Deficiency, Myelodysplastic Syndromes, Chemotherapy or Drug Effects, Bone marrow infiltrative disorders, alcohol abuse.

The combination of MACROCYTIC ANEMIA and THROMBOCYTOSIS suggests a SIDEROBLASTIC ANEMIA (a MYELODYSPLASTIC SYNDROME).

Clinical history with respect to the following conditions may be useful: Gastrointestinal Disorders, Drug or Toxin exposure, and Malignancies.

The following tests may be helpful: Reticulocyte count, Serum B12/Folate, RBC folate.

If the above tests are non-informative, then a BONE MARROW ASPIRATE/BIOPSY with material saved for potential CYTOGENETIC analysis, may be helpful.

Figure 6.1 Peripheral blood system's interpretive report in an 87-year-old female with Hemoglobin 8.4 g/dl, MCV 104.6 fl, RDW 38.2, and platelet count $668 \times 10^9/l$. The peripheral blood film showed severe macrocytosis, a dimorphic red cell population, and the presence of both hypochromic and normochromic cells. A subsequent bone marrow aspirate was diagnostic of refractory anemia with ring sideroblasts

abnormalities noted; (3) the results of cytochemical stains; (4) the interpretation of the peripheral blood or bone marrow FCM immunophenotyping results (obtained from *Professor Fidelio*'s database) and (5) a final interpretation with FAB subtype and any necessary correlation of the morphologic and immunologic findings. Since the FAB classification allows the presence of a peripheral blood monocytosis confirmed with increased serum lysozyme levels as an alternative criteria in cases of M4 with negative bone marrow staining for non-specific esterase (Bain, 1990), *Professor Belmonte* automatically looks for those findings in the database and includes them in the interpretation, if appropriate.

6.3 Systems for the blood bank, disorders of hemostasis, and other areas of hematology

Brief mention should be given to some of the expert systems which have been designed for use in transfusion medicine and coagulation services, as well as systems which are intended primarily as teaching tools in fields related to hematology.

RED is an expert system module for the interpretation of data related to red cell antibody identification (Smith *et al.*, 1985). It was intended by its authors to be one module in a more comprehensive system for

the blood bank which would be able to determine blood groups and resolve typing discrepancies, interpret results of antibody screening procedures, choose units for transfusion, and evaluate cross-match results. Systems have also been described which are useful for: (1) deciding when a donor unit should be deferred based on screening tests (Sorace, 1991); (2) providing real-time assessment of the appropriateness of platelet transfusion requests (Connelly, Sielaff and Scott, 1990) and, (3) evaluating transfusion requests for plasma, cryoprecipitate or platelets in disorders of hemostasis (Spackman and Beck, 1990).

Computer systems, some with built-in expert system modules, have been built for students of hematology, and as a source of review material or a tutorial for physicians. HEMAVID is a program that builds and maintains an object-oriented database for indexing a collection of hematology slides on videodisc (Church *et al.*, 1988). Wright–Giemsa is microcomputer-based system for simulating peripheral blood films (Healy and Buzek, 1991). The blood film characteristics are entered by the author and the system creates a simulated blood film from digitized images of individual cells. PlanAlyzer is a software package that combines elements of computer-aided instruction, expert systems, and hypermedia for teaching the workup of anemia (Beck *et al.*, 1989). FABHELP has been designed to be a concise reference of the FAB classification and a useful teaching tool in the application of FAB criteria to the diagnosis of acute leukemias and myelodysplastic syndromes (Shifmann,

1991). Finally, Intellipath is the commercial name for a Bayesian expert system and videodisc combination that are intended as teaching tools for lymph node histopathology (Nathwani *et al.*, 1990). Versions of Intellipath exist for both the 'Working Formulation' classification favoured in the United States and the 'Kiel Classification' which is used primarily in Europe.

6.4 Conclusions

Modern technology has led to an explosive growth in the amount of data generated in the hematology laboratory. Most laboratories feel a responsibility towards assisting clinicians by transforming the laboratory data into clinically useful information. This activity, known as interpretive reporting, may include marking abnormal results, printing reference values, suggesting diagnostic possibilities, and making recommendations for which additional studies may establish the diagnosis with a minimum cost, delay and discomfort to the patient.

Computer technology, which has assumed important roles in automated hematology instrumentation as well as the storage of laboratory data, can be quite useful for creating patient specific interpretive reports. These reports can improve patient care by: (1) helping to focus the attention of physicians who are presented with numerous laboratory values; and (2) providing a source of information about the interpretation of test results (Smith, Speicher and Chandrasekaran, 1984).

Harnessing the full potential of computerized expert systems has not been easy. More than two decades have been spent in basic research of fundamental topics such as knowledge representation, knowledge acquisition, problem-solving methods, and models for managing uncertainty (Shortliffe, 1993). The last few years have seen the arrival of faster and more powerful 'workstation' computers, better operating systems with graphical user interfaces, and hematologists who are developing systems that fit into the routine laboratory environment. These systems have two important features that are vital for their acceptance into the laboratory: (1) they provide consistent methods for use across many of the disciplines in the practice of hematology; and (2) they provide intelligent information for essentially every case.

The work (published in 1958 and 1961) by Dr M. Lipkin on punched card analysis and his first hematology computer system only came to our attention during the literature search for this chapter. The philosophical similarities between our hematology workstation and these 35-year-old projects are remarkable (compare our patterns to Lipkin's disease classes and the use of only the most definitive diagnostic criteria in each project). Perhaps, as physicians, laboratory administrators and knowledge-based system developers search for ever greater efficiency in the hematology laboratory of the 21st century, it would be wise to keep in mind the basic principles of good hematology practice that have been around for so many years.

References

Alvey, P. L., Myers, C. D. and Greaves, M. F. (1987a) High performance for expert systems: I. Escaping from the demonstrator class. *Med. Inform.*, **12**; 85–95.

Alvey, P. L., Preston, N. J. and Greaves, M. F. (1987b) High performance for expert systems II. A system for leukaemia diagnosis. *Med. Inform.*, **12**, 97–114.

Bain, B. J. (1990) *Leukaemia Diagnosis: A Guide to the FAB Classification*. London: Gower Medical Publishing.

Bates, J. E. and Bessman, J. D. (1987) Evaluation of BCDE©, a microcomputer program to analyze automated blood counts and differentials. *Am. J. Clin. Pathol.*, **88**, 314–323.

Beck, J. R., O'Donnell, J. F., Hirai, F. *et al.* (1989). Computer-based exercises in anemia diagnosis (Plan-Alyzer). In: Salamon, R., Protti, D. and Moehr, J. (eds), *International Symposium of Medical Informatics and Education*, pp. 177–182.

Bessman, J. D., McClure, S. and Bates, J. (1989) Distinction of microcytic disorders: Comparison of expert, numerical-discriminant and microcomputer analysis. *Blood Cells*, **15**, 533–540.

Blomberg, D. J., Guth, J. L., Fattu, J. M. *et al.* (1986) Evaluation of a new classification system for anemias using Learning System®. *Comput. Meth. Prog. Biomed.*, **22**, 119–125.

Blomberg, D. J., Ladley, J. L., Fattu, J. M. *et al.*. (1987) The use of an expert system in the clinical laboratory as an aid in the diagnosis of anemia. *Am. J. Clin. Pathol.*, **87**, 608–613.

Chueh, H. C., Barnett, G. O., Hayes, W. C. *et al.* (1989). HEMAVID: A flexible computer-based interactive video resource for hematology. *Proc. 12th Ann. Symp. Comput. Appl. Med. Care.* New York: IEEE Press. pp. 421–425.

Connelly, D. P., Sielaff, B. H. and Scott, E. (1990) ESPRE – Expert system for platelet request evaluation. *Am. J. Clin. Pathol.*, **94** (Suppl. 1): S19-S24.

Diamond, L. W., Nathwani, B. N. and Rappaport, H. (1982) Flow cytometry in the diagnosis and classification of malignant lymphoma and leukemia. *Cancer*, **50**, 1122–1135.

Diamond, L. W. and Nguyen, D. T. (1993) Communication between expert systems in haematology. In: Richards, B. (ed), *Current Perspectives in Healthcare Computing 1993*. Weybridge: BJHC pp. 111–119.

Diamond, L. W., Nguyen, D. T., Joualt, H. *et al.* (1993) Evaluation of a knowledge-based system for interpreting flow cytometric immunophenotyping data. In: Reichert, A., Sadan, B. A., Bengtsson, S. *et al.* (eds), *Proceedings of MIE 93*. London: Freund Publishing House, pp. 124–128.

Engle, R. L. Jr, Flehinger, B. J., Allen, S. *et al.* (1976) LL. HEME: A computer aid to diagnosis of hematologic disease. *Bull. NY Acad. Med.*, **52**, 584–600.

Feinstein, A. R. (1973) An Analysis of Diagnostic Reasoning: I. The domains and disorders of clinical macrobiology. *Yale J. Biol. Med.*, **46**, 212–232.

Feinstein, A. R. (1977) Clinical Biostatistics XXXIX. The haze of Bayes, the aerial palaces of decision analysis, and the computerized Ouija board. *Clin. Pharmacol. Ther.*, **21**, 482–496.

Healy, J. C. and Bozek, S. A. (1991) Wright-Giemsa: A computer-based system for the creation and presentation of peripheral blood smears. *Lab. Med.*, **22**, 728–737.

Healy, J. C., Spackman, K. A. and Beck, J. R. (1989) Small expert systems in clinical pathology. *Arch. Pathol. Lab. Med.*, **113**, 981–983.

Houwen, B. (1989) The use of inference strategies in the differential diagnosis of microcytic anemia. *Blood Cells*, **15**, 509–532.

Hughes, C. (1989) The representation of uncertainty in medical expert systems. *Med. Inform.*, **14**, 269–279.

Imbert, M., Priolet, G., Dadi, W. *et al.* (1989) An expert system applied to the diagnosis of anemia with special reference to myelodysplastic syndromes. *Blood Cells*, **15**, 563–571.

Ironi, L., Stefanelli, M. and Lanzola, G. (1990) Qualitative models in medical diagnosis. *AI in Med.*, **2**, 85–101.

Lanzola, G., Stefanelli, M., Barosi, G. *et al.* (1990) NEOANEMIA: A knowledge-based system emulating diagnostic reasoning. *Comput. Biomed. Res.*, **23**, 560–582.

Lipkin, M. (1962) Digital and analogue computer methods combined to aid in the differential diagnosis of hematological diseases. *Circ. Res.*, **11**, 607–613.

Lipkin, M., Engle, R. L. Jr Davis, B. J. *et al.* (1961) Digital computer as aid to differential diagnosis. *Arch. Intern. Med.*, **108**, 56–72.

Lipkin, M, and Hardy, J. D. (1958) Mechanical correlation of data in differential diagnosis of hematological diseases. *JAMA*, **166**, 113–125.

Nathwani, B. N., Heckerman, D. E., Horvitz, E. J. *et al.* (1990). Integrated expert systems and videodisc in surgical pathology: an overview. *Hum. Pathol.*, **21**, 11–27.

Nguyen, D. T., Cherubino, P., Tamino, P. B. *et al.* (1993). Computer-assisted bone marrow interpretation: a pattern approach. In: Reichert, A., Sadan, B. A., Bengtsson, S. *et al.* (eds), *Proceedings of MIE 93*. London: Freund Publishing House, pp. 119–123.

Nguyen, D. T. and Diamond, L. W. (1993) The concept of a computer workstation for diagnostic haematology. *Aust. J. Med. Sci.*, **14**, 71–75.

Nguyen, D. T., Diamond, L. W., Priolet, G. *et al.* (1992). A decision support system for diagnostic consultation in laboratory hematology. In: Lun, K. C., Degoulet, P., Piemme, T. E. *et al.* (eds), *MEDINFO 92*. Amsterdam: North Holland. pp. 591–595.

O'Connor, M. L. and McKinney, T. (1989) The diagnosis of microcytic anaemia by a rule-based expert system using VP-Expert. *Arch. Pathol. Lab. Med.*, **113**, 985–988.

Paterakis, G. S., Terzoglou, G. and Vasilioy, E. (1989) The performance characteristics of an expert system for the 'on-line' assessment of thalassemia trait and iron deficiency – Micro hema screen. *Blood Cells*, **15**, 541–561.

Quaglini, S., Stefanelli, M., Barosi, G. *et al.* (1986) ANEMIA: An expert consultation system. *Comput. Biomed. Res.*, **19**, 13–27.

Quaglini, S., Stefanelli, M., Barosi, G. *et al.* (1988) A performance evaluation of the expert system ANEMIA. *Comput. Biomed. Res.*, **21**, 307–323.

Shifmann, M. A. (1991) FABHELP: A rule-based consultation program for FAB classification of acute myeloid leukemia and myelodysplastic syndromes. *Lab. Med.*, **22**, 639–643.

Shiina, S., Kamci, Y. and Murakami, N. (1987) BLOOD: Expert system for data analysis in hematology. In: *MIE 87*. Rome: Edi Press. pp. 1069–1073.

Shortliffe, E. H. (1993) The adolescence of AI in Medicine: Will the field come of age in the '90s? *AI in Med.*, **5**, 93–106.

Shortliffe, E. H. and Buchanan, B. G. (1975) A model of inexact reasoning in medicine. *Mathemat. Biosci.*, **23**, 351–379.

Smith, A. G. and Gyde, O. H. B. (1992a) Leukaemia diagnosis – a challenging problem for an expert system. In: Lun, K. C., Degoulet, P., Piemme, T. E. *et al.* (eds), *MEDINFO 92*. Amsterdam: North Holland. pp. 596–601.

Smith, A. G. and Gyde, OHB (1992b) Computer-assisted bone marrow reporting – a novel use for an expert system. In: Lun, K. C., Degoulet, P., Piemme, T. E. *et al.* (eds), *MEDINFO 92*. Amsterdam: North Holland. p. 602.

Smith, J. W. Jr Speicher, C. E. and Chandrasekaran, B. (1984) Expert systems as aids for interpretive reporting. *J. Med. Syst.*, **8**, 373–388.

Smith, J. W., J. R. Svirbely, J. R., Evans, C. A. *et al.* (1985) RED: A red-cell antibody identification expert module. *J. Med. Syst.*, **9**, 121–138.

Sorace, J. M. (1991) Precedence logic in the development of a blood bank expert system. *AI in Med.*, **3**, 149–159.

Spackman, K. A. and Beck, J. R. (1990) A knowledge-based system for transfusion advice. *Am. J. Clin. Pathol.*, **94** (Suppl. 1): S25–S29.

Sultan, C., Imbert, M. and Priolet, G. (1988) Decision-making system (DMS) applied to hematology. Diagnosis of 180 cases of anemia secondary to a variety of hematologic disorders. *Hematol. Pathol.*, **2**, 221–228.

Tolmie, C. J., du Plessis, J. P., and Badenhorst, P. N. (1991) An expert system for the interpretation of full blood counts and blood smears in a hematology laboratory. *AI in Med.*, **3**, 271–285.

Part Two

Laboratory Management – Principles and Practice

7

Laboratory organization, management and economics

John Stuart and Brian S. Bull

7.1 Introduction

The management task of a head, or director, of laboratories has recently increased substantially in complexity. While national differences exist in the precise management role and the legislative constraints that apply to it, there is much common ground. This chapter is intended as a guide to the general principles of good laboratory management but highlights specific areas where national differences have an important effect.

7.2 The Management task

The task of management can be approached on more than one level and, for this reason, we do not differentiate between the terms 'administration', 'management' and 'leadership'. There is the support-function level that involves or influences all of the tasks in the laboratory. It is what managers are *expected to do* to facilitate good laboratory management. The key activities of management at this level can be summarized (Table 7.1). At this level, it is the task of management to enable all other workers in the laboratory to accomplish their tasks with a minimum of distraction. To this end it is management's responsibility to ensure a safe working environment, apportion (albeit limited) resources, and ensure that appropriate equipment and supplies are available.

A second level of management is equally important. It is what managers are *expected to be*. The key word here is integrity. Laboratory workers cannot rationally expect that the laboratory manager will solve all of the problems facing the laboratory. Some problems cannot be solved by their very nature, a solution to others may require a change in the law, and for yet others the health authority or the hospital administration may decline to provide the resources required for a solution. Workers in a laboratory,

Table 7.1 Key management activities

Provision of a timely diagnostic service
Strategic and business planning
Establishing clear lines of accountability
Establishing clear lines of communication
Monitoring workload and costs
Equipment replacement
Keeping within budget
Compliance with professional and governmental legislation
Safe working practices
Quality assurance
Staff recruitment, training and career development
Research and development
Teaching

however, have every right to expect that solutions will be sought by management with honesty and integrity. Workers can legitimately expect that they will be involved in problem solving to the extent that they are either 'part of the problem' or 'part of the solution'.

It is the fundamental task of management to develop the management skills of laboratory workers, within limits dictated by the workers' responsibilities and capabilities, and managers must always model the attributes desired. Managers who maintain their position by playing favourites, by admitting some into their clique while excluding others, or by deliberately using secrecy and unpredictability to bolster their authority are modelling management practices that will, in time, cripple the laboratory operation. Playing favourites can be done in many ways: it can be done by a salary increase, by promotion, by allocation of resources, and even by selective release of information before other laboratory staff are informed. Laboratory managers must not use these manipulative techniques personally and must ensure that all who report to them follow suit.

The management task should be approached as an integrated team effort with individuals bringing different management skills at different times to different

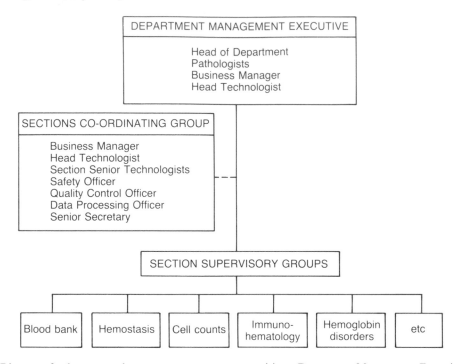

Figure 7.1 Diagram of a departmental management structure, comprising a Department Management Executive, assisted by a Sections Co-ordinating Group, and the individual departmental sections each led by a Section Supervisory Group

tasks. The team approach to management is particularly suited to hospital laboratories. This is because most workers in a clinical laboratory are well trained and have an unusually high level of responsibility to do what is best for the consumer, in this case a patient in need of their skill and expertise. The idealism of most laboratory workers, coupled with their training and expertise, makes them unusually effective as team members. Smoothly functioning teams are more effective than individuals in responding creatively to the ever changing needs of patients and health care providers.

7.3 Management structures

Effective laboratories are characterized by a number of teams operating as a network within a well-defined management structure. Typical teams will range from the most senior (Department Management Executive) (Figure 7.1) to short-term task forces that have no executive function but which are empowered to make recommendations on specific items. The management structure should be simple, clear to all staff, and with as few management layers as possible.

In the simplified example (Figure 7.1), a Department Management Executive is responsible for the function of the department and for the individual sections within it (led by Section Supervisory Groups) to which it allocates resources. Day-to-day sectional matters are dealt with by a Sections Co-ordinating Group, which may also provide service support functions (business management, computing, secretarial) to each section. Other special purpose teams (quality control, safety) are also accountable to the coordinating group. In this structure, the line of management accountability is directly from the management executive to the individual laboratory sections. The sections are encouraged to operate as a network of collaborating teams with shared resources.

The plethora of regulatory agencies that nowadays inspect and accredit hospitals and laboratories require that quality control, safety and certain other functions be strictly implemented and documented. To set up a specific committee for each required function can be disruptive to the primary function of the laboratory and be an inefficient use of the time of laboratory workers. It is often possible, however, to address two or more regulatory agency requirements in a single committee meeting if separate sets of minutes are prepared and persons with specialized knowledge and/or job titles are added/excused as the meeting progresses. It is management's task to satisfy all regulatory agency requirements, but it is also management's task to safeguard the time of laboratory workers as this is the prime and most costly resource of any hematology department.

Table 7.2 Example of a task force to make recommendations on purchase of equipment to automate a Blood Bank

Task force leader:	Blood Bank Senior Technologist
Membership:	Business Manager, Senior Technologist, Safety Officer, Blood Bank Pathologist, external adviser from Regional Transfusion Centre
Responsibility:	To complete an options appraisal for automation, making specific recommendations for types of equipment and taking into account the implications for future staffing level and skills mix, consumables budget, the emergency service, staff retraining and safety
To report to:	Department Management Executive
To report by:	2 months

Temporary teams, or task forces (Table 7.2), who answer to an executive group are a very effective means of driving forward new management initiatives and help to involve a wide spectrum of staff in decision making. Task forces have the considerable advantage over standing subcommittees of having a finite life because they are automatically disbanded once their report is complete. If unproductive, they can be restructured with a new leader or a different responsibility. Once disbanded, task force members can be used in other groupings for other management tasks. Junior members of staff gain useful management experience by serving on, and sometimes leading, task forces.

7.4 Strategic and business planning

This is a crucial management function. There is a valid distinction between strategic and business planning. Strategic planning is concerned more with the aims and direction of the department over a period of several years and may include a mission statement to encapsulate the department's philosophy. The business plan describes the objectives to be pursued over the current, or next, financial year in order to implement the strategy.

In practice, strategic and business planning are often combined in a once-yearly exercise, but the longer term view must not be neglected. Without strategic direction, a department is unlikely to develop in any purposeful way and is at the mercy of external forces for change. With agreement upon both strategy and business plan, staff within the department will have a sense of direction and of ownership of the management task.

A business plan also provides a buffer against short-term changes imposed by hospital and health authority management. For this reason it is essential that the Department Management Executive is com-

pletely familiar with the processes and methods by which the laboratory is being evaluated. Evaluation methods change over the years and it is crucial that laboratory staff understand what exactly is being monitored. Administrators at hospital or Health Authority level evaluate the laboratory and its functions, largely if not entirely, in terms of how closely laboratory output or laboratory expenditure meets some statistical goal. Should the laboratory data provided not match this goal, or not accurately reflect the true contribution of the laboratory, resources may be denied. For this reason, the laboratory management must be completely conversant with the data base that is being used and how the monitoring indices are computed. The Department Management Executive should also know how other institutions are performing. A network of laboratory managers is usually required for sharing such information since it contains sensitive business information that can rarely be obtained through official channels.

The business plan, or an edited version from which sensitive business information has been deleted, should be used as necessary to gain the commitment of other hospital bodies. The main purpose of the plan, however, is for internal use within the department.

The characteristics of good strategic and business planning include the following.

7.4.1 Analysing external factors

External factors (e.g. a competing local laboratory, a new clinical service, forthcoming government legislation) should be analysed for the opportunities and threats that they pose. This analysis must be rigorous and realistic as the departmental strategy will depend on it.

7.4.2 Analysing internal factors

Internal factors may range from past performance of departmental staff in meeting budgetary targets and quality standards to the morale and the potential for further development of the staff. Internal factors should be analysed with care to identify the true strengths and weaknesses of the department. This analysis of the department's potential must again be rigorous and realistic.

7.4.3 Planning the direction

The combination of the above two analyses, often described as a SWOT (strengths, weaknesses, opportunities and threats) analysis, should give a strong indication of the required future direction of the department. A priority order and realistic timetable for change should then be applied.

7.4.4 Setting the objectives

A list of objectives to implement the strategy over the next financial year is the core of the business plan. Each objective should be clear and purposeful, describing what is to be achieved and why, who is to achieve it and by when, and listing the end-points to be monitored to determine successful completion. While many objectives will relate to contracts with external clinical users, the business plan may also include contracts between sections of the department in relation to their provision to one another of internal services within the laboratory network.

7.4.5 Implementing the plan

All departmental staff should be involved in developing the business plan. Time devoted to this will instill a sense of ownership of the plan, as opposed to feelings of imposition from above, and the rate of implementation will be more rapid. Moreover, few plans are perfect and external factors may also change during its lifetime. Staff who own a plan will adopt a more flexible approach to its implementation and make day-to-day practical modifications to achieve the objectives desired. Individuals who feel that a plan was imposed may respond to the need for any subsequent change in the plan by 'I told you so!' Thus, time spent in building a consensus, and in explaining to those who will be disadvantaged why a particular strategy had to be adopted, is usually more than recouped by faster implementation.

The process of implementing the changes inherent in a business plan is a difficult one and requires as much attention to detail as does strategic planning. The following three principles characterize successful change management:

a. Setting clear goals and communicating them

Setting clear goals is the first step in managing change. Goals should be relevant, attainable and able to be monitored. Once agreed, the goals should be communicated to all staff in order to establish the need for change and identify who will do what. Failure to implement change often means that the original goals were not communicated effectively and should now be restated. Change will affect some members of staff more than others (the stakeholders) and they should be identified and their special requirements taken into account.

b. Monitoring progress

Progress should be monitored against agreed milestones so that all become aware of any slippage. With time, better alternatives for implementing objectives may become obvious and monitoring progress will ensure that the original objectives are adhered to

while allowing flexibility in how they are achieved. A trial-and-error basis is sometimes the best way to initiate change. Close monitoring is essential to detect wrong choices at an early stage and allow them to be corrected.

c. Reinforcing progress

Change is often led by a few enthusiasts whose achievements encourage others; there should be an active policy of looking for early progress and rewarding it. Attitudes to change are strongly influenced by recognition of a new order of things that is actively rewarded. Thus the change process should be viewed as an exponential curve based on early achievements that are positively reinforced.

The steps outlined above will suffice for most laboratories during a typical year. However, from time to time circumstances will arise requiring more fundamental change. Often these circumstances are a result of governmental directives. Sometimes such upheavals will result from changes in the space allocation or responsibilities of the laboratory. When such major changes occur, separate meetings with trained facilitators may be useful. If a series of major changes is predictable over several years, then the laboratory director or a designee can be trained for the purpose of 'in house' organizational development.

7.5 Economics

Reimbursement for health care is becoming ever more limited and good financial management is crucial for obtaining the maximum return from departmental resources. Essential requirements for management of a laboratory budget include a business manager and adequate computing power for a pathology database, spreadsheets and a costings package.

Tests which are performed in batches are often as much as an order of magnitude less costly to the laboratory than when performed one-by-one in response to urgent clinical need. While the management of the laboratory is (or should be) conversant with this cost differential, it should never be assumed that others in the health care environment are similarly well informed. Substantial budget cuts can often be absorbed without a significant reduction in the number of analyses performed so long as the users are willing to permit flexibility in the timing of those procedures. Such trade-offs are becoming an increasing fact-of-life as governments and private parties scrutinize laboratories for yet more cost savings.

7.5.1 Setting the budget

The laboratory budget depends on an accurate calculation of test costs (Table 7.3) and requires specific

Table 7.3 Factors contributing to the cost of laboratory tests

Direct costs	– consumables
	– equipment maintenance
	– staff salaries
Indirect costs	– capital assets
	– building maintenance
	– transport and portering services
	– personnel services
	– laundry services
	– telephones
	– postage
Fixed costs independent of workload	– staff salaries
	– maintenance contracts
Variable costs dependent on workload	– reagents
	– other consumables

knowledge about the rapidity with which clinicians require test results to be produced. Methods for calculating costs vary between departments and range from full-cost absorption, when all direct and indirect costs are included, to selective omission of indirect costs. The cost of replacing equipment should be included in the budget but often is not, being dependent instead on an external hospital equipment budget which is vulnerable to financial cuts.

When a budget is dependent on contracts with external users of the service, it is necessary to determine whether a block contract (fixed price irrespective of workload) or a cost-and-volume contract (price dependent on volume of work which may, however, be stratified within price bands) is the preferred option. Many budgets are fixed and based on historical levels of demand but it is sometimes better to introduce a flexible (zero based) budget in which the previous year's budget is not used as a starting point but costs are instead recovered from clinical users according to the level of clinical activity. This flexible type of budget can be useful when clinical activity is increasing rapidly and is outside the control of the laboratory. Examples include the cost of blood products and of the emergency service.

Budget rules need to be established at the beginning. Issues that should be addressed include: (1) whether or not savings can be carried forward to the next financial year; (2) the risk that a new income generation initiative will result in a proportional cut in next year's budget; (3) whether any budget deficits will be deducted from next year's budget and (4) whether any budget surplus from one laboratory area can be transferred to balance a deficit elsewhere (virement) or, alternatively, used to buy equipment. If equipment costs are to be charged against a separate budget, who is to benefit from the personnel costs saved as a result of purchase of automated equipment? How many months, or years, in advance must major equipment purchases be specified? Will replacement costs for vital equipment that has failed prematurely be charged against general laboratory

operations or has provision for such unpredictable expense been made elsewhere? Only when the ground rules for budget setting have been established, can a business plan be prepared. Depending on local financial arrangements, the budget may need to be negotiated with clinical users of the service and contracts drawn up. The business plan, modified according to the negotiated total budget, is then used to apportion resources to departmental sections according to their workload.

7.5.2 Running the budget

Efficient running of the budget again requires time to be spent by a business manager. Regular monitoring, at least monthly, is required. Computer spreadsheets are useful for predicting likely outcomes. Budget monitoring is dependent, however, on timely notification of expenditures for consumables and equipment. Each invoice needs to be validated. Some centralized finance and supplies departments fail to provide a timely service; this must be corrected. The technique of commitment (accrual) accounting, in which a provisional debit is made when the order is placed, can be useful for budget monitoring.

A built-in savings target may be required as the budget is constructed. Savings can be achieved in a variety of ways but large savings usually necessitate a reduction in number of staff (Table 7.4) as employment costs can account for up to 70–80% of total expenditure. Staff reductions require either a decrease in test output or, as already mentioned, a lengthening of the test turnaround time. The latter option may be preferable to users and to administrators. It is the responsiblility of laboratory management to give user groups and administrators sufficient information to allow an informed choice.

Table 7.4 Initiatives that may allow reduction in whole-time staff establishment

Rationalization of the service between one or more local hospital laboratories to eliminate duplication

Restructuring within a hospital laboratory to achieve cross-discipline working (e.g. between clinical chemistry and hematology)

Automation

Sub-contracting of low volume, labour intensive tests to a specialist laboratory

Employment of part-time contract staff (e.g. for the emergency service or phlebotomy service)

7.5.3 Purchasing or leasing equipment

Equipment replacement is now more often a budgetary item because of the increase in popularity of leasing, as opposed to purchasing, major items of equipment. Leasing equipment has been the preferred option in the USA for many years and has a number of advantages (Table 7.5).

Table 7.5 Advantages of leasing, as opposed to purchasing, equipment

Future costs for maintenance and consumables can be included in the contract payments and thereby predicted with accuracy

Equipment for automation can be obtained immediately

Equipment can be upgraded or replaced if workload increases substantially

No need for capital outlay

No capital charge against the asset register (where relevant)

The replacement cycle time, when equipment is purchased, is often excessively long, leading to years of struggle with sub-optimal technology

---

The decision to lease equipment must be made at an early stage of strategic and business planning because revenue savings are needed to cover the cost of the lease over the lifetime of the contract. The decision to lease or purchase must be made in relation to the economic situation at the time of the decision, but consideration should also be given to the economic situation that is likely to exist over the term of the lease. An instrument manufacturer may offer financial terms that strongly favour either lease or purchase depending on current sales performance and the stage in the production cycle of the instrument. Income to the company from a contract that ties the user to that company's reagents is also influential. While leasing is intrinsically the more expensive option, this may be largely offset by an advantageous financial package, by the potential for instant automation allowing a reduction in staff costs, or by the flexibility to upgrade or change the instrument. The latter option is particularly useful when either technology or workload is changing rapidly. If this latter reason dominates, however, the lease must be written so that termination prior to the typical 5–7-year term will not be prohibitively expensive.

7.5.4 Economies of scale

In comparison with industry, many diagnostic laboratories make inefficient use of automated equipment by using it below capacity and for only part of the 24-hour day. The requirement for readily available back-up equipment adds to the problem. Some laboratories may be forced to work inefficiently because they are tied to a stand-alone hospital. In urban locations, economies of scale can become substantial if a laboratory serves several hospitals because the increase in transport costs is far outweighed by the reduction in equipment and staff per unit of workload. While Federal legislation in the USA currently makes such collaboration between hospitals awkward, the future almost certainly will be different. Legislation that encourages the formation of consortia between large and small hospitals (including out-

patient clinic groups) to manage the health care of patient groups rather than individuals, will encourage similar sharing of laboratory facilities.

7.5.5 Centralization or near-patient testing?

Advances in instrumentation are likely to encourage two trends that are not mutually exclusive. The first is for large central laboratories to install more extensive automation with robotic-assisted handling of the pre-analytical phase of specimen identification and sample preparation. Linear robotic tracks and conveyor belt systems that feed a range of instruments are already available and may serve a combination of hematology and clinical chemistry analysers (Sasaki, 1991). The second trend is the development of small automated analysers for near-patient testing in clinical areas where turnaround time is a crucial quality requirement (see Chapter 5). Business planning in relation to the cost-versus-quality benefits of near-patient testing, compared with centralization, will therefore become increasingly necessary. It is the task of laboratory management to remind administrators that, no matter where and by whom a test is performed, a relatively large amount of quality control work (for most analyses this amounts to 15–20% of total test output) is an inevitable accompaniment. In addition, training large numbers of nurses or ward attendants will involve substantial continuing expenditures for in-service training and in-service trainers.

7.6 Setting laboratory standards

Commitment to quality in hematology laboratories has now extended beyond internal quality control and external quality assurance programs. In part, this has been a defence against falling standards as a consequence of imposed financial cuts. In addition, however, quality measures have become an integral part of the increased emphasis placed on good laboratory management. Standardization of laboratory procedures and of laboratory policies are two approaches to setting quality standards in the laboratory.

7.6.1 Standard operating procedures

Standard operating procedures (SOPs) help to maintain day-to-day quality of performance by providing stability against unauthorized variation. They help to ensure a consistent quality of work irrespective of technologist, allow procedures to be understood by everyone working in the laboratory, provide a training resource for new technologists, and facilitate rotation of technologists between departmental sections. When results fail to meet expected quality

Table 7.6 Guidelines for format of a standard operating procedure

Title and number of test procedure
Contents
Introduction
Principle of test
Specimen requirements
Reagents
Equipment
Test procedure
Calculations
Reference range
Confidence limits
Limitations of procedure
Action limits
Reporting procedure
References
Supplemental material
Authorization signatures and dates
Amendment procedure and dates

Table 7.7 Examples of policy statements

Induction of new staff
Staff development and appraisal process
Telephone answering policy (see Table 7.8)
Reporting stat specimens
Visitors – company representatives
        – service engineers
Mailing biological specimens
Using the photocopier
Use of training funds
Archiving of data

Table 7.8 Abbreviated example of a telephone answering policy

Statement of policy: The Hematology Department will ensure that all telephone calls are answered in a timely and courteous fashion

Purpose: To promote the professional image of the department and avoid confrontation by telephone

Responsibility: The head of each laboratory section is responsible for implementing and monitoring the departmental telephone policy within that section

Procedure:
1. Timeliness: Telephone enquiries should be answered promptly. If no one is present in a section to take telephone calls, the telephone must be routed to another section with that section's agreement to provide temporary cover. The last person to leave a section is responsible for arranging re-routing
2. Telephone enquiries should be answered with courtesy, the name of the section and the staff member being notified to the caller. The name of the caller should be identified clearly
3. All telephone messages should be reported on the departmental message slips
4. If the caller is confrontational, the staff member must never respond in a similar manner. It is sometimes helpful to transfer the call to a senior colleague as this indicates to the caller that the problem is being taken seriously
5. On completing the call, adverse comments in relation to the call or caller should not be made to others in the room as this can convey an attitude of unhelpfulness which influences the telephone style of other members of staff

standards, well written SOPs provide detailed instructions as to how such situations are to be handled. Indeed, it is under these circumstances that they will be most often consulted. They also provide documented evidence of working methods for regulatory authorities and demonstrate the department's commitment to high standards of documentation and performance. National guidelines for writing SOPs are used in the USA (National Committee for Clinical Laboratory Standards, 1984). A suggested format for an SOP is given in Table 7.6.

An SOP is a written standard procedure that has been approved by the section head and the departmental head. Any subsequent change in that procedure must be authenticated. Thus the precise methodology used on any one day is documented. The level of detail should be such that a moderately experienced technologist who is new to the laboratory could follow the test procedure without difficulty.

7.6.2 Laboratory policies

Laboratory policies cover a wider range of departmental activities than do SOPs, which are concerned exclusively with test procedures. Policy statements reflect the overall philosophy and standards of a department. They are a useful means of indicating to staff 'how we do things around here'. Typical topics for policy statements are listed in Table 7.7 and an abbreviated policy document is shown in Table 7.8.

Laboratory policies need to be written on what may appear to be mundane topics. However, ignoring these topics can create real problems if they are dealt with in an unstructured manner. Policies cover areas that SOPs do not reach and are particularly useful for eliminating sources of confusion and irritation. Policy statements can do much to improve a department's image and morale and they justify the management time of senior staff.

7.7 Auditing the laboratory

Audit of a laboratory's performance against set standards is an essential quality issue and extends beyond test precision. Each section of a laboratory should set itself standards by which internal performance is to be measured. The department as a whole should also set standards with regard to its effectiveness as

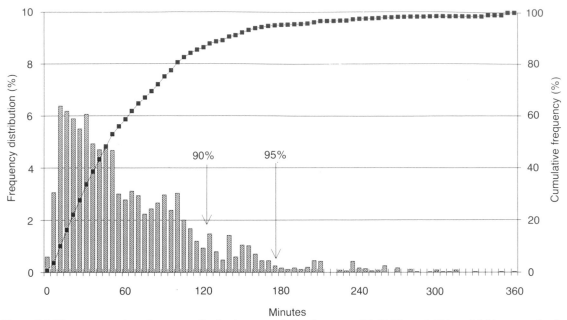

Figure 7.2 Histogram to show frequency distribution, cumulative frequency (■-■-■), and 90th and 95th percentiles for analytical turnaround time of non-urgent blood counts.

perceived externally by user clinicians and patients. Examples of laboratory audit include:

7.7.1 Test turnaround time

This parameter must be defined with care as it is not standardized between laboratories. It can be measured as the time lapse between entering a test request in the laboratory computer system to the time the result is entered and validated. A histogram plot of the frequency distribution (Figure 7.2) can then be printed for audit purposes. Useful parameters to measure include the mean or median time, the 90th or 95th percentile, and the percentage of tests reported within a pre-selected time (Valenstein and Emancipator, 1989; Westgard, Burnett and Bowers, 1990). The tail of the histogram is clearly the area of most concern.

7.7.2 Request completion time

Test turnaround time, as defined above, may bear little relationship to the total request completion time as specimen transport to the laboratory and return of the result to the clinician are both ignored. Request completion time is the more rigorous parameter, and the important one from the clinician's viewpoint. Request completion time is difficult to document unless the computer system allows booking in of requests and reporting of results in clinical areas; request completion times can then be determined for individual users of the service.

The speed with which laboratories report results is an increasingly important quality issue, particularly now that many more tests are being requested to monitor ill patients rather than make the initial diagnosis. Indeed, the time taken to report stat test results is the most visible aspect of laboratory performance to clinicians (Howanitz and Steindel, 1991). Investment in staff and equipment to provide a rapid results service increases laboratory costs but can decrease overall hospital costs per patient if there is a consequential reduction in length of stay. It is, however, difficult to quantify this cost-and-effect relationship and thus justify an increase in laboratory investment. If a very short request completion time is required by clinicians, then it may be necessary to locate equipment in a near-patient test site. Shortening the request completion time by rapid transport of specimens to a central laboratory via a computerized pneumatic-tube delivery system (Keshgegian and Bull, 1992) may be a cost-effective alternative to locating test equipment in clinical areas.

7.7.3 Appropriateness of test requesting

Laboratories should provide guidelines to clinicians as to what is appropriate use of laboratory services. This form of education may be in the form of a departmental pocket book or by computer-assisted requesting protocols (Mutimer et al., 1992). Whatever the method, it must be sustained over long periods to reduce inappropriate test requesting (Bareford and Hayling, 1990; Gama et al., 1992). Once implemented, the method should be audited, with regular feedback to users as to the volume, type and cost of their requesting habits. A zero-based, flexible budget, in which laboratory costs for test requests are recovered from clinical users according to the level of requesting, is a persuasive method of feedback.

7.7.4 User satisfaction

Questionnaires designed for out-patients to assess their satisfaction over clinic waiting time, the blood collection procedure, or the helpfulness of staff are simple means of detecting major deficiencies in quality of service. Questionnaires can also be used to assess the level of satisfaction of clinicians. However, for major users of the laboratory service, it is preferable to hold face-to-face audit meetings in which quality issues, including the need for new developments in the service, are discussed. Business managers and head technologists should be included in these meetings to ensure that awareness of customer expectations is disseminated throughout the department.

Laboratory audit must include pre-analytical, analytical and post-analytical aspects of the service. Accredited laboratories are already likely to have an analytical service of high quality and the emphasis can then be directed to completing the quality circle from blood collection to the interpretation and return of results to the clinician.

7.8 Staff development and performance appraisal

Laboratory staff are the most valuable asset of a department and represent its most expensive resource. A formal programme to enhance their skills should be given high priority by laboratory management. The programme should ensure that both the management ability and the technical ability of staff are being continuously enhanced.

Management skills that are of particular value for senior staff include interpersonal skills, team building skills and communication skills. Senior level personnel must also be able to manage budgets, delegate, interview for hiring and firing decisions and demonstrate efficient time management. To facilitate training in management, the departmental library should contain management books and training videos and attendance at selected external management training courses should be encouraged. For larger departments, it can be useful to employ management consultants to provide in-house training as part of the team building exercise. Management training of junior as well as senior staff is cost effective in that everyone then becomes aware of the need to work

as a team and subsequent management initiatives can be implemented more easily because there is a corporate sense of purpose.

Performance appraisal of staff is seldom effective unless it complements a programme of staff development. Appraisal should always be seen as secondary to, and extending, staff development as an individual cannot be appraised until clear goals have been set and the individual has developed the necessary skills to achieve the goals. There are national differences in the degree of formality and documentation required for performance appraisal and its linkage with financial reward or promotion (Stuart and Hicks, 1991, 1992). Personal development of the individual can be a stronger driving force than short-term financial reward. Linkage of performance to external awards may also reduce intrinsic motivation by lowering the staff member's freedom to manage and control his/her own job. Performance appraisal requires little in the way of formal documentation; a list of 3–4 objectives to be achieved over the next 6–12 months is often all that is required. After thorough discussion of what is expected and how compliance will be determined, the agreed list of objectives should be signed by both the appraiser and appraisee to indicate commitment.

If staff development is an integral part of the department's strategic plan, recruitment and retention of staff are likely to be enhanced. Appraisal also helps to ensure that staff activities are channelled along the agreed pathways of the strategic plan rather than allowed to follow unstructured personal agendas.

7.9 Communication

Communication pathways within a department require careful thought. Too often these pathways are unplanned, leading to confusion over what is expected from whom and resulting in loss of direction. A clear management structure, as shown in Figure 7.1, is a valuable aid to effective communication.

A useful method of communication in large departments is team briefing. This requires technical heads to arrange meetings with their section staff for briefing purposes. A short briefing document can be prepared beforehand for technical heads to ensure that staff in each departmental section are given the same message; the document can usefully include a list of actions that have been agreed upon and who is responsible for their implementation.

Leakage of information from policy-making committees can have a profoundly adverse effect on a department and should be prevented. Knowledge that unauthorized release of information is prohibited will increase candour between members of the management team. A firm refusal to comment to others until a decision has been reached and is ready to be communicated should be the rule. Managers should never leak confidential information to individual employees as a mark of favour. To use confidential information in this way violates two cardinal rules of good management: it indicates that some employees are favourites of management and it decreases trust among managers. For these reasons, whenever change in policy or formulation of new policy has been discussed by a management team, those in attendance should be briefed as to what can, and what should not, be communicated.

Management by 'walk about' is a well recognized method of communication. Communication is a two-way process, and time should be set aside in the week for the head of department to wander into departmental sections with no fixed agenda but to listen to the feed-back. This is also a good method for praising progress of individuals; however, the head of department should have done sufficient homework beforehand to know what specific initiatives are in progress for which praise will be appreciated. Praise should be timely and specific. In this connection it is always helpful for a manager to understand, at least in some small measure, the personality and temperament of each employee he or she supervises. If praise is to be most effective it must be specific to a task well done and phrased in such a fashion that it is meaningful to the deserving employee. Acquisition of such inter-personal skills requires the investment of time and effort on the manager's part. It is time well spent, for a worker who is praiseworthy deserves to be complimented about the particular aspect of the work of which he or she is most proud. Wandering around is not the time to be censorious (reprimands should be in private).

7.10 Leadership Styles

No two departments or their leaders are the same and there is no one leadership style to learn. Indeed, leaders who have a very obvious style can have limited effectiveness, particularly if the style is not a flexible one. Management training is designed to increase awareness of the style in which one operates naturally and to teach other, less obvious, styles which may be more appropriate in other contexts. For example, an individual with a predominantly informing style may find this suited to instructing medical students and new staff but less suited to negotiating with senior and experienced staff where a consultative style is likely to be more effective. Rigidity of style is to be avoided.

Performance appraisal interviews can be a useful forum for discussing the effectiveness of one's own management style as these interviews should be a two-way process with the appraisee as free as the appraiser to comment on the working relationship. Persistent use of an inappropriate style can cause an impasse which for years may limit the effectiveness of a working relationship. The open ended question 'Is there anything in my style of management that I should change to make it easier for us to work together?' is always worth asking.

It is the responsibility of management to ensure that different leadership styles are taken into consideration when teams or task forces are being put together. Most of the advantages of team working will be lost if the temperaments of the team members are not varied enough to include people with an eye for detail and feasibility as well as some who are visionary.

7.11 Laboratory Accreditation

As described in Chapter 21, an increasing number of health care systems now require that diagnostic laboratories meet national standards for accreditation. Published descriptions of national accreditation programmes include the College of American Pathologists Laboratory Accreditation Program (Batjer, 1990) and the United Kingdom voluntary scheme supervised by Clinical Pathology Accreditation (UK) Ltd (Advisory Task Force on Standards to the Audit Steering Committee of the Royal College of Pathologists, 1991).

An impending inspection for accreditation should be viewed as an opportunity to review departmental strategy, make any changes in work practices that may have been put off owing to pressure of work, and update the management process. Mock inspections, if possible by a friendly colleague from another department, are a useful way of detecting blind spots. Hospital management should also be involved at an early stage as additional resources may be needed to correct structural defects, particularly in relation to safety requirements. A checklist of 10 key points relevant to the accreditation inspection is given in Table 7.9.

Preparation for accreditation is a demanding exercise which involves many of the management issues discussed in this chapter. Successful completion of the exercise is a morale lifting event for departmental staff but, once achieved, the management process should be ongoing in order to encourage continuous renewal of the department. Individual members of staff need to be developed in new ways and departmental structures need to be modified to continuously refresh the department.

7.12 Conclusion

Good laboratory management is based on the need to treat staff with dignity coupled with the application

Table 7.9 Checklist of key points relevant to an impending accreditation inspection

1. Does the department have a clear management structure?
2. Are communication pathways effective?
3. Does the laboratory appear to be well organized, safe and pleasant to work in?
4. Are the work practices, level of equipment and repertoire of tests cost effective?
5. Is there evidence for an emphasis on quality?
6. What is the evidence for feedback from laboratory users and patients?
7. Is the laboratory user friendly?
8. What is the turnaround time for key tests?
9. Is there a programme of research and development?
10. Is there a programme of staff development?

of a few basic principles, some of which have been outlined in this chapter. Mere awareness of these principles is insufficient; they have to be applied in sufficient depth to make a difference to the way in which the department operates. The principles are not difficult, but less effective managers sometimes dismiss them as 'common sense' and proceed as before without having made the conscious decision to apply them every day. Personal development of the management skills of staff is a continuous and lifelong process. The desired outcome is to enable staff to add to their intrinsic ability so that they can work effectively with a wide range of personalities. Development of staff potential is the key factor in good laboratory management.

References

Advisory Task Force on Standards to the Audit Steering Committee of the Royal College of Pathologists. (1991) Pathology department accreditation in the United Kingdom: a synopsis. *J. Clin. Pathol.*, **44**, 798–802.

Bareford, D. and Hayling, A. (1990) Inappropriate use of laboratory services: long term combined approach to modify request patterns. *Br. Med. J.*, **301**, 1305–1307.

Batjer, J. D. (1990) The College of American Pathologists Laboratory Accreditation Program. *Clin. Lab. Haematol.*, **12**, Suppl. 1, 135–138.

Gama, R., Nightingale, P. G., Broughton, P. M. G. *et al.* (1992) Modifying the requesting behaviour of clinicians. *J. Clin. Pathol.*, **45**, 248–249.

Howanitz, P. J. and Steindel, S. J. (1991) Intralaboratory performance and laboratorians' expectations for stat turnaround times. *Arch. Pathol. Lab. Med.*, **115**, 977–983.

Keshgegian, A. A. and Bull, G. E. (1992) Evaluation of a soft-handling computerized pneumatic tube specimen delivery system. Effects on analytical results and turnaround time. *Am. J. Clin. Pathol.*, **97**, 535–540.

Mutimer, D., McCauley, B., Nightingale, P. *et al.* (1992) Computerised protocols for laboratory investigation and their effect on use of medical time and resources. *J. Clin. Pathol.*, **45**, 572–574.

National Committee for Clinical Laboratory Standards (1984) Clinical laboratory procedure manuals. Approved guideline; NCCLS publication GP2-A, **4** (2), 27–36. Villanova, Pa.; NCCLS.

Sasaki, M. (1991) An innovative conveyor belt system for a clinical laboratory. *J. Int. Fed. Clin. Chem.*, **3**, 31–33.

Stuart, J. and Hicks, J. M. (1991) Good laboratory management: an Anglo-American perspective. *J. Clin. Pathol.*, **44**, 793–797.

Stuart, J. and Hicks, J. M. (1992) Organization of a clinical directorate: Anglo-American experience from laboratory medicine. *The Clinician in Management*, **1**, 2–5.

Valenstein, P. N. and Emancipator, K. (1989) Sensitivity, specificity, and reproducibility of four measures of laboratory turnaround time. *Am. J. Clin. Pathol.*, **91**, 452–457.

Westgard, J. O., Burnett, R. W. and Bowers, G. N. (1990) Quality management science in clinical chemistry: a dynamic framework for continuous improvement of quality. *Clin. Chem.*, **36**, 1712–1716.

8

Test selection and choice of methods

R. M. Rowan

8.1 Introduction

'For the physician, there is not only a question as to what to measure and why, but equally important is the question of whether to measure or not'

(Wintrobe, 1981)

In recent years there has occurred a massive explosion in the number and complexity of medical laboratory tests and of their availability. Ready access to these has created a risk of perhaps measuring too much and not thinking sufficiently. However, that health care is increasingly dependent on laboratory findings is not in doubt.

The target of all health care laboratories is to produce reliable measurements of medically relevant analytes of proven information content in a reasonable time and at a reasonable cost. To the laboratory worker this means precision and accuracy of measurement; to the clinician it means the generation of information which is useful in diagnosis or monitoring treatment; and to the health service administrator, suitability from the cost-benefit stand-point. Laboratory data are of no value in themselves. They must be subjected to the transformation process known as interpretation and this arises in two ways. A patient's data is compared with earlier data from the same individual and management may be changed or not changed. This is referred to as longitudinal evaluation. Alternatively the patient's data is compared with that of a reference population and adjudged to represent disease or non-disease. This is transversal evaluation. To achieve these objectives requires the existence and use of standards. The process of standardization is well recognized in the laboratory sense – as the description of uniform and reproducible systems of measurement to ensure precision, accuracy, specificity and harmonization of test results. Many examples can be cited in the scientific literature. Similarly, managerial and accountancy standards are starting to be used by health care workers. Where standards are lacking is in the assessment of the clinical usefulness of medical laboratory testing. Assessment of the usefulness of laboratory tests is a complex multidimensional problem.

Many clinical laboratory tests are both technically unsound and used inappropriately. This leads to the provision of often irrelevant and inadequate information on the patient and consequently results in waste of increasingly scarce health care resources. It has been shown that high levels of laboratory testing are associated with longer patient stay in hospital. Paradoxically, recent changes in hospital policy with a view to intensifying care to shorten the length of hospital stay have resulted in the clinician requesting as many tests as possible in the shortest period of time. This latter approach still requires documented cost-benefit analysis. There are many reasons for the misuse of laboratory tests, with the clinician, the laboratory and even the patient failing to escape blame.

Many clinicians are unfamiliar with the technical and clinical limitations of the tests which they commonly order. Concepts of sensitivity, specificity and predictive value (Galen and Gambino, 1975) are not, as yet, widely used in clinical practice or alternatively are grossly misused. Clinicians also tend to add innovative tests to those already being used instead of substituting new for old. Also in this era of litigation there is a strong tendency to practise defensive medicine. There is frequently the belief that the consequences of not performing a test which may subsequently be considered, in a court of law, to be clinically useful, may be more serious than the time, effort and cost of doing it. Furthermore, reimbursement schemes may encourage maximal laboratory testing rather than the minimum consistent with good clinical care. This happens particularly where laboratories are re-imbursed on a fee per item of service basis. Medical attitudes can only be altered by improved education and this should start at undergraduate level.

8.1.1 Quality assurance

To subserve its function properly, the laboratory must have in place an exemplary quality assurance programme. The tendency to concentrate solely on analytical quality assurance must be resisted even though none will doubt the need for adequate continuous performance assessment. The non-analytical components of the quality system, however, merit equal attention. Important among the latter is communication with the user. Many laboratories have a poor record in this respect, failing to provide the clinician with detail of test imprecision and inaccuracy, of sampling and specimen transportation requirements and of interfering states and substances. Omission of these important functions can seriously impair the clinical usefulness of a test. Additionally delay in returning results to the clinician can lead to duplication of requests. The increasing use of multichannel analysers producing multiple results, many unrequested, and the newer measurements, often inadequately evaluated, add to the problem. A normal test result does not necessarily mean that the performance of a requested test is of no clinical value.

Patient attitudes can exert a major effect in the utilization of laboratory tests. Many patients have unrealistic expectations and demands. Some patients consider that the number of tests ordered is an indicator of the quality of their management and this can induce the clinician to be over-zealous in requesting diagnostic procedures. Television and the popular press also stimulate a fascination with innovative technologies. It is important to attempt to alter patient attitudes in this respect.

Clinicians and laboratorians must be induced to alter their practices, however, for other factors, e.g. organization or financial incentives, governmental or administrative intervention is necessary.

8.1.2 Basis of test selection

The preceding text describes the worst clinical and laboratory practice. Can the situation be improved? In the first instance, the appropriate selection and interpretation of diagnostic tests should be guided by diagnostic reasoning and appreciation of test characteristics (McNeil, Keeler and Adelstein, 1975; Schwartz et al., 1975). There are two fundamental criteria against which all health care programmes are judged. The first is the outcome of health care activity, i.e. the benefit not just to the individual patient but to society as a whole. The second is the cost. Based on these two criteria a hierarchical model for measuring the outcome of a test procedure can be constructed using five different levels of evaluation:

1. **Technical or analytical performance**: At its simplest, evaluation of technical performance involves assessment of method precision and how well the test results relate to truth.
2. **Diagnostic analysis**: This level of evaluation is designed to determine how well the test fulfils its objectives in terms of diagnostic sensitivity and diagnostic specificity.
3. **Diagnostic importance**: At this level the outcome is measured in terms of impact on the diagnostic reasoning of the clinician who ordered the test.
4. **Therapeutic importance**: Here outcome is measured in terms of the influence of the test on the clinician's treatment of the patient. Would the decision have been the same without the result of the test?
5. **Patient outcome**: The ultimate goal of all health service activities is to restore or improve the health of patients and thus the most important outcome measure is impact on the health status of the patient.

In using this model it should be appreciated that for a diagnostic test to be efficient at a higher level within this hierarchy, it must also have been efficient at lower levels, however, the reverse is not true. Increases in efficiency at lower levels do not guarantee commensurate improvements at higher levels. Therefore efficiency in technical outcome or diagnostic accuracy does not automatically lead to high efficiency at the patient level. In the proper evaluation of a test all five levels of outcome must be addressed; however the problem can be simplified by subdivision into three main headings, namely analytical, medical and managerial. In everyday laboratory practice three questions are constantly being asked: (1) what is the analytical quality of the test? (2) how useful is the test medically? (3) is the procedure managerially acceptable or desirable? The objective is not necessarily to decrease expenditure on laboratory services but to increase clinical effectiveness relative to the total cost of the health care service. To achieve this objective it is necessary for laboratories and clinicians to collaborate. Only prospective, rigorous, well-designed data collection and analysis can provide the correct information required for appropriate selection and utilization of tests. It must be appreciated that only properly performed evaluations, analytical, medical and managerial, facilitate the development of useful clinical guidelines and improved administrative policies.

8.2 General approach (WHO, 1989)

In attempting to determine the usefulness of a diagnostic test, certain preliminaries are essential. The first step is to define accurately and unambiguously the disease parameter (disease, stage or complication) for which the index test is being evaluated and the specific circumstances in which the test will be used. The second step is to define the pathophysiological basis of the test, the specific technical method for performing it and finally its interpretation. This should include any factors, patient or technically related, which may impair the effectiveness of the test, e.g. patient preparation, conditions of specimen collection, transport and handling, medication to be avoided. Imprecision and inaccuracy should be specified. The rules for interpretation of the test result should be defined. Critical review of the scientific literature is also required to assess what is already known about technical and diagnostic performance. This forms the basis of evaluation of the analytical process.

8.2.1 Validation standards

For evaluation of medical usefulness particular attention must be paid to the prevalence of the disease in the population being studied as well as to a validation standard to determine whether or not the disease is present. The validation standard is an independent procedure, definitive or reference, used to define the true state of the patient. The validation standard is often complex, time consuming, and costly. For certain evaluations more than one validation standard may be necessary to establish a full range of test performance. The diagnostic accuracy of the validation standard must be unchallengeable. It is important that it is independent of the index test being evaluated. Clearly the index test cannot be a component of the validation standard and must not influence the selection of the validation standard.

The population being evaluated must be specified and must be appropriate to the stage of evaluation, i.e. (1) phase 1 or preliminary evaluation (subjects with unequivocal disease and healthy controls) or (2) phase 2 evaluation consisting of clinically relevant populations (patients in whom it is anticipated that the test will be used clinically, but excluding the extremes tested in the preliminary evaluation). In the preliminary evaluation, if the index test is unable to distinguish between the extremes no further study should be undertaken. Clearly the test is unsuitable for clinical use. If, on the other hand, the index test, does distinguish between the extremes, progression to assessment of clinically relevant populations must then be undertaken. Calculations of sensitivity, specificity and predictive values must not be performed on the preliminary evaluation results since estimates of the test performance are highly biased and the test operating characteristics will be grossly overstated. For the second stage evaluation, an appropriate spectrum of diseased and non-diseased individuals should be selected. Diseased patients should comprise those in whom the index test will be used to reach a diagnosis and include minimally to moderately symptomatic patients. The non-diseased group should contain patients with similar clinical and laboratory presentations likely to cause confusion with diseased patients.

The criteria for index test interpretation and for that of the validation standard must be specified in detail and be justified. In an endeavour to avoid bias, classification of patients in the various clinical groups by the validation standard must be performed by individuals other than those interpreting the index test. Often the assistance of a statistician will be required to correct for biases inadvertently introduced.

Data emanating from this study are then analysed on four different levels:

1. Test operating characteristics (sensitivity, specificity, predictive values, receiver operator characteristic (ROC) analysis).
2. Determination of marginal test information (the greater the improvement in the estimate of the probability of disease after a test is done, the greater the value of the test).
3. Assessment of change in clinician behaviour and patient outcome.
4. Determination of the cost-effectiveness of the procedure.

8.3 Evaluation of the analytical process

Laboratory tests are not free from uncertainties or errors which impair the correctness or information content of the test result. This can result in risk to the patient. For this reason, as well as the considerable cost to the resources of the health care system of false test results, careful evaluation of the methods employed in the laboratory is mandatory. Evaluation is designed to establish the validity or otherwise of an analytical process. In other words, the evaluation process assesses the coincidence between the test result and what the test was intended to determine. Test validity is restricted by uncertainties inherent in the procedure and by technical errors arising during its performance.

8.3.1 The measuring process

To understand where uncertainties and errors arise it is useful to examine the test (method of measurement) as a process involving three basic elements (Mandel, 1959). The first is the object of the measurement (Q), an unknown quantity, which enters the measuring process as the sample. The second is the numerical value (M), which is obtained by performing the measuring process in accordance with a given set of instructions. While M is always a function of Q there are inevitably other factors, usually related to environmental conditions (C) which have an effect on the measurement (M). C is the third element involved in the measurement process and is not a single variable, but a vector in a space with a large number of dimensions. For any given value of C,

Analytical result = true result

+

bias

+

assignable causes

of error

+

random error

+

blunder

Figure 8.1 Additive Model for Analytical Error: Bias and assignable causes of error together constitute the systematic error

e.g. C_x, the measurement M is a mathematical function of Q, represented by:

$$M = f(Q/C_x)$$

As C varies, there corresponds to each value of C a curve representing the relationship between M and Q. It is the totality of these curves which constitute the measuring process. Measurements which correspond to the same value of Q will not necessarily agree since they may lie on different M,Q curves. The variability is the 'experimental error' and is partly random and partly systematic. The experimental error may be large or small depending on the extent to which environmental conditions can be controlled. To this model must be added the problem of interference. Analytical interference is any systematic error of a measurement caused by a sample component other than the analyte. Interfering properties (I), often drugs, commonly affect medical laboratory tests. It is impossible or impractical to correct for all known interfering factors. It has been demonstrated that interference can depend on the quantity either of the analyte or the interferent or that several interferences can influence each other. Inclusion of interfering properties leads to a more general representation of the measuring process:

$$M = f(Q, I/C)$$

This relationship specifies that the measurement, for any given environmental conditions is a function of the property to be measured, and of the interfering properties.

Interferences are divided into endogenous and exogenous. In the case of endogenous interference this arises: (1) in the sample during the pre-analytical

phase, e.g. red cell hemolysis resulting in the release of hemoglobin; (2) physiologically in the healthy state, e.g. proteins or (3) *in vivo* in pathological conditions, e.g. bilirubin. Exogenous interfering substances are drugs, anticoagulants, foods or substances degrading from the environment. The Société Française Biologie Clinique (1986) has defined a protocol for studying interferences.

8.3.2 Classification of uncertainties and errors

Uncertainties and errors arise at three distinct levels, technical, biological and nosological. At a technical level measurements can be impaired by unavoidable imprecision and inaccuracy, the latter particularly from drug interference with the analytical reaction. At the biological level, food, exercise and diurnal rhythms can all vary with the measurement. This can apply both when comparing a current measurement with a previous one in the same patient (delta check) or when comparing a patient with a reference population for diagnostic purposes. It is at the disease classification or nosological level, however, that the greatest uncertainties arise perhaps because at this level mathematical statistical methods are much less easy to apply.

To describe analytical errors in a quantitative test it is conventional to use an additive model. An operationally defined model such as that proposed by Buttner (1993) is employed (Figure 8.1). As previously stated these deviation components may be systematic (constant deviation or bias) or random (variable). Systematic deviation can comprise a constant component but, in addition, may contain variable components which can be assigned to specific causes (Shewhart, 1931), the so-called assignable causes of error. A final error is the 'blunder' which should be avoided by meticulously following the procedure protocol.

8.3.3 The analytical evaluation procedure

This is described in detail in Chapter 16; however some general points require to be made.

Clinical interpretation of the quantitative laboratory data depends on: (1) the calibration of instruments; (2) inherent fluctuation of the analytical measurements; (3) biological variation within an individual; and (4) inherent differences in values among individuals. Overall evaluation of a laboratory test is based on an anlysis of these sources of variation so that tolerance limits can be set for both analytical and clinical performance. These tolerance limits represent boundaries within which the analytical variation has an effect on the clinical performance of the test.

Procedures for the evaluation of analytical methods and instruments have evolved rapidly in recent years. Analytical evaluation procedures are designed primarily to ensure that manufacturer's claims can be substantiated in routine laboratory practice.

Targets for precision and accuracy should reflect 'state of the art' methodology and instrumentation potential available. Such performance goals then require evaluation to determine whether or not they satisfy a clinical need in terms of assisting in the diagnostic process, monitoring of treatment or providing prognostic information. At the same time, however, they also form a quantifiable basis for the internal quality control of the procedure. This approach has recently been adopted by NCCLS (1989) in a protocol on performance goals for analytical precision and accuracy of indirect and therefore calibratable particle counting multichannel hematology analysers. The ideal performance goal is defined as the range of the maximal allowable error in laboratory results that can be permitted without degrading medical usefulness and this range is bounded by tolerance limits. A compromise must be reached, however, between this 'ideal' and what is attainable with modern instrumentation. Imprecision and inaccuracy are the two major causes of assay variation. Performance goals for these should be set at three levels: low range, mid-range and high range.

Zero imprecision is not attainable. All procedures and instruments possess some inherent imprecision and therefore performance goals must allow for this. In addition to analytical imprecision, there is also biological variation. Whichever is larger becomes the limiting factor. Where, for example, biological variation exceeds analytical imprecision, further improvement in the analytical variation will not produce measurable improvement in clinical utility. However, reduction in analytical imprecision is still useful in setting performance goals for the analytical procedure.

Inaccuracy must also be evaluated and quantified for the influence it imparts on clinical decision making. Analytical inaccuracy has a number of independent components namely: (1) error in value assignment to a calibrator; (2) error in transference of the calibration value to the instrument; (3) drift of an instrument following calibration and (4) the Poisson counting error (indirectly through calibration accuracy). Each of these possess a number of subcomponents. Most instruments are calibrated only at one level with the assumption that errors at all other levels are linearly proportional. For this reason the identification of non-linearity in any part of the range of value encountered in clinical practice forms an important part of the evaluation. Non-linearity produces its greatest effects at the extremes of the measurement range rather than at the calibration point, and can cause major change in measurement sensitivity and specificity. The Poisson counting error relates to any measurement based on particle counts. When large numbers of cells are counted, this error becomes negligible; however, this error dominates when only small numbers of cells are counted. Inaccuracy causes a major problem in shifting patient's test values relative to fixed decision levels. For analysis with clearly defined upper and lower decision limits, shift in values will alter test operating characteristics. There will be a major decrease in clinical specificity and either a decrease or increase in clinical sensitivity depending on the direct of the shift.

Adoption of the concept of defined performance goals will address a particular criticism of evaluation protocols in that few encourage comparison of the imprecision and inaccuracy data generated with objective quality specifications.

The use of a reference method as an accuracy base to resolve discrepancies highlighted in the comparability component of the evaluation requires prior thorough validation of the capability of the laboratory staff to perform the analysis and also validation of volumetric glassware, instrument, reagents and any other materials used in its performance.

Until recently the standard manner in which laboratory methods were evaluated was by one-at-a-time protocols in which a single characteristic was evaluated in depth, e.g. effect of dilution, carry-over. Such procedures although often lengthy, provide good estimates of single analytical characteristics, but do so quite independently of other characteristics. This approach contrasts very markedly with the multifactor experimental designs now being introduced in clinical chemistry. The first multifactor experimental design for use in laboratory medicine was reported by Daniel (1975) for the evaluation of large batch-type analysers. The aim was to estimate intercept, slope, sample to sample carry-over, non-linearity, drift and error in one analytical run and was accomplished using multiple regression. Whereas linear regression is a statistical calculation which results in parameters describing the relationship between two sets of measurements, usually on the same specimens, multiple linear regression is a statistical calculation that provides multiple slope parameters responding to different factors. Multifactor experimental designs provide the maximum amount of information with only minimum expenditure of time and materials. Designs are selected to provide near orthogonality. Orthogonal designs have uncorrelated factor effects which make them easier to interpret. Statistically, orthogonality is a very desirable feature since it simplifies the least squares calculations and causes the covariance between any two contrasts to be zero. A result of this is that if the experimental errors of the observations are normally distributed and have all the same variance, the orthogonal contrasts will all be statistically independent of each other. Data analysis procedures are designed so that each point serves several purposes and all possible information is extracted from the selected sequence of results. The reader interested in this form of evaluation is referred to the recent review by Goldschmidt and Krouwer (1993). Although multifactor designs are suitable for tests and instruments used in hematology, to date the one-at-a-time protocol is still mainly being used. A current limitation of the multifactor approach is the relative difficulty in calculating effects. The development of suitable computer software will facilitate such data analysis and interpretation. The multiple factor design protocol is simple to perform. In general, estimates from multifactor and one-at-a-time protocols are in agreement. Any differences are usually only of minor importance in routine practice. Not all characteristics are obtainable from the multifactor factor design. For example, expected values, clinical specificity and sensitivity correlation and interference by specific compounds can only be assessed by one-at-a-time protocols.

Various standardizing bodies have produced recommendations for the evaluation of analytical systems including the International Council for Standardization in Hematology and the European Committee for Clinical Laboratory Standards (ECCLS) (Haeckel *et al.*, 1986). The ICSH Protocol has been revised to include automated differential leukocyte counting, reticulocyte counting and cell marker studies (ICSH, 1994). The essential difference between these evaluation protocols lies in the single multicentre evaluation model favoured by the chemists and the multiple single centre evaluations favoured by the hematologists. It is conceded (Rowan and England, 1993) that the multicentre approach for hematology would produce certain benefits, such as access to patients from a variety of ethnic groups and therefore patterns of inherited diseases. On the other hand, however, the multicentre approach would add both to the logistic problems of the evaluation and to its costs.

With both protocols there is agreement on the various levels of evaluation: the manufacturer's evaluation to establish performance criteria; a laboratory (or laboratories) acting of behalf of a consumer organization to verify that the instrument meets the performance claims; and finally an evaluation by intending users using an abbreviated protocol.

The National Committee for Clinical Laboratories Standards has recently published a protocol designed exclusively for the preliminary evaluation of quantitative clinical laboratory methods (NCCLS, 1993) to assess their suitability for operation in an individual laboratory. This is designed to allow the laboratory to make a preliminary decision about acceptability of a new method or instrument. It is designed as a quick check to exclude major problems and is neither a rigorous characterization of long term performance nor an evaluation of the many factors which can affect results. The protocol aims to produce a preliminary evaluation of linearity, precision and accuracy performance. Although intended for automated instruments it can be modified for use in evaluating manual procedures, kits and other *in vitro* diagnostic devices. Performance characteristics, as described previously, may be evaluated simultaneously by repeating a sequence of only eleven samples, plotting the data and performing some simple calculations. By using multiple linear regression analysis additional factors affecting imprecision can be obtained such as carry-over and drift. This procedures does not replace formal evaluation, merely serving to determine whether or not the method has grossly unacceptable performance.

The general scheme for an evaluation protocol which follows, should be taken as the minimum requirement and describes only the basic principles. Full details for the evaluation of an analytical process are described in Chapter 16. Evaluation protocols fall into a number of component parts each of which must be followed in a logical order. The following sequence is common to all:

1. Collection of preliminary information
2. Planning of technical assessment
3. Preliminary assessment
4. Performance assessment
5. Efficiency assessment

The preliminary assessment serves the multiple functions of allowing staff the opportunity to become familiar with the test procedure, to screen out products or systems unacceptable for use in the laboratory environment and to identify major components of variance of results. The performance assessment is a more rigorous process of measuring the performance of the system under test by analysing specimens from a representative sample of the usual subject population in parallel with the routine method. Where discrepancies arise between the two, these are resolved by comparison with reference methods. Specimen selection can be difficult. Ideally, selection should be random but this usually does not guarantee representation from all parts of the range encountered in clinical practice. A quota is required for specified concentration ranges: about one-third straddling the range found in non-diseased subjects, one-third beyond the upper decision level and one-third below the lower decision level. Statistical analysis of randomly selected specimens should be quite separate from selected patients with identifiable pathologies or potentially interfering conditions that are recognized to interfere with the analysis.

8.4 Evaluation of medical usefulness

8.4.1 Principles of test selection

Laboratory tests should only be performed when the information from the clinical history and physical examination is inadequate to answer the clinical question being asked or to quantify an anemia. The decision to perform a test is made on the assumption that the result will appreciably reduce uncertainties.

Tests and procedures are used for a variety of clinical purposes and these must not be confused. In general, tests are used: (1) in the diagnosis of disease; (2) in screening asymptomatic individuals to detect certain categories of disease; (3) to make treatment decisions and (4) in making a prognosis.

a. Diagnosis of disease

The diagnostic process requires two steps. First the clinician establishes a differential diagnosis and reduces this by progressively ruling out specific diseases. This procedure requires tests which are very sensitive. Sensitivity is defined as the probability that a test result will be positive when the disease is present. A sensitive test, when normal, therefore, permits the clinician to exclude the disease with confidence. Having narrowed the differential diagnosis, the next step is the pursuit of a strong clinical suspicion, this requiring a very specific test. Specificity refers to the probability that the test result will be negative when the disease is not present. Therefore, such a test, when abnormal, should essentially confirm the existence of the disease. Thus, intelligent selection of a laboratory test depends on a choice appropriate for the purpose intended. The purpose should accurately reflect the clinician's likely estimate of the disease based on available clinical evidence. A test is used to exclude a diagnosis when the disease is unlikely and conversely to confirm the diagnosis when a disease is probable.

b. Screening for disease:

The screening of asymptomatic individuals by means of laboratory tests has the primary objective of detecting diseases whose morbidity and mortality can be reduced by early detection and treatment. It also serves the secondary role of reassuring individuals found not be suffering from the disease. The basic principles underlying the philosophy of screening are that the benefit of the procedure outweighs cost in terms of risk to patient and expense to the healthcare system (Griner et al., 1981). Guidelines for the selection of the population to be screened and the tests used for early disease detection have been described by the Canadian Task Force on Periodic Health Examination (1979) and include:

1. The disease should be sufficiently common to justify the effort and expense in detecting it
2. The disease should create sufficient morbidity if not treated
3. Effective treatment must be available to alter the natural history of the disease
4. Detection and treatment of the presymptomatic

patient should result in benefit beyond that obtained by treatment of the early symptomatic state

An acceptable screening test will be one that will be abnormal in virtually all patients with the disease and will give the clinician the confidence that the disease is not present when the test result is normal. Specificity is very important when screening for rare diseases because of the implications of false-positive results when the test is not specific.

c. Treatment of patients:

During the course of patient treatment, laboratory tests are commonly repeated, therefore the reproducibility of a test is one of its most important characteristics. Repeat test are used for the following purposes:

- to monitor disease process status: is it progressing, stable or resolving?
- to identify and monitor reversal of complications of treatment
- to ensure adequacy of drug levels
- to assist in defining prognosis
- to check an unexpected test result

d. Making a prognosis:

Laboratory tests are used for making a prognosis for a specific patient. This involves the derivation from the occurrence of a certain test result or pattern of test results a conclusion about future events. These future events constitute the 'outcome'. The starting point is the current observation and the 'outcome' or prognosis is a probability statement usually on how a patient will respond to a particular form of treatment or whether or not the patient will survive and, if so, for how long. The statistical methods used for defining a valid rule are more complicated than for the diagnostic process. This is because time variation must be taken into account. Detail of statistical treatment is given in Buttner (1993) and Cox and Oakes (1984).

The vast majority of laboratory tests are performed for the purpose of patient management. The optimal frequency with which a test is repeated for the purpose of patient management requires both knowledge and experience. To do this correctly, the clinician must understand the expected rate of change in the disease process concerned as well as the limitations of the test procedures. There is no simple rule to circumvent these problems.

8.4.2 The reference range in health

A normal quantitative test result can exclude certain groups of diseases. A good example of this is the

Table 8.1 Binary table

		DISEASE PRESENT	ABSENT	TOTAL
TEST	POS	TP	FP	TP + FP
	NEG	FN	TN	FN + TN
	TOTAL	TP + FN	FP + TN	

TP = number of patients with the disease with a positive test result (true positive); FP = number of patients without the disease with a positive test result (false positive); FN = number of patients with the disease in whom the test result is negative (false negative); TN = number of patients without the disease in whom the test result is negative (true negative).

finding of a normal 2-hour postprandial blood sugar level which virtually excludes diabetes mellitus as a diagnosis. There are, however, two major difficulties in defining the normal, or, better expressed, reference range in health. The first problem arises in the definition of a healthy population. The second lies in the results distribution model on which the calculation of the reference range is made.

Major problems arise from the lack of clear and unequivocal definitions of the words 'normal' and 'healthy'. Most often, it would appear that 'healthy' is defined as the most convenient, ostensibly disease-free group of individuals available. These may be laboratory personnel, medical students, blood donors, hospital outpatients in apparently good health or certain categories of hospitalized patients in whom there is no reason to suspect hematological abnormality. There is little or no knowledge about the subject's origins, about the population from which the subjects are derived; nor about the measurement technique applied. This is unacceptable; values must be measured in well-defined and adequately categorized populations: the technique of measurement must be known together with its imprecision and inaccuracy. Reference ranges, so defined, will then be acceptable provided similar techniques are used in a patient from a similar population. Dybkaer and Gräsbeck (1973) proposed the term 'reference values' for such population-based results. The International Federation of Clinical Chemistry (IFCC) and the International Council for Standardization in Haematology (ICSH) have published standards on the use of reference values (IFCC/ICSH, 1983/84; IFCC/ICSH, 1987a,b.). Sunderman (1975), in an excellent editorial on the subject, lists five major specification categories to accompany reference values:

1. The reference population, and the way it is selected.
2. The physiological and environmental conditions under which specimens were obtained.
3. The technique and timing of specimen collection, transport, preparation and storage.

4. The analytical method used, its imprecision, inaccuracy and quality assurance requirements.
5. The data set that was observed and the reference intervals derived.

This subject is described in detail in Chapter 15.

8.4.3 Test operating characteristics

To fully understand the derivation of evaluation methods, distinction must be drawn between qualitative and quantitative tests. The qualitative test provides a single 'yes/no' response. Provided interpretation of a quantitative test result can be reduced to a similar yes/no response, i.e. normal or abnormal, the procedures for determining test operating characteristics are identical. In laboratory practice, however, most tests are quantitative in nature, the determination of quantities being on a difference or ratio scale. Determination of the validity of these tests is more difficult since instead of the discrete probabilites inherent in the qualitative test, continuous probability density functions are now encountered. The solution to this problem for quantitative tests rests in the definition of decision criteria ('limiting values' or cut-off points). If this can be accomplished, then a fourfold decision scheme, similar to that used for qualitative tests, can be used to define the test operating characteristics.

a. Sensitivity and specificity

Every laboratory test possesses a set of characteristics which reflect the information expected in patients with and without the disease in question. This leads to two fundamental questions:

1. If the disease is present, what is the likelihood that the test result will be positive? The answer to this question determines the sensitivity of the test.
2. If the disease is not present, what is the likelihood that the test result will be normal? The answer to this question determines the specificity of the test.

These characteristics can be displayed by a simple binary table (Table 8.1).

From this table various probabilities can be calculated. These are described below and illustrated by examples based on the data in Table 8.2, where in 1000 cases, TP = 400, TN = 370, FP = 130 and FN = 100.

1. Probability that the test will be positive when the disease is present, i.e. the **sensitivity** of the test:

Table 8.2 Use of the binary table to determine the predictive values of positive and negative test results

		DISEASE	
		PRESENT	ABSENT
TEST	POS	400	130
	NEG	100	370

(Adapted from Griner et al., 1981) Sensitivity = 80%; specificity = 74%. Positive predictive value is 400/400 + 130 = 75% and negative predictive value is 370/370 + 100 = 79%

$$\frac{\text{True positive results}}{\text{Total patients with disease}} =$$

$$\frac{TP}{TP + FN} \text{ (e.g. } \frac{400}{400 + 100} = 0.80).$$

2. Probability that the test will be negative when the disease is not present, i.e. the **specificity** of the test:

$$\frac{\text{True negative results}}{\text{Total patients without disease}} =$$

$$\frac{TN}{FP + TN} \text{ (e.g. } \frac{370}{130 + 370} = 0.74).$$

The relationships between the magnitude of the analytical inaccuracy and the sensitivity and specificity of a test depends on where the decision values lie on the curve of the distribution of test values and the slope of the distribution at that position (see Section 8.4.4(a)). Tests with steeper distribution curves at the decision level are more affected by assay drift than are tests with flatter distribution curves. Clinical specificity is much less dependent on assay imprecision than on assay accuracy.

3. Probability that the test will be positive when the disease is absent, i.e. the false positive rate for the test:

$$\frac{\text{False positive results}}{\text{Total patients without disease}} =$$

$$\frac{FP}{FP + TN} \text{ (e.g. } \frac{130}{130 + 370} = 0.26).$$

4. Probability that the test will be negative when the disease is present, i.e. the false negative rate for the test:

$$\frac{\text{False negative results}}{\text{Total patients with disease}} =$$

$$\frac{FN}{TP + FN} \text{ (e.g. } \frac{100}{400 + 100} = 0.20).$$

These four test characteristics can be considered to be constant provided: (1) they have been determined from a large sample of individuals with and without the disease; (2) the test procedure does not deviate and (3) the same criteria are used to define a positive result. On their own, however, these test operating characteristics cannot determine the presence or absence of disease unless the sensitivity is 100% and the specificity is 100% and this seldom pertains. An integrative process is necessary to resolve this problem combining the test operating characteristics with the clinician's prior estimate of the probability of disease (prior possibility or pre-test probability). This introduces the concept of disease prevalence in the community.

b. Predictive values

Since the task of the clinician is still to determine whether or not a disease is present, two questions must be asked:

1. Given a positive test, what is the probability that the disease is present? This probability reflects the predictive value of a positive test result.
2. Given a negative test, what is the probability that the disease is absent? This probability reflects the predictive value of a negative test result.

Predictive values can also be illustrated with reference to the simple binary Table. From Table 8.2 a positive value is derived from:

$$\frac{\text{True positive}}{\text{True positive + true negative}} =$$

$$\frac{TP}{TP + FP} \text{ (e.g. } \frac{400}{400 + 130} = 0.75),$$

and a negative predictive value from:

$$\frac{\text{True negative}}{\text{False negative + true negative}} =$$

$$\frac{TN}{FN + TN} \text{ (e.g. } \frac{370}{100 + 370} = 0.79).$$

To complete the calculation, however, an estimate of the likelihood of disease before the test must be combined with the known operating characteristics of the test. To illustrate this consider a pre-test likelihood of disease of 50:50 but for simplicity express in absolute numbers rather than percentages, i.e. disease present, n = 500; disease absent, n = 500 (Table 8.2).

The application of the test operating characteristics to these numbers results in an increase in the likeli-

Table 8.3 Influence of prior estimates of likelihood of disease on the predictive values of positive and negative results. All values expressed as per cent

Prior estimate of likelihood	Test positive Predictive value	Test negative Predictive value
90	97	29
80	92	48
70	88	61
60	82	71
50	75	79
40	67	85
30	57	90
20	43	94
10	25	97

(Adapted from Griner et al., (1981)

hood of the disease from 50% to 75% when the test is positive, an incremental ruling-in gain of 25%. A normal test result, on the other hand, has reduced the likelihood of disease from 50% to 21% (probability of no disease = 79%) an incremental ruling-out gain of 29%. The effect of differing prior estimates of likelihood of disease is shown in Table 8.3.

The calculation of the predictive values of positive and negative results for any test, whose sensitivity and specificity are known, by varying prior probabilities may help to show in which circumstances the test is most useful.

Likelihood

The concept of variation in a test's diagnostic performance over the entire analytical range has already been introduced. The value of the diagnostic performance of a test can be enhanced by evaluating the sensitivity and specificity for specific ranges of results. Calculation of the likelihood ratios (e.g. true positive to false positive ratio) for test results intervals provides more information than merely treating a test result as positive or negative. The likelihood ratio is a measure of discrimination by a test result. A test result with a likelihood ratio greater than 1.0 raises the probability of disease and is referred to as a positive test with this method. A test result with a likelihood ratio less than 1.0 lowers the probability of disease and, using the same rules, is called a negative test result.

Likelihood ratio =

$$\frac{\text{frequency of positive results in diseased}}{\text{frequency of positive results in non-diseased}}$$

$$(\text{e.g. } \frac{400}{130} = 3.07),$$

or it can be calculated from:

$$\frac{\text{sensitivity}}{1 - \text{specificity}} \quad (\text{e.g. } \frac{0.80}{1 - 0.74} = 3.07).$$

or

Likelihood ratio =

$$\frac{\text{frequency of negative results in non-diseased}}{\text{frequency of negative results in diseased}}$$

$$(\text{e.g. } \frac{370}{100} = 3.7),$$

$$= \frac{\text{specificity}}{1 - \text{sensitivity}} \quad (\text{e.g. } \frac{0.74}{1 - 0.80} = 3.7).$$

An alternative formula, the Youden index (Youden, 1950), is as follows:

sensitivity + specificity − 1
(e.g. (0.80 + 0.74) − 1 = + 0.54).

Values range from − 1 to + 1; tests with positive values are considered to be positive.

d. Test selection when alternatives exist

Test operating characteristics are also of value in determining which test of a number of alternatives is the most appropriate for selection. Clearly the purpose for which the test is being used will determine the required operating characteristics. When two or more tests are available to confirm the presence of a disease, that with the highest specificity should be preferred. When used to exclude a diagnostic possibility, the test with the higher sensitivity is usually preferred. It must be remembered, however, that the operating characteristics of a test vary according to the criteria used to define an abnormal result. If the criteria are made more stringent the specificity will be greater but at the expense of reduced sensitivity. Less stringent criteria produce the opposite effect; sensitivity becomes greater at the expense of specificity.

e. Operating characteristics of combination testing

It is only in rare situations that a disease is diagnosed on the basis of a single feature, be that a pathognomonic clinical sign or laboratory result. Two or more tests are usually performed to evaluate a diagnostic possibility. Each test exhibits false classifications to a greater or lesser degree. When several tests are combined, accepting that the reference interval for each is the central 95% of the values of its reference population, the expected values for all the events lying within the respective univariate reference intervals are much lower. This reduction increases as the number of tests increases. This problem can only be avoided if multivariate reference regions are defined instead of multiple univariate reference intervals. Once again the fact that many biological quantity distributions are not Gaussian compounds the statistical solution. The reader interested in pursuing this in greater detail should consult Buttner (1993) both for statistical treatment of the issues and for a

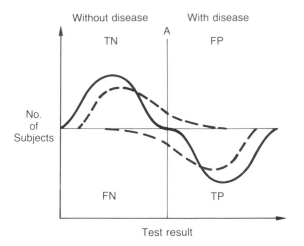

Figure 8.2 The decision criterion dilemma for the quantitative test. (TN = true negative, FN = false negative, FP = false positive and TP = true positive)

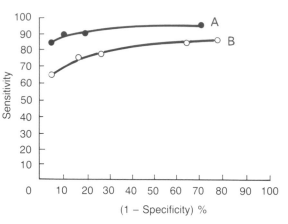

Figure 8.3 Receiver operator characteristic curves for two tests (A and B) making the same measurement

description of theoretical methods which are independent of distribution.

8.4.4 The special problems of the quantitative test

a. Decision criterion

Ideally there should be no overlap in ranges of test results for those individuals with and without a particular disease (Figure 8.2: solid line). Line A defines the cut-off point (decision criterion) to the right of which the result is 100% sensitive and to the left of which the result is 100% specific. There are no false positive or false negative results. This is an ideal test but unfortunately no such quantitative tests occur in practice. The broken line in Figure 8.2 shows the usual relationship in practice, i.e. there is overlap between the range in health and the range in disease. High imprecision of a test procedure leads to high levels of false positive and false negative results compared with a test whose level of imprecision is low. Likewise, analytical inaccuracy influences the validity of a test. The cut-off point (decision criterion) will shift with increasing inaccuracy, e.g. when there is erroneous calibration of an instrument. False positive and false negative findings are dependent on the location of the cut-off point in a quantitative test.

When developing a test which possesses a numerical range for clinical use, it is customary to define the reference range in health as being limited to ± 2 standard deviations from the mean thus encompassing 95% of test results among disease-free subjects. Therefore approximately 2.5% of subjects fall either above or below this range. In the example given in Figure 8.2 the choice of cut-off point A results in

high specificity but low sensitivity. This is adequate to confirm a suspected diagnosis but could not be used to screen for or exclude a disease because of its low sensitivity. To improve performance with the latter, the cut-off point requires to move to the left thus improving sensitivity but reducing specificity. Each cut-off point defines a set of operating characteristics for the test. Some tests, therefore, can be used either to confirm or exclude disease by altering the criteria for an abnormal test result according to the purpose of the test. Decision limits used in the clinical interpretation of test results depend on the reference ranges established for the test. If the instrument drifts the test values will not correspond to the clinician's reference points and this leads to incorrect interpretation.

b. Receiver operator characteristic analysis (ROC analysis)

The optimization of decision limits is important for quantitative laboratory tests. Although various methods exist for accomplishing this, the most widely adopted technique is that of receiver operator characteristic analysis (ROC analysis). A graph is constructed which correlates true positive rates (sensitivity) with false positive rates (1-specificity) for a series of cut-off points for any test. This graph is called the Receiver Operator Characteristic of a test. The method originates from the statistical theory of signal detection from noise (Swets, 1964), the ROC curve representing the probability of true positive results as a function of the probability of false positive results (Figure 8.3). The graph can be used to determine the optimum decision criterion for the purpose for which the test is being used. In addition ROC analysis can be used to define which of two tests should be selected for a particular use. In Figure 8.3, two hypothetical tests, A and B, may be used for diagnosing the same disease. For both tests, as the criteria for a positive test are made more stringent, the curves move to the left and down, i.e. the specificity becomes greater and the sensitivity lower. If either test A or test B is used to confirm a strong clinical suspicion that a disease is present, these stringent criteria will be appropriate. However, as the criteria for a positive test are made more liberal, the curves move to the right and upwards resulting in greater sensitivity and lower specificity. These liberal criteria are appropriate if the purpose of the tests is to exclude the disease in question. Comparison of these two tests shows that, regardless of the purpose, test A is always superior to test B. Such comparisons are useful in determining the best test for a particular purpose.

8.4.5 Determination of marginal test information

In clinical practice, laboratory test results are interpreted in conjunction with clinical and other diagnostic information. It follows that the greater the improvement in the estimate of the probability of disease after a test is performed, the greater the clinical value of the test. This is the generally accepted definition of marginal test information. Models to discriminate among alternative diagnoses or outcomes can be developed, the simplest being one constructed without the index test and then with the index test included. The difference between these models reflects the contribution of the index test to the outcome. Methods for determining marginal test information include multivariate and Bayesian analysis. Multivariate analysis is made possible by the availability of statistics software packages which are simple to use but the experimental design is very important. Two statistical procedures are suited to this purpose. These are discriminant analysis and cluster analysis. The difference between the two is that the former requires a group assignment for each element used to calculate the coefficient of the discriminant function. It is thus evident that the result of a discriminant analysis depends on how accurately the respective grouping is reflected by the information contained in the data. Normal distributions as well as identical covariance matrices are assumed within the different groups in the case of linear discriminant analysis whereas skewed distribution and unequal covariance matrices are assumed for quadratic discriminant function. Use of Bayes' Theorem for calculating the post-test probability of disease is provided by Sox (1986).

Alternatively, Bayesian analysis can be used to estimate marginal test information. With this method, the probability of a diagnosis is calculated using: (1) estimated disease prevalence in the population being studied; and (2) the sensitivity and specificity of the relevant clinical findings and laboratory tests available prior to the introduction of the index

test. The probability of disease is then recalculated after performance of the index test and the difference between pre-and post-test probability of disease is a measure of the marginal test information. If the probability of disease after the index test is very similar to the probability of the disease before the index test, then this test is unlikely to affect management. A worked example of the use of Bayes' Theorem for calculating the post-test probability of disease is provided by Sox (1986).

Both statistical approaches require prospective, uniform data collection following a carefully planned and structured protocol. In order to determine the correlation among alternative laboratory tests it is necessary to perform each test independently either on the same specimen or on specimens collected simultaneously from the same patient. Only in this way can the validity of the analysis be assured since none of the techniques used for handling missing data can correct for resulting bias.

8.4.6 Significant change in laboratory data

This is a difficult area governed by two factors, namely the experience and intuition of the clinician on one hand and the dictates of the laboratory on the other.

In an attempt to establish medically useful guidelines Skendzel, Barnett and Platt (1985) invited randomly selected physicians to assess a number of clinical problems and select those changes in test results which would cause them: (1) to alter their diagnosis; (2) to change their treatment of patients or (3) to stimulate further analysis of the patient's clinical status. Responses to this survey were used to calculate goals for laboratory precision which would satisfy the requirements of the average clinician and from this three important findings emerged. In the first place most clinicians required substantial change in test results before they changed their diagnosis or treatment and the imprecision present in laboratory testing fell within these limits. Secondly since the clinician makes a complex judgement when analysing test results, what consitutes significant change depends on the clinical situation. With asymptomatic patients the change necessary to generate clinician concern is greater than in patients with acute illness or in monitoring therapeutic regimes. Finally clinicians, irrespective of specialty appeared to react intuitively in very similar ways to change in test results. The magnitude of changes in test results that trigger clinical actions depend on the clinician's assessment of the combined analytical and biological variations. Changes which exceed this are considered unusual and merit further investigation.

The observation that present levels of laboratory imprecision for many tests more than satisfy clinical requirements prompts the suggestion that further improvements in clinical and laboratory practices may be served better by attempting to control non-analytical causes of variation particularly during the pre-analytical phase of laboratory procedures.

In the laboratory traditionally and quite arbitrarily, significant change in the measurement of an analyte is defined as difference from a previous measurement which is greater than 3SD. The standard deviation is determined following replicate analysis performed on multiple aliquots of a single pool. Examples for hematology analytes cited by Koepke and Koepke (1987) are:

Hemoglobin concentration	0.9 g/dl
Hematocrit	0.037
Red cell count	$0.18 \times 10^{12}/l$
White cell count	$3.6 \times 10^{9}/l$

Clearly, however, the magnitude of significant change will vary slightly from laboratory to laboratory because of methodological differences.

8.5 Economic evaluation

8.5.1 The techniques available

An increasingly important part of health care technology assessment is economic evaluation or appraisal. This is the generic term for a range of techniques devised to assist decision making when choices require to be made between several courses of action. There are four main approaches to economic appraisal each involving systematic identification, measurement, and where appropriate, evaluation of all the relevant costs and consequences of the options under review (Robinson, 1993). These approaches are:

1. Cost-minimization analysis

This is used when there is evidence to indicate that the outcomes of the procedures under consideration are the same. Since there is no difference in clinical outcome, the analysis can concentrate on identifying the least cost option.

2. Cost-effectiveness analysis

This is used when the outcomes of different procedures may be expected to vary but these outcomes may be expressed in common natural units, e.g. per life saved, per symptom-free day. With a common unit of outcome, different procedures can be expressed in terms of cost of unit of outcome.

3. Cost-utility analysis

This is used when the outcomes do vary. In the health care context, 'utility' refers to the subjective level of well-being that individuals experience in different states of health. To measure 'utility' various quality of life scales have been developed, e.g. quality adjusted life years (QALYs). QALYs are based on the concept that a health care programme is more effective when health improvements are increased, patients enjoy these improvements longer and more patients are helped. This is referred to as the health status index approach (Patrick, Bush and Chen, 1973). This concept has proved unpopular since it focuses on life years rather than individuals as the recipients of health improvements. Recently Nord (1992) has outlined an alternative procedure – saved young-life equivalent (SAVE) – which is suggested as a unit of value. Both QALY and SAVE allow comparison in terms of cost utility ratios.

4. Cost-benefit analysis

This is used when a monetary value is being placed on services received. The term should be restricted to those forms of evaluation used to place a monetary value on outcomes.

The appropriate method of economic evaluation will depend on the context in which choice requires to be made. Clearly when outcomes are identical the most straight-forward form of cost-minimization can be applied. Cost-effectiveness analysis has certain limitations which have led to greater interest in measurement of cost-utility. Beyond this, cost benefit analysis offers the most comprehensive and theoretically sound form of economic evaluation but its application in the context of health care is fraught with practical problems.

8.5.2 Option appraisal

Option appraisal (DHSS, 1988) is a useful management tool which has many applications in health care services. It is strongly recommended that option appraisals should always be undertaken before significant investment decisions are made about equipment. Such appraisals should cover the full range of options, should include expert advice (often multidisciplinary) on the implications of each option and should consider the views of the professional user. The process involves a systematic approach to expenditure decisions which incorporates:

- the objectives (user requirements, equipment specifications and performance)
- the various ways of meeting the objectives (draw up a short list)
- the cost of each option (appraisal of these options; development of arguments for and against particular choices)
- the benefits of each option

The process can be used for both major and minor equipment acquisitions. It should be appreciated that even small items, used in large enough numbers, can have high total cost and benefit consequences.

The process of option appraisal falls into two phases. Phase I is concerned with whether or not to provide a service and, if the response is affirmative, how best to provide it. This may involve consideration of health care service strategic planning and becomes relevant when purchasing a very expensive item of equipment, introducing a new technology or a new service or equipping a new hospital. In such a situation full option appraisal should be undertaken. Phase II is the 'best buy' appraisal and is concerned with identifying best value for money. In the case of replacement of routine equipment, Phase II only is required. Good option appraisal combines estimates of costs and benefits with appropriate professional judgement.

a. Assessing costs

It is necessary to assess the resource consequences of both capital and running costs. Certain principles must be followed in assessing the resource consequences of options:

- **Opportunity costs**: This should be used in appraisal. When resources are committed to a particular use, the opportunity to put them to another is lost. The value of the next best use is the opportunity cost of resource use.
- **Incremental costs**: In most instances it is the incremental not average costs that measure true economic cost.
- **Irretrievable costs**: Generally past expenditures and other cost irrevocably committed should be ignored in the appraisal. Instrument resale value may, however, have a bearing on certain options.
- **Price basis**: All cost values should be expressed in prices ruling in one particular year, the so-called 'base year'. Revaluation may be necessary so that all prices are expressed in the base year.
- **Inflation**: If it is anticipated that general inflation will affect all cost components equally then it should be ignored. If, however, some costs rise by more or less than general inflation, such costs are described as rising or falling in 'real' terms. In such circumstances it is the cost after allowing for inflation that should be used in the calculations.
- **Use of charitable funds**: Whilst the initial acquisition may be purchased from charitable funds it is most likely that running costs and the cost of replacement equipment will fall on the health care service. The future funding consequences of purchase from charitable funds must be considered as part of the appraisal. The overall cost to the health care service may be such as to render the project not worthwhile.
- **Alternative financing of purchases**: 'Alternative'

or 'unconventional' finance are terms used to embrace a wide range of arrangements enabling assets to be acquired immediately but at the same time permitting the cost to be spread over a period. Such arrangements include deferred payment or purchase, hire purchase, leasing and sale and leaseback. These schemes only work because the supplier is able to finance the purchase of the asset. Thus part of the charge to the user will be a financing cost. These schemes must be carefully analysed since they usually turn out to be more expensive in the end than outright capital purchase.

b. Capital costs

The principal aims in the assessment of capital costs are to compare alternative ways of using assets and investment resources both for developments within the service and for improving efficiency and to compare the non-recurrent costs of the different options. The main capital cost categories are those for the basic equipment, additional peripheral equipment, space to accommodate the new equipment and any consequential costs associated with refurbishment or modification of buildings. Any additional installation costs must be included in the capital costs. Future costs beyond the base year should be discounted to indicate present value of the costs. It is necessary to calculate the equivalent annual cost where options have different lifespans.

Since forecasting events and costs is involved in the procedure it is necessary to conduct a sensitivity analysis. Sensitivity analysis is the process of assessing how the appraisal will be influenced by variation in the major assumptions which underlie it and may necessitate a series of calculations illustrating the financial impact of such variations. This process is designed to provide managers with some indication of the effect of uncertainties on the choice of options.

c. Revenue costs

Detailed assessment of running costs is mandatory for any option appraisal not just to compare relative running costs of the different options but to assess whether or not they are affordable. The principal components are staff, consumables, maintenance contract and spares costs, not forgetting out of hours use and additional costs incurred during the transition period.

d. Assessing benefits

Ideally options should be appraised in terms of their anticipated contribution to improvement in health of individual patients or to a population at large. Such benefits are classed as ultimate. Usually, however, it is difficult to identify such benefits particularly in relation to laboratory tests. With the latter only an assessment of intermediate benefits is possible and these define volumes of service activity and quality, both of which are highly relevant since they describe, *inter alia*, diagnostic accuracy, analytical throughput and speed of reporting results. Non-monetary benefits and disadvantages must be included in the appraisal and these should be quantified using a weighting system. It has been suggested that a group of experts, users and managers construct the weighting system by means of a questionnaire on perceived desirable attributes. The grounds on which values are assigned to the weighting system must be recorded in the option appraisal. In the assessment of benefits the hierarchical model for evaluation described in the introduction to this chapter forms a useful basis for compilation. Benefits can therefore be suggested in terms of:

1. Technical performance
2. Diagnostic accuracy
3. Diagnostic impact
4. Impact on treatment
5. Impact on patient outcome

e. Types of appraisal

Various types of appraisal exist depending on the availability of financial resources. When a fixed quantity of resource is allocated, then appraisal can be restricted to the relative benefits of those options falling within the financial limit. The aim here is to select the option which maximizes benefits. Where there exists a fixed service requirement, the appraisal need only address the relative costs determining that option which minimizes costs. Where neither the resource allocation nor the service objective is fixed, full benefit-cost appraisal must be undertaken seeking that option which give the greatest excess of benefits over costs.

8.5.3 Factors involved in cost analysis of equipment.

a. Capital cost

The capital cost of a new instrument includes depreciation and interest; however, if the instrument is leased, the capital cost should be replaced by the leasing charge. Depreciation may be linear (cost divided equally over the anticipated life of the instrument) or non-linear (depreciation greater during the early life of the instrument). The period of depreciation is usually taken as 7–10 years. Interest costs can be included in the calculation.

b. Maintenance cost

The cost of the maintenance contract is usually ob-

tained from the manufacturer although in certain cases an in-house tender may be more competitive. It is usual to use the adjusted cost of the maintenance contract which allows for the warranty period within the anticipated lifetime.

c. Labour costs

Direct personnel time includes preparation, analysis and recording of results for a defined procedure at a defined workplace. Short waiting periods which cannot be utilized for other work are included in direct personnel time measurements. Longer periods which can be used for alternative duties are excluded. A system of unit values has been used to record this both in Welcan UK (1993) and in the Laboratory Workload Recording Manual of the College of American Pathologists (1992) (see Chapter 9). Indirect personnel time should be registered at an auxiliary cost centre and then subsequently distributed across the main cost centres.

d. Cost of materials

It is important to appreciate that the cost of instrument preparation including calibration usually remains constant regardless of workload and thus direct proportionality between material costs and workload is not maintained. Cost of materials should be divided into fixed costs, i.e. those costs associated with preparing the instrument for use, for calibration and for quality assurance, and the variable costs, i.e. those costs directly associated with the analysis of patient samples. The costs of reagents, calibrators and control materials should also reflect the unavoidable wastage which occurs.

e. Other costs

These include necessary services, i.e. electricity, water, etc., data processing and laboratory management.

8.6 Conclusion

Economic evaluation covers only one dimension of the overall evaluation process and must be linked to clinical or other health care studies which establish the efficacy and effectiveness of the procedures under consideration. This provides information on the production-function relationship; that is, how the inputs are related to outcomes.

Cost   Benefit

Inputs ⟶ Procedure ⟶ Outcomes

Economic evaluation should always be undertaken

alongside clinical trials so that appropriate data collection can be built in as an integral part of the assessment. Unfortunately this is rarely done.

However, laboratory performance is not just an exercise in economies but an integral and highly important function in patient care. There are many occasions when investment in a procedure which, at first sight, may appear to be expensive but which, because it reduces diagnostic error or uncertainty, may well be justified since it leads to more rapid and precise determination of patient status, shorter hospitalization and improved patient outcome.

References

Büttner, J. (1993) Evaluation of diagnostic and prognostic measures, In: Haeckel, R. (ed.), *Evaluation Methods in Laboratory Medicine*. Weinheim: VCH. pp. 1–46.

Canadian Task Force on the Periodic Health Examination (1979) The periodic health examination. *Can. Med. Assoc. J.* **121**, 1193–1254.

College of American Pathologists (1992) *Workload Recording Method and Personnel Management Manual*. Northfield, ILL: College of American Pathologists. 60093–2750.

Cox, D. R. and Oakes, D. (1984) *Analysis of Survival Data*, London: Chapman and Hall.

Daniel, C. (1975) Calibration designs for machines with carry-over and drift. *J. Qual. Techn.* **7**, 103–108.

DHSS: NHS Procurement Directorate (1988) *Option Appraisal of Medical and Scientific Equipment*. London: HMSO. p. 60.

Dybkaer, R. and Gräsbeck, R. (1973) Theory of reference values, *Scand. J. Lab. Invest.*, **32**, 1–7.

Galen, R. S. and Gambino, S. R. (1975) *Beyond Normality – the Predictive Value and Efficiency of Medical Diagnosis*, New York: Wiley.

Goldschmidt, H. M. J. and Krouwer, J. S. (1993) Multifactor experimental designs for evaluations, In: Haeckel, R. (ed.) *Evaluation Methods in Laboratory Medicine*. Weinheim: VCH, pp. 71–86.

Griner, P. F., Nayawski, R. J., Mushlin, A. I. *et al.* (1981) Selection and interpretation of diagnostic tests and procedures: Principles and applications. *Ann. Intern. Med.*, **94**, 553–563.

Haeckel, R., Busch, E. W., Jennings, R. D. *et al.* (1986) Guidelines for the evaluation of Analysers in Clinical Chemistry, ECCLS Document 3, No. 2, Berlin: Beuth, Verlag.

ICSH (1994) Guidelines for the evaluation of blood cell analysers including those used for differential leucocyte and reticulocyte counting and cell marker applications. *Clin. Lab. Haemat.*, **16**, 157–174.

IFCC/ICSH (1983/84) The theory of reference values. Part 5: Statistical treatment of collected reference values. Determination of reference limits. *J. Clin. Chem. Clin. Biochem.*, **21**, 749–760.

IFCC/ICSH (1987a) Approved recommendation (1986) on the theory of reference values. The concept of reference values. *J. Clin. Chem. Clin. Biochem.*, **26**, 337–342.

IFCC/ICSH (1987b) The theory of reference values. Part 6: Presentation of observed values related to reference values. *J. Clin. Chem. Clin. Biochem.*, **25**, 657–662.

Koepke, J. A. and Koepke, J. F. (1987) *Guide to Clinical Laboratory Diagnosis*. East Norwalk, CN: Appleton and Lange.

Mandel, J. (1959) The measuring process. *Technometrics*, **1**, 251–267.

McNeil, B. J., Keeler, E. and Adelstein, S. J. (1975) Primer in certain elements of decision making, *N. Engl. J. Med.*, **293**, 211–215.

National Committee for Clinical Laboratory Standards (1993) Preliminary evaluation of quantitative clinical Laboratory Methods, 2nd edn. Tentative guideline. NCCLS document EP10-T2, NCCLS, Villanova, PA.

National Committee for Clinical Laboratory Standards (1989) Performance goals for the internal quality control of multichannel hematology analysers. Proposed Standard, NCCLS, Villanova, PA, Vol.9, No.9, 621–641.

Nord, E. (1992) An alternative to QALYs: the saved young-life equivalent (SAVE). *Brit. Med. J.*, **305**, 875–877.

Patrick, D. L., Bush, J. W. and Chen, M. M. (1973) Methods for measuring levels of well-being for a health status index. *Health Serv. Res.*, **8**, 229–244.

Robinson, R. (1993) Economic evaluation and health care: What does it mean? *Brit. Med. J.*, **07**, 670–678.

Rowan, R. M. and England, J. M. (1993) Special aspects in haematology. In: Haekel, R. (ed.), *Evaluation Methods in Laboratory Medicine*, Weinheim: VCH. pp.141–151.

Schwartz, W. B., Gorry, G. A. Kessirer, J. P. *et al.* (1975) Decision analysis and clinical judgement. *Am. J. Med.*, **55**, 459–472.

Shewhart, W. A. (1931) *Economic Control of Quality of Manufactured Product*, Toronto: Van Nostrand Co.

Skendzel, L. P., Barnett, R. N. and Platt, R. (1985) Medically useful criteria for analytic performance of laboratory tests. *Am. J. Clin. Pathol.*, **86**, 200–205.

Société Française Biologie Clinique (1986) Expert panel for the validation of methods. Protocol for the validation of methods (document B, stage 3). *Ann. Biol. Clin.*, **44**, 686–745.

Sox, H. C. (1986) Probability theory on the use of diagnostic tests. *Ann. Intern. Med.*, **104**, 60–66.

Sunderman, F. W. Jr (1975) Current concepts of 'normal values', 'reference values' and 'discrimination values' in clinical chemistry. *Clin. Chem.*, **21**, 1973–1877.

Swets, J. A. (1964) Signal detection and recognition by human observers. *Contemporary Readings*. New York: Wiley.

Welcan, U. K. (1993) *Workload Measurement System for Pathology*, Cardiff, UK; Welsh Office.

WHO (1989) Meeting on the assessment of clinical usefulness of laboratory tests. WHO/LAB/89.4.

Wintrobe, M. M. (1981) To measure or not to measure? That too is a question, In: Ross, D. W., Brecher, G. and Bessis, M. (eds), *Automation in Haematology*. Berlin: Springer-Verlag, pp. 3–5.

Youden, W. J. (1950) Index for rating diagnostic tests. *Cancer*, **3**, 32–35.

9

Workload and performance indicators

Laurence P. Skendzel

9.1 Introduction

At a time of rising health care costs, demands for more services, and government intervention, laboratory directors no longer can rely on subjective and somewhat haphazard systems for management. There is significant pressure on laboratories to control costs and at the same time, improve services. Laboratories have become cost centres instead of revenue producers. There is even more at stake. A probable change in the system for financial reimbursement on a per-capita basis (in the USA) will require a better understanding of laboratory productivity. At the same time, questions arise about the quality of laboratory services and the effectiveness of laboratory tests in patient care. In this setting, pathologists and laboratory managers will place greater emphasis on the efficiency of the laboratory as a workplace, the effectiveness of the laboratory in meeting requirements for service and, the efficacy or appropriate use of laboratory tests to produce the intended benefit to the patient.

This is a laudable mission statement but achieving these goals may be extremely difficult. While computerization of the laboratory has improved fiscal control, much remains to be done. Vendors of software for laboratory computers have been slow in developing or expanding their management programs. For most laboratory computer systems, cost accounting programs are not available because they are complex and frequently not adaptable for use in every laboratory. At the present time, studies to evaluate the effectiveness of laboratory service requires time-consuming manipulation of data. While the efficacy of laboratory tests has been studied in pilot programs, the concept of comparing test results with patient outcomes has not had widespread application. In time, the demand from hospitals, physicians and government will stimulate the design and implementation of advanced computer programs to achieve the new goals of laboratory management.

While the task is considerable, some programs are in place to guide laboratory managers in deriving reasonable estimates of labour costs. The majority of laboratories keep track of productivity and data collected nationally permits comparison with peer laboratories. The evaluation of effectiveness and efficacy remains in the early stages of development. This report reviews the current status of laboratory management systems. While literature reports generally consider the entire laboratory operation, the concepts have direct application to the hematology section.

9.2 Measures of laboratory efficiency

9.2.1 Workload indicators

The College of American Pathologists (1992) Workload Recording System is the predominant system for tabulation of labour productivity. Based largely on a program originally designed by the Canadian Association of Pathologists, the CAP published the first edition of a workload recording method in 1970. They released the latest and the last revision in 1992. The Canadian and American groups stayed in close communication and complemented each other's programs.

In an attempt to capture technical, clerical and support services (aide-time), the CAP system defines laboratory functions as 'activities' or 'procedures.' For each activity, the CAP relies on the support of a handful of clinical laboratories to perform cumbersome time studies of technical, clerical and aide functions relating directly to testing. Using these data, each laboratory activity acquires a unit number representing the average minutes of personnel time required for completion. Activities relating to quality control testing, repeat testing, proficiency testing, etc., receive the same unit value assigned to patient specimens. Productivity is the sum of the raw count for each technical, clerical or aide activity multiplied by their unit value. In the CAP system, productivity may be determined for the entire laboratory, its individual sections, or for a specific test.

In the original design, the CAP used total or 'paid' hours of the laboratory staff to define productivity. Over time, the program became more sophisticated and more complicated when the CAP offered the option of describing productivity based on paid hours, worked hours (paid hours minus paid time off), and productivity after subtracting time for education, training and other activities not directly related to testing (non-workload hours). In my experience, productivity expressed in terms of paid hours served as the best indicator for establishing the cost of a test.

For the hematology section, the CAP took on the almost herculean task of measuring unit values for virtually all cell counting instruments. The latest edition of the workload manual lists over thirty instruments which perform automated blood count profiles (hemogram). The time assigned for testing extends over a wide range but the most popular instruments show unit values of approximately three minutes. Coagulation tests represent a second major activity in the hematology section. For the prothrombin and partial thromboplastin time tests, unit values range from 3.0 to 6.5 units. Specific procoagulant factor assays are assigned unit values in the 40–60 minute range. The assignment of workload units for pretransfusion testing illustrates the complexity of the system. For ABO cell, serum and Rh_o (D) typing the unit value of 7.0 minutes per specimen. ABO cell and serum typing only, receive a unit value of 5.0 minutes per specimen. Antibody detection performed as a procedure that is part of the type and screen or in conjunction with a cross-match is assigned a unit value is 7.0 minutes. If the same procedure is applied to processing a large group of specimens at the same time, i.e. screening blood donors, the workload is 20 units/batch.

The British adopted a version of the Canadian workload measurement system under the title of 'Welcan' in 1988, based largely on pilot studies conducted by pathologists in Wales (Bennett, 1991). The Welcan system, like the Canadian and American versions, provides a schedule of unit values by testing procedure to reflect the average technical, clerical and aide time required to perform a laboratory test.

Besides providing a manual of workload units, the CAP offered a subscription program in which laboratories submit their workload data for comparison with other participants. The CAP reported a median productivity over a three-year period of 38–42 units/hour for the hematology section (Figure 9.1). The range of productivity, extending from 10 to 70 unit/hour, illustrates one deficiency with the workload recording system: some laboratories fail to update and monitor the use of units. It is time-consuming and requires almost constant attention to details.

In our laboratory, the CAP workload program provides a reasonable estimate of productivity. All technical activities in the hematology section have CAP workload units. For clerical services not directly related to a specific test, and phlebotomy and glassware cleaning services we calculate workload units and allocate them to each section of the laboratory based on utilization. As an illustration, the collection of blood specimens for hematology section comprise 35% of the services of the phlebotomists and the section is assigned that proportion of workload units. Similar allotments are made for clerical and glassware services. The sum of units for technical and other support services represents the total productivity of the hematology section. Using data from the hospital financial department we calculate the total expense, salary, supply and indirect expenses per workload unit for the hematology section (Table 9.1). The average cost of a test performed in the hematology section over a three-year period ranged from $1.14 to $1.26. For a hemogram with a workload of three units, the cost estimate is $3.42 to $3.78.

The CAP workload system allows us to compare changes in productivity among sections of the laboratory. Tests in hematology require more workload hours than those performed in chemistry and radioisotopes. This information serves as a guide for acquiring new automated instruments and additional computerization of instruments or prompts study of workflow to reduce workload units.

Use of workload systems is not universal. In a 1989 survey of laboratories (Hallam, 1989), only half of respondents measure staff productivity, a striking decrease from a participant rate of 76% in 1984. The larger the hospital, the greater the likelihood of using this system. Reactions to the CAP program were mixed but the majority of laboratories use the computations in budget planning, projecting staffing needs and comparing productivity with peers.

The workload system had its greatest popularity in the 1970s and 1980s. The increasing complexity of the system coupled with the difficulty in updating the workload units has led the CAP to discontinue time studies of instruments and tests. Our experience supports this decision. In a busy clinical laboratory, the task of updating workload files receives low priority. Another contributing factor to loss of popularity is the lack of universal acceptance by hospital administrators. The laboratory setting favoured a unit system that was not adaptable to other hospital services. Comparative data from programs like those of the CAP are of limited value. Some of the histograms displaying the distribution of workload units reported by CAP participants failed to display a distinct mean or median. Participating laboratories apparently have different applications of the workload system. Although the CAP withdrew this service, the Canadian Association of Pathologists in association with the Management Information Service Group of Canada, persevere in the project they originally designed and have released a 1991 update

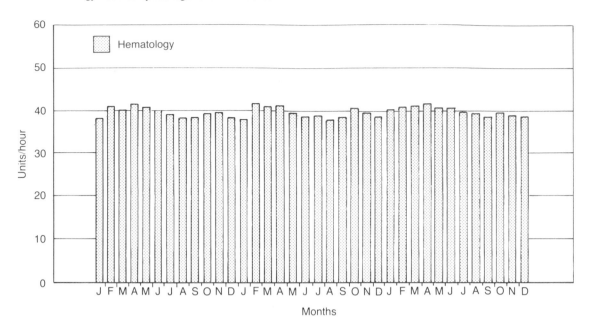

Figure 9.1 Median productivity for the hematology section over a 3-year period (Jan. 1989–Dec. 1991) reported by CAP workload recording method subscription participants

(MIS Group, 1991). The Welcan system is in the early stages of program development and its contribution to laboratory management has not been established (Bennett, 1991). Laboratories which have used workload units effectively (in the USA) will have to rely on their own time studies or refer to data from the Canadian and British programs.

Travers (1989) describes in detail a model for measuring labour productivity. The objective of her program is not only to assign units of activity for the technical portion but to identify each component of the work process. Attention is given to such items as 'preparing the work place', 'scheduling daily laboratory work'. The times required for these processes are tabulated along with time required for the technical procedure. This system gives a laboratory director detailed information on how the staff spends their time. Using a process flow chart, some repetitive

steps may be improved, reassigned or eliminated. The task of 'preparing the work place' may be assigned to an aide, or 'scheduling daily laboratory work' may be standardized and simplified. Although the measurement of each step in the testing sequence, including administrative tasks, is also time-consuming, the laboratory staff gains the advantage of reviewing the entire testing process. Travers includes tabular listing of causes and solutions for low labour productivity in her report.

Several reports describe the application of the workload recording method in the laboratory setting. Kosinski and Klevinski (1990) developed a system that records and calculates workload data with Lotus 1-2-3. Employees from each laboratory department enter their daily test totals on a worksheet and the computerized program converts number of tests into workload units. Updating the system does not require extensive experience with computer programming. If the workload system is used to answer the question of personnel needed for laboratory operation, Maffei (1990) points out to managers the importance of constant attention to maintaining reliable data. Using the Welcan workload measurement system, Tarbit (1990) noted only a moderate correlation between analytic time per test and the direct cost of assay and concluded that the system failed to reflect total resource consumption.

9.2.2 CAP Laboratory Management Index Program for the entire laboratory

In an environment of changing payment and delivery

Table 9.1 Productivity of the Munson Hematology Section over a three-year interval

Indicator	1989	1990	1991
Workload units, total	588,000	653,000	639,967
Workload units/paid hr	27	33	30
Total expense, dollars/workload unit	$1.25	$1.14	$1.26
Salary expense/workload unit	0.50	0.42	0.48
Supply expense/workload unit	0.13	0.15	0.17
Indirect expense/workload unit	0.62	0.57	0.64
Proportion of direct expense			
Salaries	80%	73%	74%
Supplies	20%	27%	26%

PRODUCTIVITY

$$\frac{\text{On-site total billable tests}}{\text{Tech FTE}}$$

$$\frac{\text{On-site total billable tests}}{\text{Total FTE}}$$

$$\frac{\text{Technical FTE}}{\text{Total FTE}}$$

$$\frac{\text{Worked hours}}{\text{Paid hours}}$$

$$\frac{\text{On-site total billable tests}}{\text{Paid hours}}$$

UTILIZATION

$$\frac{\text{Inpatient on-site billable tests}}{\text{Discharge}}$$

$$\frac{\text{Outpatient on-site billable tests}}{\text{Outpatient visit}}$$

COST-EFFECTIVENESS

$$\frac{\text{Nonpatient on-site billable tests}}{\text{On-site total billable tests}}$$

$$\frac{\text{Total expense}}{\text{On-site total billable test}}$$

$$\frac{\text{Total labour expense}}{\text{On-site total billable test}}$$

$$\frac{\text{Total expense}}{\text{Discharge}}$$

$$\frac{\text{Total expense}}{\text{Outpatient visit}}$$

Figure 9.2 Three major indicators to monitor laboratory efficiency and test utilization. (FTE; full-time equivalents)

systems, laboratory managers need a set of critical measures that monitor laboratory efficiency and test utilization. With the prevailing attitude that laboratory organizations are too diverse for any single set of indicators to be applicable for all, laboratory directors have developed individualized management systems but without the benefit of peer comparison.

The CAP, recognizing the importance of a national set of indicators for peer comparison, has assembled a Laboratory Management Index Program (1992).

In the first phase, they set guidelines on how to evaluate the productivity, utilization and financial performance of the entire laboratory. The second phase will define a set of indicators for the sections of the laboratory including hematology. At the time of this report, the peer comparison statistics for the entire laboratory are fairly well established while guidelines for the hematology section are in the testing and evaluation stage.

In a move designed to remove some of the pitfalls of the workload reporting system, the CAP took the time to carefully define each indicator. Billable tests, i.e. those billed to the patient or third party payer, become the cornerstone of the new program. Individual tests or profiles of tests performed on one sample of body fluid with one piece of automated equipment represent one unit. Since multitest profiles arc grouped around the instrument used for assay and require little additional effort, they count the profile as a single billable unit. Quality control, proficiency testing and repeat tests are counted as non-billable tests. For the calculation of management indices, the CAP relies on the number of full-time equivalents, salaries, supply and equipment costs. The program specifies exactly how to calculate depreciation expense.

Three major indicators to monitor laboratory efficiency and test utilization are shown in Figure 9.2. Productivity ratios describe how the laboratory uses its workforce. Employee numbers expressed as full-time equivalents (FTE) and paid hours serve as denominators while the numerators are the total billable tests, number of technical employees and worked hours. Utilization ratios measure how medical staff physicians order laboratory tests. There are two ratios: one measures the number of billable tests per discharge; the other rates the mean number of outpatient billable tests for each outpatient visit. This ratio also gives a measure of the efficacy of laboratory tests. Cost-effectiveness ratios look at the utilization of personnel, consumables and equipment. These ratios provide answers to questions on the relationship of quality control, labour expenses and total expenses to billable tests.

Using data supplied by participants in their program, the CAP provides peer comparison data based on: (1) number of billable tests and (2) the complexity of testing performed by the laboratory. Only fragmentary information is available at this time on the issue of rating laboratories by complexity because the system is in the evolutionary stage. First, participants provides this information on the extent of these services:

A. Complexity of laboratory information system
B. Extent of phlebotomy services
C. Extent of research and development
D. Extent of training programs
E. Use of laboratory courier service

F. Extent of laboratory services to nursing homes, industry, veterinary offices, etc.
G. Agencies/associations inspecting laboratory
H. Ratio of medical technologists to total laboratory staff
I. Extent of testing in blood bank, chemistry, toxicology, hematology, urinalysis
J. Special tests including blood gases, cytogenetics, flow cytometry, stat services.

Then, the CAP assigns a numerical value depending on complexity. The total point count for each participant serves as the basis for classification. Laboratories with a total point score of 0–13 fall in complexity Group I; 13–24 in Group II; 24–45 in Group III; and 45–57 in Group IV.

As an illustration, our laboratory falls in complexity Group IV. The laboratory information system is 'state-of-the-art', laboratory services reach out to extended care facilities and nursing homes, veterinarians and physicians' offices, and complex tests are performed in hematology, chemistry and blood bank including blood gas analyses and stat services.

Table 9.2 Fiftieth percentile productivity ratios for the total laboratory, laboratories classified by complexity of testing.* (CAP Laboratory Management Index Program, Quarterly Report, October–December 1992)

Ratios	Group I	Group II	Group III	Group IV
BT/FTE/Quarter	1747	1598	1681	1446
BT/Technical FTE/Quarter	2565	2578	2747	2505
BT/Paid Hour	3.38	3.00	3.22	2.82
Total labour/BT ($)	3.38	3.92	3.24	3.85
Depreciation Exp/BT ($)	0.32	0.31	0.26	0.37

BT = Billable test.
* Classification based on type of laboratory instrumentation, skill required and extent of testing.

Figure 9.3 Fiftieth percentile utilization ratios for the total laboratory, laboratories classified by complexity of testing.* (CAP Laboratory Management Index Program, Quarterly Report, October–December, 1992)

Ratios	Group I	Group II	Group III	Group IV
Inpatient BT/Day	2.77	3.64	3.50	4.29
Inpatient BT/Discharge	20.36	22.63	26.88	29.35
Inpatient BT/Bed	150.98	217.07	245.44	254.69

BT = Billable test.
* Classification based on type of laboratory instrumentation, skill required, and extent of testing.

Tables 9.2 and 9.3 display productivity and utilization ratios for laboratories participating in the CAP program. An edited summary of one participant's

Table 9.4 Laboratory Management Index Program. Simulated Participants Summary Listing of Derived Indices

Derived index	Your Data 4th quarter	Peer rank, percentage
Productivity comparison		
BT/FTE	1867	69
BT/Technical FTE	4544	91
BT/Paid hourly	3.56	64
Total labour/BT ($)	3.42	—
Depreciation exp/BT ($)	0.17	11
Utilization comparison		
Inpatient BT/Day	3.95	55
Inpatient BT/discharge	22.99	50
Inpatient BT/bed	260.33	41
BT Stat/BT (%)	8.06	11
Cost-effectiveness		
Total expense/discharge ($)	163.77	24
Total expense/patient day ($)	28.13	31
Direct expense/BT ($)	5.66	38
Total expense/BT ($)	7.12	28

BT = Billable test.

performance is shown in Table 9.4. This laboratory shows high productivity of patient tests, a high ratio of tests performed by technologists, a labour force with fewer technologists than laboratories in the peer group. The laboratory is more cost-effective when compared with its peers. Physicians fall into the midrange for utilization of laboratory services although stat requests are infrequent.

9.2.3 Cap Management Index Program for the hematology section

While this phase of the program is in the early stages of development, the CAP generously provided preliminary data for inclusion in this report. The calculation of productivity and utilization ratios of the hematology sections are identical to those used for the entire laboratory. Summary reports shown in Tables 9.5 and 9.6 give an indication of the information provided by this management program. The CAP did not provide reports performance for individual laboratories.

Once laboratory managers become familiar with the information supplied by this program, they can gauge how their laboratory compares with its peers. Using CAP data the productivity ratios for the hematology section indicate higher output when compared with the ratios for the total laboratory. These results appear valid since the complete blood count and coagulation screening tests are now automated and among the most frequently ordered tests. Utilization ratios for hematology show increased use of inpatient billable tests per day. When viewed from the perspective of hematology tests performed during the entire hospital stay (billable tests/discharge) the ratio is lower than utilization for the entire laboratory.

Table 9.5 Fiftieth percentile productivity ratios for the hematology section. Laboratories classified by complexity of testing.* (CAP Laboratory Management Index Program, Pilot Study)

Ratios	Group I	Group II	Group III	Group IV
BT/FTE/quarter	2692	3927	4555	4162
BT/paid hour	4.45	7.68	7.96	7.96
Total labour/BT ($)	2.41	2.36	2.41	3.09
Depreciation exp/BT ($)	0.52	0.29	0.17	0.10

BT = Billable test.
* Classification based on type of laboratory instrumentation, skill required and extent of testing.

Table 9.6 Fiftieth percentile utilization ratios for the total laboratory. Laboratories classified by complexity of testing.* (CAP Laboratory Management Index Program, Pilot Study)

Ratios	Group I	Group II	Group III	Group IV
Inpatient BT/day	3.19	3.62	3.79	5.18
Inpatient BT/discharge	15.61	20.34	23.55	54.47

BT – Billable test.
* Classification based on type of laboratory instrumentation, skill required, and extent of testing.

9.3 Measures of laboratory effectiveness and efficacy

The current focus in management of the hematology section and the entire laboratory centres on programs which extend beyond evaluation of analytical performance. All factors involved in test ordering and utilization come under scrutiny. The term 'quality assurance' describes efforts to evaluate all aspects of laboratory service. Savage (1989) identifies three phases: *process* quality assurance or quality control to ensure that analytical runs have no greater degree of variation than would be expected; *interface* quality assurance dealing with an assessment of laboratory service in collection and handling of specimens and return of test results; and, *outcome* quality assurance to evaluate indicators for ordering clinical laboratory procedures.

While the term 'quality assurance' serves as an overall descriptor of the new management programs, the literature on this topic contains a confusing mixture of poorly-defined phrases including 'performance indicators', 'quality indicators', 'quality care', 'interface/outcome assurance', etc. To avoid further ambiguity, the following definitions are proposed to clarify the intent of these programs:

Effectiveness is the extent that the laboratory meets requirements for service. Patients, physicians, laboratory staff and payers set the guidelines for effectiveness.

Efficacy is the appropriate use of laboratory tests to achieve the intended benefit to the patient. Determining efficacy requires evaluation of patient out-comes.

Current literature reports largely explore measures to improve the effectiveness of laboratory services and only an occasional reference examines the efficacy of tests.

An axiom in management states that, before you can improve, you have to know where you are. For this reason major emphasis (in US laboratories) focuses on establishing indicators of how effectively the laboratory meets requirements. Quality care is defined as meeting the expectations and needs of patients, doctors and payers. The programs used to define quality generally follow the guidelines established by W. Edwards Deming, the American statistician who helped rebuild Japanese industry. First, define the customer. Second, determine what the customer wants. Third, establish indicators to measure the effectiveness of the laboratory in meeting the needs of the customer.

In an informal survey conducted by Statland (1989) clinicians list these requirements: an adequate test menu to meet clinical needs; information about tests; instructions on patient preparation and collection of specimens; analytical procedures with appropriate precision, accuracy, sensitivity and specificity; results reported within an appropriate turn-around time; and a laboratory consultation when needed. Examples of indicators a laboratory may use to measure effectiveness include the incidence of timely reporting of test results, the accuracy of test reports and the incidence of repeat phlebotomy because of improper specimen collection. Collecting data on these aspects of laboratory service is frequently performed manually and consumes much time. More important to success is education of staff in the process of how to define indicators and measure performance.

A recent project in our laboratory illustrates the approach used in a quality assurance program that focuses on effectiveness of service. The first step is to define requirements jointly with the customer or user. In our case, the laboratory staff and physicians jointly established a requirement of reporting prothrombin times and partial thromboplastin time tests to the nursing station by 8.00 a.m. on samples collected in the early morning. The laboratory monitors how the physicians, nurses and laboratory fare in meeting the specified goal. The frequency of success or failure is recorded along with reasons why the system breaks down. When the requirement is not met, the entire process beginning with the ordering of the test by the physician to the return of test results to the nursing station is reviewed. Using measurement data, the group of physicians, nurses and laboratorians identify root causes for failing to meet the requirement. These are illustrations of factors affecting the process: physicians do not write orders legibly or clearly; nurses fail to submit orders to laboratory in a timely fashion; nurses fail to order test; phlebotomists overlook requests; laboratory is short-staffed. After taking steps to improve the system, performance is measured again. This sequence may be repeated until the requirement is met. These quality improvement programs place emphasis on involving all parties (physicians, nurses, laboratory staff) in the process of establishing goals, defining root causes for failure, and interpretation of measurement data. In contrast to other management systems, these programs concentrate on the processes involved in ordering tests, collection of samples, testing and the return of results rather than on the people involved. Communication and collaboration with physicians and nurses receives major attention even though it is a time-consuming process.

For the hematology section, the delivery of laboratory test results has received major attention. In a national survey of physicians and nurses, they expect a turn-around time of approximately two hours, for the CBC, cross-match and prothrombin time tests in a non-emergent setting (Hallam, 1988a,b). The participants in the survey reported a turn-around time in the 1–3 hour range. Measures used by these laboratories to meet the requirements set by clinicians include acquisition of instruments which analyse specimens faster, education of the laboratory staff on how to handle test requests and computerization of test ordering and reporting. Another survey by Steindel and Jones (1991) indicated that the best laboratories have a turn-around time of 22 minutes for hemoglobin assays in an emergent setting.

Studies of the efficacy of laboratory tests are unfolding but remain at an early stage of maturation. The relationship between patient outcome and laboratory test is explored only superficially. In a report by Schifman (1990), his medical and laboratory staffs worked together to set guidelines for appropriate laboratory utilization. In hematology, the maximum number of complete blood counts and platelet counts per hospital patient is twice weekly if the results are within the reference range; the frequency increases to up to twice daily when results are abnormal. Similar guidelines were established for white cell differential count, sedimentation rate and other commonly used coagulation tests. A computerized laboratory data handling system serves to provide feedback swiftly to clinicians when guidelines are exceeded. The program has reduced the demand for laboratory services.

Another laboratory group used the guidelines established by Schifman (1990) to measure the impact of standing orders on laboratory utilization (Studnicki et al., 1992). Prohibition of standing orders resulted in a 55% decrease in test volumes. They conclude that a major cause of excessive laboratory testing is the practice of repetitive ordering by physicians in the absence of a significant change in test values.

A strategy for achieving improvement in laboratory practice that is receiving more attention is *benchmarking* – comparing performance with laboratories who have high marks in quality assurance programs. The CAP, through its Q-Probes programme, gathers data from participants in the subscription program on issues of effectiveness and efficacy and ranks them on how they fare compared with their peers. Performance of the 'best' laboratories becomes the benchmark or goal others may strive to achieve. Emphasis of the program is on measuring the outcomes of specimen collection and transportation, tests interpretation and results reporting (Bachner and Howanitz, 1991).

Two CAP-Q Probes deal with testing in the hematology section. Jones and Meier (1992) reported the results of a study on the acceptability of specimens for complete blood count analysis. In the best laboratories, the rejection rate was 0.12%. The poorest performance occurred when non-laboratory persons collected the specimens. Ten per cent of laboratories reported a rejection rate exceeding 1.25% of specimens up to a maximum of 28%.

A second Q-Probes program studied the utilization of prothrombin time and activated partial thromboplastin time tests (Meier and Reiner, 1990). Opinions were obtained from physicians who indicated that these tests were appropriate in monitoring heparin or warfarin therapy, in evaluating evidence of bleeding and as preoperative tests in patients with specified risk factors relating to bleeding tendencies. Laboratories participating in the program provided information to the CAP on how these tests were used in their hospitals. Only 60% of these tests were associated with appropriate clinical indications. The major reason for inappropriate ordering was the use of tests as additional precautionary measures before a surgical operation.

9.4 Commentary

The replacement of the workload recording system by the management index program will provide laboratory managers with better information on the efficiency of the laboratory as a workplace. One advantage of the new program is the ready availability of data. All hospital accounting departments keep records of the number of billable tests, supply and reagent costs and employee salaries and hours worked. Laboratory departments must maintain some records of non-billable tests but the cumbersome task of maintaining the workload system has been eliminated. Using data from the index program, we were able to develop a comprehensive description of our laboratory compared to peer groups. The ratios pointed out 'weak' areas that required improvement but it also brought to light our strengths. This degree of description was not achieved when the workload system alone was in place. Further refinements in the CAP program will provide insight into the operation of specific sections of the laboratory including hematology.

Pathologists are adapting to a significant change in laboratory practices. The new model for health care delivery emphasizes patient care and meeting the needs of physicians and nurses. Evaluation of analytical performance no longer serves as the sole basis measuring the quality of laboratory service. The 1990s will be characterized as the decade when the efficacy and effectiveness of laboratory services became the leading issue. Why the driving trend toward quality management? One reason is the realization that meeting the needs of patients, physicians and nurses requires laboratory performance that eliminates retesting or rework. Efficiency leads to lower costs. Curiously, a report in 1978 on how physicians use laboratory tests in the clinical setting met with considerable resistance from laboratory managers and some pathologists who regarded analytical performance as the sole measure of quality (Skendzel, 1978). Today, the physician is regarded as the 'customer' and asking questions on test utilization is entirely appropriate. The next step in laboratory management will attend to the issue of the efficacy of laboratory tests. Which tests are appropriate for diagnosis and treatment of specified disorders? What is the frequency of testing? What level of abnormality in test results prompts a clinical decision?

This is an interesting period for clinical laboratories. A spirit of co-operation and collaboration is replacing the traditional barriers that have existed within the health care system (in the USA). The effect of this startling change in direction is not entirely known but it is exciting to be part of an evolution that places more attention on patient care.

Acknowledgements

Patricia Champion, of the College of American Pathologists Central Office, provided information on the Laboratory Information Management Index Program and released data from pilot studies.

Linda DeWitt graciously prepared numerous revisions of the manuscript.

References

Bachner, P. and Howanitz, P. J. (1991) Q-Probes: A tool for enhancing your lab's QA. *Med. Lab. Observer,* **23** (Nov), 37–42.

Bennett, C. H. (1991) Welcan UK: Its development and future. *J. Clin. Pathol.,* **44**, 617–720.

College of American Pathologists (1992) Laboratory Management Index Program, Northfield, ILL: College of American Pathologists

College of American Pathologists (1992) Workload Recording Method and Personnel Management Manual, Northfield, ILL: College of American Pathologists.

Hallam, K. (1988a) Turnaround Time – Part I: Speeding up, but is it fast enough? *Med. Lab. Observer,* **20**, 28–31, 34.

Hallam, K. (1988b) Turnaround Time – Part II: How labs improve their performance. *Med. Lab. Observer,* **20**, 39–41, 44–46.

Hallam, K. (1989) Laboratory Productivity, Part I. Active efforts prevail. *Med. Lab. Observer,* **21**; 22–27.

Jones, B. A. and Meier, F. A. (1992) Q-Probes™ 92–05. *Hematology Specimen Acceptability. Data Analysis and Critique.* Northfield, ILL: College of American Pathologists.

Kosinski, D. S. and Klevinski, C. (1990) Simple workload recording system that your entire staff can use. *Med. Lab. Observer,* **22**, 65–66.

Maffei, L.-M. (1990) New approach to workload recording. *Clin. Lab. Management Rev.,* **4**, 105–108.

Meier, F.A. and Renner, S.W. (1990) Q-Probes™ 90–19A. Coagulation test utilization. Data analysis and critique. Road, Northfield, ILL: College of American Pathologists.

MIS Group (1991) Canada, Mercury Court, 377 Dalhousie Street, Suite 200, Ottawa, Ontario, Canada K1N9N8.

Savage, R.A. (1989) Suggestions for quality assurance routines in the clinical hematology laboratory. *Lab. Med.,* **20**, 556–559.

Schifman, R.B. (1990) Quality assurance objectives in clinical pathology. *Arch. Path. Lab. Med.,* **114**, 1140–1144.

Skendzel, L.P. (1978) How physicians use laboratory tests. *JAMA,* **239**, 1077–1080.

Statland, B.E. (1989) Quality Management: Watchword for the '90's. *Med. Lab. Observer,* **21**, 33–35, 38–40.

Steindel, S.J. and Jones, B. (1991) Q-Probes™ 91–05A. Routine test turnaround time. Data analysis and critique. Northfield, ILL: College of American Pathologists.

Studnicki, J., Bradham, D.D., Marshburn, J. *et al..* (1992) Measuring the impact of standing orders on laboratory utilization. *Lab. Med.* **23**, 24–28.

Tarbit, I.F. (1990) Laboratory costing system based on number and type of test: its association with the Welcan Workload Measurement System. *J. Clin. Pathol.* **43**, 92–97.

Travers, E.M. (1989) Strategies for improving laboratory productivity: in managing costs in clinical laboratories. New York: McGraw-Hill Information Services Inc; pp. 123–129 and 203–219.

10

Blood samples and reagents: hazards and risks

D. A. Kennedy

10.1 Introduction

In many countries official authorities and professional organizations have published codes of safe laboratory practice and while these documents may differ in some technical detail and in degree of emphasis they all appear to be based on the same fundamental principles. Generally, the information is presented as a set of specific instructions and extrapolation to different circumstances is not a straightforward task. Moreover, most of these documents fail to give examples or case studies to support the need for the guidance that is given, despite the fact that it is known that understanding is greatly facilitated by such material.

A laboratory manager who has a thorough knowledge of the hazards of blood, reagents and other substances hazardous to health (SHH) and the management of risks is in a better position to convince sceptical scientific colleagues of the benefits of a change in a working practice or to justify the introduction of a new control measure which they have perceived to be unnecessary and irksome. Similarly, administrative and financial officers are more likely to sanction expenditure in the name of safety if they can be convinced of the benefits to staff and the reduction in civil liability that can accrue. Further-

more, national laws may create certain obligations. Thus, e.g. in the UK, an employer is required to carry out risk assessments and to demonstrate the operation of a safe system of work, whilst in the USA, a bloodborne pathogens exposure control plan or a chemical hygiene plan must be written. It is conjectured that a visiting health and safety inspector, or other law enforcement officer, will have more confidence in the proposals and arguments of a laboratory manager who can demonstrate a real knowledge of the issues in question. The object of this chapter is to provide an introduction to the general principles that need to be understood in order to devise and operate a safety management system for workplaces where blood and other SHH are handled.

First, because the concepts are sometimes confused, it is necessary to distinguish what is meant by the words 'hazard' and 'risk'. For convenience a hazard can be defined as a particular inherent harmful property, e.g. is infectious, toxic or corrosive, while risk is the likelihood of exposure to the harmful property. Currently it is considered that the most significant hazard of working with blood is disease caused by the transmission of a bloodborne virus such as hepatitis B (HBV), hepatitis C (HCV) and the human immunodeficiency virus (HIV). However, there may be other etiological agents present in blood samples (Table 10.1) and blood should always be handled as though there is an inherent risk of transmission of pathogens. Figure 10.1 is a simple general

Micro-organisms [from a blood sample] enter the body
↓
The internal environment permits replication
↓
Phagocytosis is ineffective
↓
Micro-organisms overcome or are not susceptible to the immune system
↓
There is cell and tissue damage

Figure 10.1 Simple general model of the pathogenesis of infectious disease (based on Mims, 1982)

Table 10.1 Bloodborne pathogens that may present an occupational risk of transmission

HAV (NCCLS, 1991)
HBV (NCCLS, 1991)
HCV (NCCLS, 1991)
HIV (NCCLS, 1991)
HTLV I/II (NCCLS, 1991)
Delta hepatitis virus (UK Health Depts, 1990)
Salmonella typhi (Collins, 1993)
Brucella species (Collins, 1993)
Plasmodium falciparum (Collins and Kennedy, 1987)

Table 10.2 Basic information on HBV and HIV

HBV

10^8–10^9 infectious particles/ml of blood
0.04 μl infected blood can cause hepatitis B disease
1 : 1000 people in the UK are carriers
Risk of infection after needlestick with HBV blood is
   6–30%
Survives in dried blood for at least one week
Immunization available

HIV

10^0–10^4 infectious virions/ml of blood
At least 100 μl of blood probably needed to produce HIV
   infection
1 : 2000 people in the UK are carriers
Risk of seroconversion after needlestick with HIV blood is
   0–0.9%
Stable for 'long time' in frozen or lyophilized state
Survives in dried blood for about one week
No immunization available

Based on data from BMA (1990); NCCLS (1991); UK
Health Depts (1990).

**Table 10.3 Portals of entry for substances hazardous to
health**

Respiratory tract, i.e. via nose and mouth breathing
Alimentary system, i.e. ingestion via the mouth
Eye, i.e. via the conjunctiva and cornea
Mucous membranes, e.g. via the lining of the mouth and
   nose
Skin – undamaged skin, and
   – damaged skin, e.g. via cuts and needlesticks with
      contaminated devices and via existing skin lesions

model of the pathogenesis of infectious disease. This
illustrates the fact that the risk of development of
disease amounts to the likelihood of the conjunction
of certain essential factors. Table 10.2 gives some
basic information on HBV and HIV that may be
found useful in risk assessments.

In this chapter, the focus is on the mechanisms
whereby in occupational settings micro-organisms
can enter the body by exploiting unguarded portals
of entry (Table 10.3). In the light of this information,
preventive measures are addressed and some of the
risks that accompany these are considered. In view
of their general importance in occupational hygiene,
special attention is paid to airborne exposure (gases,
vapours and aerosol), percutaneous exposure (e.g.
needlestick, with particular reference to bloodborne
micro-organisms). It is important to appreciate that
micro-organisms share common portals of entry with
other SHH, e.g. chemicals. To illustrate this, sodium
azide is a very toxic chemical that may be used as a
preservative for laboratory reagents and was once
present in reagents in automated blood cell counters.
In small doses it can cause transient headaches, hypo-
tension or nausea. Large doses can be fatal, with no
effective treatment. In the workplace sodium azide

**Table 10.4 Role of the hand in transmission of
contamination**

Hands and fingers frequently injured
Hands become contaminated with workplace materials
External contamination of gloved hand
Contacts*   hand – face in general
            hand – mouth
            hand – eye
            hand – nose
Habits*   nose picking
         nail biting

* These may be involuntary.

can be ingested, inhaled (as the fumes of hydrazoic
acid) or absorbed transcutaneously (Abrams, El-Mallakh and Mayer, 1987). In addition, sodium azide
also forms very unstable compounds with copper
and other metals and explosions have occurred in
laboratory wastepipes that were used to dispose of
cell counter effluent (Kennedy, 1988a).

It is a basic principle of occupational hygiene that
wherever possible safe substitutes should be found
for hazardous substances that are used in the
workplace. Accordingly, manufacturers have found
alternative reagents for blood cell counters. But
where the specimen is hazardous, as may be the case
with blood, this solution is not possible. Thus the
principles that are discussed in the context of
bloodborne pathogens are applicable generally to all
SHH that must be handled in the haematology laboratory.

10.2 Portals of entry for SHH, exposure mechanisms and control measures

10.2.1 Introduction

The portals of entry for SHH, for micro-organisms
as well as chemicals, are listed in Table 10.3. In
addition, it is important to recognize that the hand
may be implicated in the occupational transmission
of SHH as a result of normal human behavioural
traits (Table 10.4); many studies have demonstrated
ubiquitous environmental surface contamination
with materials present in workplaces, including blood
(Table 10.5). A hand that is itself contaminated by

**Table 10.5 Studies demonstrating workplace blood
contamination**

Lauer *et al.* (1979)	clinical laboratories
Holton and Prince (1986)	clinical laboratories
Piazza *et al.* (1987)	dental surgeries
Beaumont (1987)	autopsy suite
Kennedy, Stevens and Horn (1988)	clinical laboratories
Evans, Henderson and Bennett (1990)	clinical and research laboratories

contact with a contaminated surface can in turn transfer SHH as a result of natural unconscious contacts with the nose, eye and mouth. These aspects will be referred to below.

10.2.2 Respiratory system

As breathing is a vital process any substance hazardous to health, including micro-organisms, that can become airborne as a gas, vapour or aerosol cloud can gain a big advantage by exploitation of the respiratory portal of which the alveolar region is the most vulnerable. Toxic gases and vapours may arise in the hematology laboratory and little more needs to be said about these. Bloodborne pathogens would only be a threat to the respiratory portal if the carrier blood does become aerosolized. Deposition in the alveolar region of the lung of fine particles that are present in aerosol clouds is maximal in the range 3–5 μm aerodynamic diameter. Whether fine particles of this order can occur as a result of normal laboratory manipulations of blood has been a much-debated topic. Some people have taken the view that blood is very difficult to aerosolize and some have claimed that whole blood cannot be aerosolized at all. This is discussed below. There is little doubt that toxic chemical liquids can become aerosolized by laboratory manipulations.

Aerosol production

There is, unfortunately, a tendency to use the word 'aerosol' to denote any airborne droplets that arise as a result of handling liquids in the workplace. An aerosol is more correctly defined as a biphasic system in which fine solid or liquid particles, of the order of < 10 μm aerodynamic diameter, are dispersed in a gaseous phase. From the occupational hygiene viewpoint the most important property of very low mass particles is that they settle out very slowly in still air; indeed, for practical purposes they have no motion independent of the gas in which they are suspended. This means that they can easily diffuse or move with local air currents some distance away from the site of production. On the other hand, droplets (sometimes erroneously called aerosols) are much larger particles that have a definite, sometimes visible, trajectory. This means that they are deposited close to the site of production giving rise to surface contamination. Fine airborne particles, if inhaled, can lodge in different parts of the respiratory system, depending upon the aerodynamic diameter, where they can cause infection, irritation or be absorbed if water soluble. Those < 5 μm in diameter are considered to pose the greatest risk to the respiratory system because they can become lodged in the alveolar regions of the lungs where gas exchange takes place.

In order to produce droplets or aerosol particles, energy must be introduced into the starting material to overcome the cohesive forces, e.g. viscous forces in a liquid. The amount of energy that is required is roughly proportional to the new surface that is formed. Production of a water aerosol illustrates the principles involved.

If 1 ml of water is converted into particles with an aerodynamic diameter of:
(1) 5 μm, more than 1.5×10^{10} particles are produced and the surface area is approximately 1.2×10^4 cm².
(2) 2 μm, about 2.4×10^{11} particles are produced and the surface area is 3.0×10^4 cm².
Evaporation from the new surfaces that result from aerosolization is rapid, e.g. the life of a droplet of water 2 μm in diameter is 6×10^{-3} s in dry air at approximately 20 °C. After evaporation of aerosol particles, droplet nuclei composed of the non-volatile residuum (micro-organisms or chemicals) remain suspended in the air.

Aerosols are formed by two events in sequence (Hemeon, 1963):

1. Pulvation: a mechanical or pneumatic process that projects fine particles a high velocity from the coagulated state into the air of the immediate vicinity as individual particles; and
2. Secondary air currents which transport the localized particles away from the site of formation.

The simplest and commonest pulvation mechanisms for liquids are formation of ligaments or sheets from the parent liquid followed by break up of the ligament or sheet to smaller particles. Table 10.6 lists some basic laboratory processes that may result in aerosol production.

Whole blood aerosol

The debate on whether a true aerosol can be produced from whole blood may have been originated by a paper in which it was conjectured that, in the absence of any other definite cause, a cluster of hepatitis B cases in a hemodialysis unit may have been spread by airborne droplets (Almeida *et al.*, 1971). In fact, a number of studies have demonstrated that blood can be aerosolized by laboratory manipulations, probably by either break up of very thin sheets or fine ligaments of blood (Table 10.7). Plasma and serum can also be aerosolized, perhaps

Table 10.6: Some laboratory processes that produce aerosols

Shaking
Pouring
Blowing the last drop from a pipette
Removal of wetted plug and screw caps
Bursting bubbles and films of liquid
Centrifugation
Ultrasonic cell disruption
Vibration of a fine capillary

Table 10.7. Reports of whole blood aerosol

Rutter and Evans (1972)	Microhematocrit centrifuge with leaking tube, microtonometer, removal of blood-wetted plug and screw caps
MRC (1975)	Insertion into and withdrawal of hypodermic needle from rubber tubing, spraying from an unspecified nebulizer, bursting of bubbles
Peterson (1980)	Insertion into and withdrawal of hypodermic needle from rubber tubing
Harper (1981)	Use of blood film spinner

Table 10.8. Risk of airborne infection – factors

Micro-organisms would have to survive:
1. Energy injection needed to produce tiny airborne droplets
2. Rapid drying of droplets leaving suspended micro-organisms
3. Prevailing environmental conditions
4. Entry and transport in the respiratory system
Then, they would have to find a niche from which to establish an infection site

with greater ease than whole blood. Notwithstanding the evidence that a whole blood aerosol has been demonstrated (Table 10.7), the question remains whether at present this amounts to a significant occupational health risk in hematology laboratories. Currently there appears to be a worldwide consensus that HBV and HIV are not transmitted in occupational settings, or in the community, by the aerosol route and that the percutaneous route of transmission (see below) presents the greatest risk. But other micro-organisms, e.g. Brucellae (Table 10.1) may be present in large numbers in blood and these may be transmittable via the respiratory system as well as via the alimentary route and by needlestick. However, virtually no relevant information is available on brucellosis risks in the hematology laboratory. Brucellosis appears to be the commonest laboratory-acquired infection (Collins, 1993) and is reported to have an infectious dose of $< 10^2$ organisms by the respiratory route (Kaufmann *et al.*, 1980). Table 10.8 lists some factors that would have to be considered in assessing the risk of an airborne occupational infection.

10.2.3 Alimentary system

Any substance hazardous to health that is ingested has the potential to be absorbed from any part of the alimentary system from the mouth downwards, although some micro-organisms may not be able to survive a low gastric pH. In the laboratory, three possible exploitation mechanisms can be postulated.

1. Droplets containing SHH coming to rest on the lips followed by ingestion.
2. Transfer of SHH to the mouth *via* the fingers (see Table 10.4) or *via* other contaminated objects.
3. When mouth pipetting, sucking liquid containing SHH into the mouth, followed by the entry of the contaminated liquid into the gastro-intestinal tract.

Mouth-pipetting, along with drinking, eating, smoking and applying cosmetics and the like is universally prohibited in clinical laboratories. In the hematology laboratory use of the traditional sucker would appear to present the greatest risk.

Salmonella typhi which may be present in blood [Table 10.1] is normally transmitted via the alimentary portal. Over 25 years ago, a colleague of the author was infected when handling a blood sample which, unknown to him, contained *Salmonella typhi*. His only known exposure was to carry out a manual hemoglobin determination. It is conjectured that perhaps the mouthpiece of his sucker became contaminated with the blood or, as was common practice at the time, after he had pipetted the blood into ammoniated water, he mixed the contents of the tube by using a finger as a closure and thereafter there was unconscious hand–mouth contact (Table 10.4).

10.2.4 Eye (conjunctiva and cornea)

While in a strict anatomical sense the conjunctiva may be classified as a mucous membrane (see below), it is convenient to consider it separately. The conjunctival membrane covers the outer surface of the white portion of the eye and the inner aspect of the eyelids. Its superficial circulation is such that a suction effect can be observed which may play a part in absorption through the surface (Papp, 1959). An SHH that can find its way into the tears can pass into the nasolacrimal duct and thence enter the nose and can drain into the throat. Unless damaged, the cornea provides an efficient barrier against microbial invasion. On the other hand, non-polar chemicals (i.e. those that are fat soluble) easily penetrate the corneal epithelium. Except for the cornea, the conjunctiva is the portion of the eye that is most exposed to SHH. Local damage to the eye, possibly very serious, can be caused by contact with corrosive chemicals and eye surfaces damaged by microbially-contaminated objects tend to become infected. HBV was experimentally transmitted when the corneal surfaces of a chimpanzee were inoculated with 50 μl of hepatitis B surface antigen [HB$_s$Ag] positive plasma (Bond *et al.*, 1982). Seroconversion occurred when HB$_s$Ag-positive blood was squirted into an eye which was rubbed with a hand (Kew, 1973). Other laboratory-acquired infections, although not blood-borne, have been associated with sprays and droplets hitting the face or eye. Hand-eye contact (Table 10.4) is common. When surreptitious observations were made of two doctors in the course of 30 min, one touched his face 27 times and the other rubbed his eyes 15 times (Collins, 1993). This illustrates the potential for infection *via* the hand–eye route. There is a report of a cluster of eye infections in which the eyepieces of shared industrial microscopes were implicated as vectors (Olcerst, 1987). Here it is possible that conjunctival infections followed contamination of eyelids by contact with contaminated fingers via the eyepieces. Safety spectacles (see below) with toughened glass or plastics lenses, especially when fitted with side shields, and full face visors offer very good protection against droplets, sprays, splashes and missiles containing SHH. Ordinary prescription spectacles which are worn by many laboratory workers to correct visual defects must provide, incidentally, a degree of protection against projected droplets.

10.2.5 Other mucous membranes

Mucous membranes line all those passages by which the internal parts of the body communicate with the outer parts. They are continuous with the skin at the various orifices of the surface of the body and are soft, velvety, are very vascular and are coated with mucus which is of a tenacious consistency. They line both the gastro-pulmonary and genito-urinary tracts and may be classified as belonging to, and continuous with, one or the other of these tracts. HBV has been transmitted experimentally in human volunteers *via* the oral mucosa (Peterson, 1980) and mucous membranes are considered to be sites of entry for HIV [NCCLS, 1991]. It is conjectured that the inner surface of the nose is perhaps the most vulnerable mucous membrane in occupational settings, and can be exploited by SHH present in impacting droplets or on contaminated fingers (see Table 10.4).

10.2.6 Skin

The body surface is covered with skin which has a relatively impermeable dry horny outer layer. Normal undamaged skin is a natural barrier to micro-organisms but can be breached at the site of naturally-occurring breaks in its continuity such as at hair follicles or at the nail fold. Micro-organisms can exploit uncovered skin lesions such as cuts or abrasions and those deposited upon sharp or penetrating surfaces, e.g. needles, blades and broken glass (i.e. 'sharps'), can gain entry when the skin is breached.

Toxic chemicals can undoubtedly penetrate unbroken skin. With increasing lipid solubility and decreasing molecular weight, the absorption of non-polar substances increases through the outer layer of skin, although further transport into blood vessels is promoted by water solubility. Abrasion of the skin increases absorption for both polar and non-polar compounds. In the workplace, some skin contact with chemicals is almost unavoidable. Such percutaneous exposures may not necessarily constitute a risk, but seemingly minimal skin contact can sometimes produce a toxic effect. Percutaneous absorption may be difficult to detect and the effects may not be readily apparent. Thus its significance in the workplace has probably been underestimated. The subject is dealt with comprehensively by Grandjean (1990). Corrosive chemicals used in the hematology laboratory, e.g. strong acids and bases, can cause skin burns.

10.2.6 Needlestick and other 'sharps' injuries

A survey in the USA showed that 25% of all occupational injuries were finger injuries; 10% of these, and ranked first, were lacerations caused by knives. Ranked second, 9.4% of the injuries, were puncture wounds caused by hypodermic needles (CDC, 1983). A review (Collins and Kennedy, 1987) of data from 12 surveys of occupational needlestick injuries, 9 from the USA and 3 from the UK, indicated that nurses are the most at risk, followed by domestic staff who handle waste. The incidence of needlesticks in laboratory workers was 2.4–17.9% of the total reported in the surveys. In 4 surveys the incidence per 100 employees years was 10.8–18.0. Twenty-one types of infection and two malignancies have been ascribed to occupational breaches of the skin (Collins and Kennedy, 1987) but most of these were not associated with blood. It is generally accepted that in laboratories needlestick injuries, where there is transfer of contaminated blood, present the biggest occupational risk of transmission of HBV, HCV and HIV, although other micro-organisms may be present in blood [see Table 10.1]. Phlebotomy must present a significant risk of occupational needlestick injury, e.g. the UK market for phlebotomy needles in 1992 was estimated to be 54 million. In the USA, with a bigger market, it was estimated that in 1990 there would be 800 000 occupational needlesticks (Anon., 1990).

It has been argued (Kletz, 1976) that there is a need to predict accidents before they occur and that by collecting information on human failure rates it is possible to do this so that preventative action can be taken. In order to understand the occurrence of needlestick a systematic approach based on an event tree (Kennedy, 1988b) can be used. Phlebotomy using an evacuated sample collection system is a good model on which to base studies of opportunities for needlestick injuries.

Fig 10.2 illustrates the principles. It has been argued that resheathing needles causes 40% of all occupational needlesticks and therefore needles should not be resheathed before disposal into a

Fit needle to holder

↓

Unsheath needle

↓

Insert needle into vein*

↓

Insert collection tube into holder – draw blood*

↓

Remove collection tube from holder*

↓

Remove needle from vein*

↓

Re-sheath needle*

↓

Remove re-sheathed needle from holder* [re-use holder]

↓

Dispose of sheathed needle into sharps box*

↓

Handle/dispose of sharps box*

* represents an opportunity for blood-contaminated needlestick

Figure 10.2 Phlebotomy with evacuated blood collection system

sharps container. On the other hand, there is evidence that hospital cleaning and portering staff are at risk from needlestick which may indicate improper disposal of unsheathed needles. In turn, this argument is used to justify a policy of resheathing needles before disposal. Development and study of an event tree such as is illustrated by Fig. 10.2 can provide a simple and easily understood model of what is actually happening in practice. In the light of accident statistics this can enable identification of areas which require the manager's particular attention. Furthermore, the approach can be very helpful in a cost-benefit analysis when considering the introduction of 'safety needles', safe resheathing devices or other engineering control measures (Anon., 1991).

Phlebotomy needles are not the only sharps found in the hematology laboratory. Table 10.9 lists some sharps, other than needles, that were noted in a survey of the causes of skin injuries in a large hematology laboratory carried out by the author.

10.2.7 Sharps risks to patients

During nuclear medicine procedures, one patient was inadvertently injected with fresh whole blood from an HIV-infected patient after a used syringe containing the blood was mistaken for another syringe containing red cells labelled with a radionuclide. In a similar case there was inadvertent injection of radio-nuclide labelled white cells taken from an HIV-infected patient. In a third case, there was re-use of a

syringe resulting in injection of residual blood from an HIV-infected patient.

These cases have been reviewed by the Center for Disease Control (CDC, 1992). In another case, in Canada, a patient with no apparent risk factors developed *Plasmodium falciparum* malaria in circumstances which indicated possible re-use of an evacuated blood collection system needle (Varma, 1982). Given the very large number of phlebotomy needles that must be used worldwide *per annum*, perhaps these cases indicate the tip of an iceberg. A cluster of hepatitis B cases was associated with a spring-loaded finger stick device that was used for capillary blood sampling. A subsequent investigation indicated that the platform of this device which was intended for single use only was not routinely changed after each use. This suggested that contamination of the platform by HBV-infected blood was the mechanism of percutaneous transmission of HBV (Polish *et al.*, 1992). Clearly the hematology laboratory manager who is responsible for a blood collection or a diagnostic radionuclide service must exercise the greatest care to prevent re-use of blood-contaminated needles and other single use devices.

10.3 Limitations and inherent hazards of control measures

Control measures may have limitations and some may have inherent hazards, the risk assessments of which should always be taken into account.

10.3.1 Fume cupboards safety cabinets

Fume cupboards (fume hoods) should be used to contain work which presents a risk of exposure to toxic gas or vapour. These are described in detail by

Table 10.9 Sharps causing hand and finger injuries

Component of blood cell counter
Centrifuge
Stapling machine
Scalpel

Glass fragment
Glass slide – unbroken
Glass slide – broken
Glass pasteur pipette
Plastic pasteur pipette
Glass test tube
Glass capillary tube

Edge of locker
Autoclave tin
Inside of sharps container
Metal sealing ring of vial
Metal tube rack
Edge of seat
Paper in office

Stricoff and Walters (1990). Where very toxic substances have to be handled, it is necessary to use a
glove box containment system in which the material
being worked on is separated from the worker by
means of a full physical barrier which includes glove
ports. Microbiological safety cabinets are designed
to capture and retain infected airborne particles released in the course of certain manipulations and to
protect the laboratory worker from infection which
may arise from inhalation (Collins, 1993). Class I-
type cabinets are open fronted and offer a degree of
protection to the user. Class 2-type cabinets, also
open fronted, offer a degree of protection to the
worker and to the material being handled which
is bathed in a stream of HEPA-filtered air. The
highest level of containment is afforded by Class 3-
type cabinets which are similar in design to glove
boxes. Containment systems require proper management to ensure that efficient protection is afforded at
all times. The recently updated British Standard BS
5726 illustrates the preferred management approach
(Table 10.10).

It should be borne in mind that work may involve
exposures to substances hazardous to health (SHH)
via other portals of entry as well as the respiratory

**Table 10.10. Factors in the management of containment
systems**

Choice of system with regard to limitations (Table 10.11)
Specification of proper design, construction and
    performance prior to installation (BSI, 1992a)
Information to be exchanged between purchaser, vendor
    and installer and proper installation (BSI, 1992b)
Demonstration of required performance after installation
    (BSI, 1992c)
Proper use and maintenance (BSI, 1992d)

Table 10.11. Protection afforded by containment systems

Portal	Enclosure	
	Open-fronted	Full physical barrier
Respiratory	yes	yes
Alimentary	no[1]	yes
Eye	possible[2]	yes
Undamaged skin	no	possible[3]
Damaged skin	no	no[4]
Mucous membrane	possible[5]	yes
Hand contacts (see above)	no[6]	yes

Notes
1. Mouth pipetting possible (see above).
2. Partial barrier – droplets in eye possible (see above).
3. Chemical may diffuse through glove material (see
   below).
4. Possible for needlestick following penetration of glove.
5. Partial barrier – droplets in nose possible (see above).
6. Partial barrier – hand contamination possible (see
   above).

portal (see above). In the light of this, Table 10.11
outlines the limitations of the open fronted and full
barrier type of containment systems. It should be
noted that while barrier-type containment systems
offer the best protection of all, the thick rubber
gloves that are integral features of glove boxes and
Class 3 microbiological safety cabinets cannot protect against needlestick and may allow diffusion of
some chemicals (see below).

In addition, containment systems may expose users
to the risk of electric shock, fire, explosion, traumatic
injuries from falling sashes, cuts from sharp metal
edges, glass viewing panels that may shatter spontaneously and eye injuries caused by exposure to ultraviolet light (Kennedy, 1988a).

10.3.2 Gloves

Some people who wear gloves for phlebotomy may
complain of a loss of tactile sensitivity with subsequent increase of needlestick risk. This may be
averted by training (NCCLS, 1991). In use, the protection offered by disposable rubber gloves may be
reduced as a result of 'pin-holes' and even thick
rubber gloves offer no significant protection against
needlesticks. Chemicals may diffuse through glove
materials and inside gloves the increased temperature
and vapour pressure, sweating and softening of the
epidermis provide the most favourable conditions
for absorption of toxic chemicals. Accordingly,
gloves need careful selection with regard to the materials being handled. The increase in wearing of gloves
by health care workers has demonstrated the prevalence of latex allergy. A survey carried out in the US
Army Dental Corps demonstrated that approximately 9% of dentists were affected by latex allergy
(Berky, Luciano and James, 1992). Fortunately, hy-
poallergenic materials are available (Hamann, 1993).
Importantly, it should be borne in mind that while
gloves may protect a laboratory worker's hands
against contamination, if worn thereafter they may
transmit contamination to surfaces including computer keyboards, telephones and door handles (Beaumont, 1987) and can thereby present a risk to unsus-
pecting workers not wearing gloves. Phlebotomists
should always change gloves between patients
(NCCLS, 1991). Disposable gloves must never be
washed and re-used.

10.3.3 Safety spectacles

Common-use items may be vectors of infection (Olcerst, 1987) and if eye protection is to be shared
there should be a system of cleaning and disinfection
before re-issue to another member of staff. Single-
person-use eye protectors are preferable and some
workers will require prescription spectacles. It should
be remembered that short-sighted staff may remove
spectacles for close-up work and for microscopy

while long-sighted staff will wear spectacles only for close-up work. Hence in both cases, staff will lose the benefit of eye protection unless plain lens spectacles are also provided. A solution to this problem is to provide varifocal lens protective spectacles but this will increase costs. Other important factors are that prescriptions change and that fashions change. Both of these will militate against the continued wearing of eye protection. The provision of eye protection requires careful management and a budget sufficient to fund necessary changes of spectacles in the interest of safety.

10.4 Universal precautions

This is an approach to health care workplace infection control in which, because it is impossible to know the potential for infectivity in every case, *all* human blood and certain other body fluids are treated as if they are known to be infectious for HBV, HIV and other pathogens. In the USA, adoption of this approach is a requirement of the Occupational Safety and Health Administration's [OSHA] Bloodborne Pathogens Standard (OSHA, 1991). Similar practices are recommended by the World Health Organization and by the Department of Health in the UK. Universal precautions have replaced the earlier practice of adopting special precautions, i.e. extra precautions, where there was evidence or suspicion that HBV, HIV and other bloodborne pathogens presented a risk of infection. Table 10.12 summarizes universal precautions in the context of the hematology laboratory. It is not exhaustive and is based on the requirements of OSHA and guidance from other official bodies. With reference to the model of the pathogenesis of infectious disease (Figure 10.1), the object is, in the light of general agreement on cost-benefits, to minimize opportunities for exploitation of portals of entry by bloodborne pathogens, to provide immunization against HBV, and to be prepared with prophylaxis for accidental exposures, e.g. following needlestick. While the contamination control and sharps management measures are likely to provide a high degree of protection against transmission of blood-

Table 10.12 Universal precautions in the hematology laboratory

Control of contamination

Require handwashing after exposures, after removing gloves and before leaving the laboratory.

Prohibit eating, drinking, smoking, application of cosmetics and lip balm, handling of contact lenses and storage of food and drink.

Use robust and leakproof sample containers and centrifuge in sealed buckets if the patient is known to be a carrier of HBV, HCV or HIV.

Laboratory work – require wearing of gloves, eye protection and face shields where there is a risk of direct contact with splashes, spray, spatter or droplets of blood or blood-contaminated surfaces.

Phlebotomy – do not discourage the routine wearing of gloves; require that they be worn when a patient is known to be a carrier of HBV, HCV or HIV, when a member of staff has cuts, scratches or other breaks in the skin, when there is an extra risk of blood contamination, e.g. an un-cooperative patient, and when the member of staff is receiving training.

Require that all splashes and spills be dealt with immediately and the area be decontaminated.

Require regular cleaning and decontamination of all environmental surfaces and all devices after use.

Sharps

Provide training in safe use and disposal.

Require that a syringe and needle should never be used as a pipetting device and avoid the use of sharp objects or glass wherever possible.

Require that contaminated needles and other sharps should never be bent, recapped, or removed unless there is no other option.

If contaminated sharps must be handled, it must be by mechanical means or a one-handed technique which minimizes the risk of injury.

Provide, as close to the site of use as possible; adequate puncture-resistant, leakproof and adequately-labelled sharps disposal containers, institute measures to ensure that they are not overfilled, and require their safe use and disposal.

Immunization

Offer and make arrangements for hepatitis B immunization and follow-up.

Offer and arrange for other appropriate immunization, where available, and follow-up.

First aid provisions

Make arrangements for immediate cleaning and dressing of cuts and other skin lesions.

When there is a risk of a transmission of HBV, ensure that trained staff are available to administer combined active immunization and passive immunization with hepatitis B immunoglobulin and to provide follow-up.

When there is a risk of transmission of HIV, ensure that medical or other trained staff are available to provide counselling and to administer AZT prophylaxis if considered necessary.

Where there is a risk of transmission of other pathogens, medical or other trained staff should be available to administer appropriate prophylaxis or therapy.

borne pathogens, they should be seen as the basic requirements for routine hematology laboratory work that may have to be supplemented, e.g. by use of a microbiological safety cabinet to carry out manipulations known to produce droplets and aerosol, in situations where there is a special risk. At present, a vaccine for HBV, together with hepatitis B immunoglobulin, is the only immunological protection that is routinely given and there is no vaccine for HIV infection. While AZT can be given prophylactically following accidental exposure to HIV, there are doubts about its effectiveness (Lange *et al.*, 1990). It is considered that the best management approach is to put maximum effort into maintaining at a high level the measures designed to prevent transmission of bloodborne and other pathogens. In should be borne in mind that where effective immunization, prophylaxis or therapy is available for other pathogens that are likely to be encountered as a result of exposure to blood, provision of these should be considered. It is recommended that the adoption of universal precautions, without supplementary control measures, should always be supported by a detailed and fully-documented risk assessment. Risk assessments should always take into account limitations and inherent hazards of control measures that are proposed.

10.5 Conclusions

It is generally accepted that human life can never be entirely free of risk and it follows that however well equipped and well managed a hematology laboratory may be, there will always be a residual occupational risk of transmission of SHH and in particular pathogenic micro-organisms present in blood.

'Know your enemy' is a good maxim and the laboratory manager is advised to adopt an anthropomorphic approach in which an attempt should be made to imagine, with regard to the local circumstances, what an SSH would have to do in order to enter the body. The words 'exploit' and 'exploitation' are usually used with reference to opportunistic humans rather than micro-organisms or chemicals; their use in the context of this chapter is an illustration of the above approach. A laboratory manager who is prepared to think like this should be in an excellent strategic position to keep SHH fully under control.

The opinions expressed above are those of the author and do not necessarily reflect those of the UK Department of Health.

References

Abrams, J., El-Mallakh, R.S. and Mayer, R. (1987) Suicidal sodium azide ingestion, *Ann. of Emerg. Med.*, **16**, 1378–1380.

Almeida, J.D., Chisholm, G.D., Kulatilake, A.E. *et al.* (1971) Possible airborne spread of serum-hepatitis virus within a haemodialysis unit. *Lancet*, **2**, 849–850.

Anon. (1990) *AIDS Newsletter*, 5(10), 14.

Anon. (1991) Special report and product review. Needlestick-prevention devices. *Health Devices*, **20**, 154–180.

Beaumont, L. R. (1987) The detection of blood on non-porous environmental surfaces: an approach for assessing factors contributing to the risk of occupational exposure to blood in the autopsy suite. *Infection Control*, **8**, 424–426.

Berky, S. T., Luciano, W. J. and James, W. D. (1992) Latex glove allergy: a survey of the US Army Dental Corps. *JAMA*, **268**, 2695–2697.

Bond, W. W. *et al.* (1982) Transmission of type B viral hepatitis via eye inoculation of a chimpanzee. *J. Clin. Microbiol.*, **15**, 533–534.

British Medical Association (BMA) (1990) A code of practice for the safe use and disposal of sharps. London: British Medical Association.

British Standards Institution (BSI), (1992a) BS 5726: Part 1, Microbiological safety cabinets; Part 1, Specification for design, construction and performance prior to installation. London: British Standards Institution.

British Standards Institution (1992b) BS 5726: Part 2, Microbiological safety cabinets; Part 2, Recommendations for information to be exchanged between purchaser, vendor and installer and recommendations for installation. London: British Standards Institution.

British Standards Institution (1992c) BS 5726: Part 3, Microbiological safety cabinets; Part 3, Specification for performance after installation. London: British Standards Institution.

British Standards Institution (1992d) BS 5726: Part 4, Microbiological safety cabinets; Part 4, Recommendations for selection, use and maintenance. London: British Standards Institution.

Centers for Disease Control (CDC) (1983), Current trends in occupational finger injuries – United States. *Morbidity and Mortality Weekly Report*, **32**, 589–591.

CDC (1992) Patient exposures to HIV during nuclear medicine procedures. *Morbidity and Mortality Weekly Report*, **41**, 575–578.

Collins, C. H. (1993) *Laboratory Acquired Infections*, 3rd edn. London: Butterworths.

Collins, C. H. and Kennedy, D. A. (1987) Microbiological hazards of occupational needlestick and 'sharps' injuries. *J. Appl. Bacteriol.*, **62**, 385–402.

Evans, M. R., Henderson, D. K. and Bennett, J. E. (1990) Potential for exposure to biohazardous agents found in blood. *Am. J. Publ. Health*, **80**, 423–427.

Grandjean, P. (1990) *Skin Penetration: Hazardous Chemicals at work*, London: Taylor and Francis.

Hamann, C. (1993) Alternatives to health care workers with latex glove allergies. *JAMA*, **269**, 2368.

Harper, G. J. (1981) Contamination of the environment by special purpose centrifuges used in clinical laboratories. *J. Clin. Pathol.*, **34**, 1114–1123.

Hemeon, W. C. L. (1963) *Plant and Process Ventilation*, 2nd edn, New York: The Industrial Press.

Holton, J. and Prince, M. (1986) Blood contamination

during venepuncture and laboratory manipulation of specimen tubes. *J. Hosp. Infect.*, **8**, 178–183.

Kaufman, A. F., Fox, M. D., Boyce, J. M. *et al.* (1980) Airborne spread of brucellosis, *Ann. NY Acad. Sci.*, **353**, 105–114.

Kennedy, D. A. (1988a) Equipment-related hazards. In: Collins, C. H. (ed.) *Safety in Clinical and Biomedical Laboratories*, Ch. 2, C. H., London: Chapman and Hall Medical, pp. 11–46.

Kennedy, D. A. (1988b) Needlestick injuries: mechanisms and control. *J. Hosp. Infect.*, **12**, 315–322.

Kennedy, D. A., Stevens, J. F. and Horn, A. N. (1988) Clinical laboratory environmental contamination: use of a fluorescence/bacterial tracer. *J. Clin. Pathol.*, **41**, 1229–1232.

Kew, M. C. (1973) Possible transmission of serum (Australian antigen positive) hepatitis via the conjunctiva. *Infect. Immuni.*, **7**[5], 823–824.

Kletz, T. A. (1976) Accident data – the need for a new look at the sort of data are collected and analysed. *J. Occup. Acc.*, **1**, 95–105.

Lange, J. M. A., Boucher, C. A. B., Hollak, C. E. M. *et al.* (1990) Failure of zidovudine prophylaxis after accidental exposure to HIV-1. *N. Engl. J. Med.*, **19**, 1375–1377.

Lauer, J. L., Van Drunen, N. A. and Washburn, J. W. (1979) Transmission of hepatitis B surface antigen in clinical laboratory areas. *J. Infect. Dis.*, **140**, 513–514.

Medical Research Council (MRC) (1975) Experimental studies on environmental contamination with infected blood during haemodialysis. *J. Hyg. Camb.*, **74**, 133–148.

Mims, C. A. (1982) *The Pathogenesis of Infectious Disease*, 2nd edn, London: Academic Press.

National Committee for Clinical Laboratory Standards (NCCLS) (1991) Protection of laboratory workers from infectious disease transmitted by blood, body fluids and tissue. 2nd edn. NCCLS Document M29–T2, Vol. 11, No. 14, Villanova: NCCLS.

Occupational Safety and Hygiene Administration (OSHA), (1991) Bloodborne Pathogens Standard, *Federal Register*, **56** (235), 64175–64182.

Olcerst, R. B. (1987) Microscopes and ocular infections. *Am. Indust. Hyg. Assoc. J.*, **48**, 423–431.

Papp, K. (1959) The eye as a portal of entry of infections, *Bull. Hyg.*, **34**[10], 969–971.

Peterson, N. J. (1980) An assessment of the airborne route in hepatitis B transmission. *Ann. NY Acad. Sci.*, **353**, 157–166.

Piazza, M., Guadagnino, V., Piccotto, L. *et al.* (1987) Contamination by hepatitis B antigen in dental surgeries. *Br. Med. J.*, **295**, 473–474.

Polish, L. B., Shapiro, C. N., Bauer, F. *et al.* (1992) Nosocomial transmission of hepatitis B virus associated with the use of a spring-loaded finger-stick device, *N. Eng. J. Med.*, **236**, 721–725.

Rutter, D. A. and Evans, G. G. T. (1972) Aerosol hazards from clinical laboratory apparatus, *Bri. Med. J.*, **1**, 594–596.

Stricoff, S. R. and Walters, D. B. (1990) *Laboratory Health and Safety Handbook*, New York: Wiley Interscience.

UK Health Departments (1990) Guidance for clinical health care workers: Protection against infection with HIV and hepatitis viruses, London: HMSO.

Varma, A. J. (1982) Malaria acquired by accidental inoculation, *Can. Med. Assoc. J.*, **126**, 1419–1420.

Further reading

Advisory Committee on Dangerous Pathogens (1990) *Categorisation of pathogens according to hazard and categories of containment*, 2nd edn, London: HMSO.

Advisory Committee on Dangerous Pathogens (1990) *HIV – The Causative Agent of AIDS and Related Conditions*, 2nd revision of Guidelines, London: Department of Health.

Center for Disease Control (1984) *Biosafety in Bio-Medical Laboratories*, Washington, U.S. Government Printing Office.

Health Services Advisory Committee (1985) *Safety in Health Services Laboratories: Hepatitis B*. London: HMSO.

Health Services Advisory Committee (1991) *Safe Working and the Prevention of Infection in Clinical Laboratories*. London: HMSO.

Luxon, S. G. (ed.) (1992) *Hazards in the Chemical Laboratory*. London: Royal Society of Chemistry.

Working Group of the Royal College of Pathologists (1992) *HIV infection: Hazards of Transmission to Patients and Health Care Workers during Invasive Procedures*. London: Royal College of Pathologists.

World Health Organization (1991) *Biosafety Guidelines for Diagnostic and Research Laboratories Working with HIV*. Geneva: World Health Organization.

World Health Organizational (1993) *Laboratory Biosafety Manual*. Geneva: World Health Organization.

Laboratory liability and risk management

Mark D. Koepke and Willard E. Boyd III

11.1 Introduction

The hematology laboratory actually produces two kinds of outputs – quantitative data and qualitative information. For quantitative data the laboratory relies to a great degree upon the manufacturers of the instrument, reagents, controls and kits, all of which are necessary for the production of the data, but the laboratory personnel are responsible for procedures that may develop any problems with these several factors. Technologist errors of omission as well as commission are examples of quantitative errors. Therefore the laboratory, at least to some degree, has a shared responsibility for the accuracy of its data.

But another aspect of liability – that associated with the production of qualitative information – probably poses a greater liability risk to the laboratory. Examples in the hematology laboratory include the interpretation of blood film morphology with differential counts, bone marrows and other tests that depend upon the expertise and experience of the technologists and clinical pathologists or hematologists. Errors of this type are more often thought to be the responsibility of the clinical pathologist or hematologist, even though he/she may only supervise the operation. A recent article (Somrak, 1992) reviews testing liabilities in cytopathology which in several ways are similar to qualitative hematology laboratory testing.

11.2 The modern laboratory – changes in structure and function

Hospital laboratories are frequently organized with two distinctly different groups of individuals. Technologists are hospital employees who take at least part of their direction from a second group, the clinical pathologists and medically-qualified hematologists. In many instances clinical pathologists and hematologists consider themselves independent practitioners who 'consult' in the laboratory on a fee-for-service basis. Alternatively, there is a growing trend in the USA and common practice in the UK for the pathologist to be salaried hospital employees. A detailed description of the various relationships of pathologists with hospitals can be found in a recently published manual (College of American Pathologists, 1993). Suffice it to say that the structure of a modern laboratory is highly variable and in a state of flux in this period of health service reform.

In addition to the structural changes occurring in the modern laboratory, it is apparent that the function of the laboratory has been changing rapidly. This is clearly illustrated in the increasing prominence of point-of-care testing in America today. It is now increasingly viewed that the laboratory in a hospital is responsible for a whole host of laboratory studies wherever they are done in the institution.

For example, in hematology, several hand-held devices are now being marketed that perform hematology tests. While earlier devices for the estimation of hemoglobin/hematocrit employed the concept of whole blood conductivity and a calculation of the hematocrit, significant problems were noted when such devices were used with 'sick' patients. This problem was undoubtedly due to deviations from normal in electrolyte and protein concentrations of the plasma. Newer devices concurrently measure electrolyte concentrations (e.g. plasma sodium) and appropriate corrections are automatically made. Hand-held hemoglobinometers have been used for a number of years and their performance is comparable to central laboratory measurements. Finally, devices to measure the prothrombin time and even the partial thromboplastin time are now available; initial evaluations have shown these to be quite acceptable in terms of reliability.

The measurements done by non-laboratory personnel present an increased risk for the laboratory. Since the laboratory service often is responsible for all laboratory testing, in-house evaluation of such devices is required to ensure their comparability of the tests results with the standard laboratory methods. In addition, quality control procedures must be in place and continually monitored in order to ensure continuing acceptability of these studies. These aspects are discussed in greater detail in Chapter 5 (see also Chapter 1).

Acceptable point-of-care testing is best provided if it is directly controlled by the laboratory service and included in its quality control/quality assurance network. In this way, studies done in the central laboratory and the outlying areas can be harmonized, thus avoiding potential confusion for the clinicians as they interpret the laboratory results.

11.3 Risk management and standards of care

Given the dynamic state of hospital laboratories, the risk management process to identify risks before they become liabilities is essential for all areas of the organization. In the laboratory, the personnel from director to phlebotomist all have a responsibility to identify and analyse potential problem areas. These discussions usually result in the initiation of educational programmes including the implementation of preventive measures by which it is hoped to avoid any difficulties. But laboratory practice, even under the best of circumstances, may still result in untoward effects on patient care. Therefore, liability insurance is the final requirement in the management of risk (Cooney, 1992).

With the increasing realization of the liabilities of the laboratory (as well as most other segments of the health care industry) most health care providers have established formal or informal risk management/ quality assurance programmes. A primary component of such programme is the determination of and adherence to the so-called standards of care. In the past these standards were implied, and at times argued in court. More recently, they have been codified in federal as well as state and local regulations (Foster, 1990).

In 1988, the United States Congress enacted and President Reagan signed into law, the Clinical Laboratory Improvement Amendments of 1988 (CLIA '88) which, when fully implemented, subject all clinical laboratories operating in the USA to these regulations. The Health Care Financing Administration (HCFA), the federal agency responsible for the regulatory process, has issued regulations governing personnel, quality control, proficiency testing and other aspects of quality assurance (Federal Register, 1993).

Finally, the different states in the USA and many other countries have regulations for clinical laboratories through regulatory programmes that have varying standards depending upon the laboratory's location, e.g. hospital, independent or physician's office

(Foster, 1990). Chapter 20 provides an insight into these requirements.

As noted above, such items as personnel requirements and their relationship to the complexity of the various tests, quality control and quality assurance programmes as well as proficiency testing requirements have all been included in these voluminous regulations. Although the federal regulations more or less restate practice guidelines that laboratories were following for years, the amendments extend the authority of the government into the many thousands of physicians' office laboratories that previously were unregulated. As a result many American laboratories have been busy preparing for these changes.

11.4 Laboratory cases with medicolegal aspects

Several short case studies outlined in the following paragraphs help illustrate the types of liabilities to which laboratories are continually subjected. The rules of law that may pertain are outlined and methods to avoid the problems are discussed. While the arguments presented in this section are pertinent to American law, they are also of interest to laboratory workers in other countries where similar situations are equally likely to occur. Table 11.1 defines a number of the legal terms that are found in these hypothetical cases.

Cross-match specimen for emergency transfusion (Case Study 1)

One day a specimen for an emergency cross-match was received in the transfusion service. It was identified with the patient's first initial and last name, hospital ID number and date. Two units of blood were set up for this pediatric patient who was scheduled to go to surgery for an emergency procedure. A short time later, the operating room technician came to the transfusion service requesting a unit of blood for a patient with the 'same' name, this time with a full first name. Since the transfusion service technologist had just completed the cross-match on the patient with this name, and knowing that the patient was scheduled for surgery, he issued the unit. All of the required checks were not done since this was an emergency even though specimen identification procedures are a standard of laboratory practice.

What had happened was there were actually two patients with the same last name and first initial. One was an adult (Type O) who had been in the operating room for some time and the other was a pediatric patient (Type A) who was still on the pediatric unit. The transfusion service employee mistakenly assumed that the pediatric patient had gone to surgery and needed the blood. An acute hemolytic

Table 11.1 Definitions of relevant legal terms

Borrowed Servant Rule: The doctrine holds that where an employee is directed or connected by his employer to perform services for another, the employer is not responsible legally for the employee's conduct while performing such services

Breach of Duty: The failure to discharge a duty to the appropriate legal standard

Direct Duty: The doctrine which imposes a non-delegable duty of care on the hospital that is owed directly the patient. Under this duty the hospital is required to discharge certain duties for the patient. This direct duty is distinct from vicarious liability and exists concurrently with the duties owed by members of the hospital's staff

Standard of Care: The standard to which a duty of care must be discharged. This is determined by reference to professional standards though the final determinant rests with the court

Negligence: This is a term of art which has at least two distinct meanings. One meaning refers to the tort of negligence. The second meaning refers to the lack of care giving rise to a breach of duty which is part of the tort of negligence

Res Ipsa Loquitur: Latin for 'the thing speaks for itself'. A rule of evidence which applies when the situation was within the control of the defendant and the occurrence of the accident would be highly unusual in the absence of negligence on the part of the defendant

Tort: A civil wrong giving rise to an action for damages. The principal tort in the context of medical malpractice is that of negligence though trespass may also be relevant. In order for a plaintiff to succeed in the tort of negligence five elements must be proven:
1. The existence of a duty of care,
2. The breach of the duty of care (i.e. negligence),
3. The plaintiff suffered an injury,
4. Causation, i.e. that the injury sustained by the plaintiff caused by the breach of duty of the defendant,
5. The loss or injury is of a type giving rise to damages which are recoverable in law.

Vicarious liability: The doctrine which imposes liability upon a master for the tortious acts of his servant which are committed in the course of his employment. The master is not liable for the acts of the servant which are unauthorized and which are carried out 'on a frolic of his own'

transfusion reaction occurred and the patient subsequently died.

This is a case referred to in legal parlance as *res ipsa loquitur*, i.e. the case speaks for itself, because it is obvious to a layman that the wrong blood was issued and the patient died as a result. Indeed, in cases where the occurrence of the event are highly unusual in the absence of negligence and the occurrence of the events are within the sole control of the defendant then negligence is readily inferred by applying this doctrine. The courts have established a major exception to the requirement that all five elements of a negligent tort (see Table 11.1) must be proven for a party to prevail in a negligence claim. Therefore, it can be quite easy for an attorney to convince a jury that there was an actionable tort, or wrong, done to the patient in the operating room. Indeed, since these cases are thought to be so obvious that they almost always lead to a jury verdict in favour of the plaintiff.

Risk management techniques to avoid such problems include the use of sophisticated, fail-safe systems for patient and specimen identification as well as fool-proof methods for the issuing of blood from the transfusion service. The larger and more complex the institution, the greater is the problem. Fortunately, laboratory and hospital information systems are being developed to prevent such tragedies as far as possible. However, the cost for a truly adequate information system is considerable.

A case of mistaken identity (Case Study 2)

A middle-aged woman went to an emergency room

of a hospital complaining of severe neck pain and headache as well as a fever. The physician who examined her ordered a number of laboratory tests including a blood count. The band cell count was reported to be abnormally high, i.e. '24%; normal 0–3%'. Pain medication was prescribed and the patient was sent home.

On the following day, the patient returned complaining of the same but even more severe symptoms. Again a blood count was ordered. This time the 'white cell measure' had dropped from '24%' to '6%'. This report was interpreted as good news and a different pain killer was prescribed and the patient was again sent home.

But two days later the patient was found collapsed at the entrance of another hospital in the area. She was quickly admitted. A diagnosis of toxic shock syndrome due to a streptococcal infection was made. Despite heroic treatments, including hyperbaric chamber therapy, the patient underwent multiple amputations of fingers as well both lower legs.

A subsequent re-evaluation of the second blood film showed a '50%' and not a '6%' band count as originally reported. What apparently happened was that while the first blood count revealed a significant 'left shift' in the neutrophils, the repeat blood film examination performed by another technician was reported as almost normal. As a result the patient's doctor felt there was considerable improvement and acted accordingly. The review of the second film showed in reality a considerable increase in the left shift. If this had been reported appropriately, i.e. a 'left shift' indicating a severe infection, the doctor would undoubtedly have admitted the patient when seen on the second visit to the emergency department.

In this case, the individual technologist's differences in the morphologic criteria for band neutrophils resulted in the problems noted above. Had the technologist's work schedules been reversed an entirely different course of events would probably have ensued. However, an error was made and the five elements of a negligence suit could be proven. The only legal questions therefore that warrants discussion is determining *who* is liable.

Under traditional concepts of liability, a hospital laboratory might be held vicariously liable for the conduct of its employee. Under this common law doctrine, the negligence of an employee may be imputed to the employer if the employer has some control over the employee's work and if the negligent act is committed within the scope of the employee's work. The doctrine is inapplicable where the conduct of the employee is outside the scope of his/her employment (Keeton, 1984).

Despite the negligence of a laboratory employee, the doctrine of vicarious liability might be deemed inapplicable where the conduct of the employee was directed by a third party who is not an employee of the institution, i.e. the traditional clinical pathologist or hematologist. Depending upon the circumstances, the clinical pathologist or hematologist might be treated as an independent contractor over which the laboratory (or hospital) has very little control. Where this is the case, the hospital laboratory might shield itself from liability resulting from the negligence of its employee pursuant to the *borrowed servant* rule. Under this rule (also known as the '*captain of the ship*' doctrine) the pathologist would be the liable party (Stricklen and Ballard, 1991) because he/she had the control over the technologist. However, even with the independence of the clinical pathologist, the hospital laboratory still might be deemed liable under the doctrine of *ostensible agency* (Boyd v. Albert Einstein Medical Center, 1988) which holds that where the injured party is led to reasonably believe there exists an employer–employee relationship, such an apparent relationship will be deemed to exist, thus leaving the employer liable (Stern, 1991).

Furthermore, even where the *borrowed servant* rule is deemed applicable, the hospital laboratory might still be deemed liable for negligence if it does not prevent the pathologist's negligence. Under the doctrine of *direct duty*, the hospital laboratory has a legal duty to meet certain standards of care to protect its patients (Simonson, 1986). Included in these standards may be the obligation to ensure it has competent employees as well as competent pathologists working for it. Thus, instead of just being a **hotel** for practising physicians, the hospital has, in fact, been deemed an institution which **houses** only competent physicians (Stern, 1991).

Finally, the concept of *enterprise liability* has emerged as a possible alternative to traditional theories of liability where blame is identified with a particular individual. Under the theory of enterprise liability, individual hospitals as well as other health care organizations would be solely liable for medical malpractice by their affiliated health care providers. This would be true even where the health care providers were not technically employees of the organization. An exception to this doctrine would be made for injury resulting from intentional misconduct, where individuals would remain liable for their conduct. With the imposition of enterprise liability, individual physicians and other health care providers would be relieved from legal liability for medical malpractice (Abraham and Weiler, 1992).

In the case presented, risk management techniques would include continuing education for all persons performing blood film evaluations in order to assure uniform reporting of this important study. Both quantitative and qualitative aspects of this very common hematology test come into play. The identification of a 'left shift' in neutrophils has been the subject of a continuing debate for many years. While some (Mathy and Koepke, 1974) have shown that this phenomenon has been quite useful in the identification of patients, particularly elderly and pediatric patients, with early inflammation and/or infection others have not been convinced. The automated hematology analysers have been variably successful in flagging for the presence of less mature neutrophils. Thus, the debate continues.

Can coagulation testing predict bleeding problems? (Case Study 3)

A 44-year-old man was admitted to the hospital for an evaluation of a persistent yet mild jaundice. It was decided to perform a percutaneous liver biopsy since many of the other laboratory studies were equivocal. But prior to the biopsy, a prothrombin time was done which was reported as 16 s. The liver biopsy was performed. However, after the procedure the patient developed a tachycardia and fall in his blood pressure. Blood transfusions were given and the patient went to the operating room where a large hepatic hematoma was found. The lacerated liver was sutured and the bleeding was controlled.

Subsequently the patient's physician questioned the laboratory director about any causal relationship of the prothrombin time of 16 s with the patient's bleeding episode. The physician admitted that at a recent seminar on hepatic disease the nationally-recognized speaker had stated that a prothrombin time should be '16 seconds or less before doing a liver biopsy'.

Here again, a potential plaintiff would attempt to establish the various elements of a negligent tort. But as opposed to the two previous cases presented where the standard of reasonableness was clearly violated, in this situation, the validation of the standard of care will be difficult to establish.

In such a situation, the courts will look to expert testimony and published standards such as licensure requirements, accreditation standards and institutional rules to determine the standard of care. And with the establishment of state legislation in a minority of states, courts are beginning to permit the use of practice guidelines as evidence of a standard of care. For example, in the state of Maine legislation has been enacted which establishes medical practice guidelines as an affirmative defence to certain malpractice suits. This five-year demonstration project, begun in April 1990 has created committees largely composed of physicians which have developed practice parameters for obstetrics and gynecology, radiology, anesthesiology and emergency medicine. After agreement on the guidelines was achieved, physicians in the state who agreed to participate had the right to use the guidelines as a defence in cases brought to trial if they adhered to the relevant guidelines. Both the State Bureau of Insurance as well as the Board of Registration in Medicine will also evaluate the effect of this project on medical liability claims, insurance premiums and defensive medicine. By 1997 the results of this trial must be reported to the governor and the legislature at which time expansion, modification, continuation or discontinuation of the project will be debated.

In this case it is apparent that the significant differences in the systems used for the measurement of prothrombin time may have confused the patient's physician. Was the expert who gave the seminar interpreting a shorter prothrombin time system, or a longer one? While the implementation of the INR system presumably has solved this problem for patients on long-term anticoagulant therapy, there is yet no consensus for prothrombin time comparisons in patients with other prothrombin time abnormalities. Nevertheless, physicians must be aware of these differences and be cautious in the interpretation of results as well as transfer of data from published studies into their own practices. Here again, the education of the medical staff regarding these problems is an important role for the laboratory director. The increasing implementation of point of care prothrombin time testing will undoubtedly accentuate the problem (see above).

11.5 The clinical pathologist/ hematologist in court

Laboratory directors can be named in professional liability claims jointly with other physicians or sometimes with an institution. Litigation may arise from a variety or sources such as the use of transfusions or provision of blood products or in connection with a misdiagnosis or misinterpretation of a blood film, bone marrow or lymph node preparations or even peer review activities.

Litigation is frequently the result of a miscommunication or poor communication. Therefore, laboratory directors should try to communicate with the clinicians clearly and concisely, and document such communications. Such documentation will ensure that proper testing procedures and protocols were followed and a record of such has been made.

Despite the best of laboratory practices the possibility of litigation remains and it is therefore essential that adequate insurance coverage be obtained for both the laboratory directors as well as all personnel at risk for such litigation. When the responsibility for the case is not clear there must be assurance that at least the 'enterprise' is adequately covered.

Conversely, a clinical pathologist or hematologist may give expert opinion as a witness in a professional liability action such as the case discussed in the previous section. In such cases it is important that the pathologist carefully reviews all laboratory reports as well as other medical documents and have the facts in order so that a logical and lucid discussion of a case can be given. One or more pretrial conferences with the attorney may be necessary. At that time the physician should be made aware of the salient facts and should acquaint the attorney with the points and extent of his testimony. Testimony should always be limited to one's areas of expertise. Finally, consultation with physicians having experience in the area of controversy may be helpful (College of American Pathologists, 1993).

Acknowledgement

The authors wish to thank Professor Dame Rosalinde Hurley, LLB, MD, FRC Path who kindly reviewed the manuscript and provided many helpful comments and clarifications.

References

Abraham, K. S. and Weiler, P. C. (1992) Organizational Liability for Medical Malpractice: An Alternative to Individual Health Care Provider Liability for Hospital-related Malpractice. Robert Wood Johnson Foundation.

Boyd v Albert Einstein Medical Center (1988) 547 A. 2d 1229 (Pennsylvania Superior Court).

College of American Pathologists, 10th Edition (1993) *Professional Relations Manual*, Northfield, ILL. pp 1–178.

Cooney, M. M. (1992) A collaborative approach to managing risk. *Med. Lab. Observer*, Suppl. **24**, September 36–41.

Federal Register (1993) Regulations implementing the Clinical Laboratory Improvement Amendments of 1988 (CLIA '88) 42 Code of Federal Regulations Part 493.

Foster, H. S. (1990) Governmental quality assurance regulation of haematology laboratories. *Clin. Lab. Haematol.* **12**, (Suppl. 1), 143–155.

Keeton, W. P. (1984) *Prosser and Keeton on Torts sos* 69, Saint Paul, MN: West Publishing Company.

Mathy, K. A. and Koepke, J. A. (1974) The clinical usefulness of segmented vs stab neutrophil criteria for differential leukocyte counts. *Am. J. Clin. Pathol.* **61**, 947–958.

Simonson, P. (1986) Corporate Negligence: An Evolving Theory of Hospital Liability. Practicing Law Institute.

Somrak, T. M. (1992) Legal liability in the cytopathology laboratory. *Lab. Med.*, **23**, 648–651.

Stern, J. B. (1991) Malpractice in the Managed Care Industry. *Creighton Law Review*, pp. 1285–1287.

Stricklen, M. M. and Ballard, F. L. Jr (1991) Representing Health Care Facilities. Practicing Law Institute, pp. 26, 29.

Part Three

Analytic Methods and Systems

12

Specimen collection, handling, storage and variability *

O. W. van Assendelft and A. Simmons

12.1 Introduction

The necessity for accurate and precise methodology in the clinical laboratory is repeatedly stressed and quality-control monitoring of the analytical process has become a way of life for laboratory staff. In general, however, little attention has been devoted to establishing quality assurance measures for collecting, handling, processing and storing blood specimens. Highly controlled, sophisticated laboratory technology is of no avail if the specimens are error-ridden due to faulty identification or poor collection techniques. Proper specimen collection and handling are, therefore, of the utmost importance; the likelihood for error in these areas is probably greater than the likelihood of errors that may occur during the laboratory determinations themselves.

Collection errors range from incorrect identification of the patient specimen to hemolyzed specimens or the use of inappropriate anticoagulants. Studies have indicated that as many as 8% of errors in patient's name, age, sex and identification numbers go undetected, even with extensive manual checking procedures (Taswell et al., 1974). Standards and guidelines for proper specimen collection and handling can reduce, and have reduced or alleviated many of these problems. The International Council for Standardization in Haematology (ICSH) has published guidelines for standardization of blood specimen collection for establishing reference values (ICSH, 1982). This chapter reviews these and other guidelines and recommendations for specimen collection, handling and storage, primarily oriented towards specimens for the hematology laboratory. The recommendations and guidelines are equally valid for collection and processing in a blood-bank environment (AABB, 1987, 1990).

---

* The use of trade names is for identification only and does not constitute endorsement by the Public Health Service or the US Department of Health and Human Services.

12.2 Intra-individual variability

Variations in analyte concentration within one and the same individual can be divided into: (1) analytical variation and (?) variation related to the subject or to the time of specimen collection. Analytical variation will not be considered in this chapter.

12.2.1 Physiological variation

Subject variation includes all sources of non-analytical error. Factors influencing variation include the use of medications or (illegal) drugs, physical activity, emotional stress, patient posture, diurnal variation and other miscellaneous causes.

Certain drugs and medications influence some hematological test results (Elking and Kabat, 1968; Sunderman, 1972) and there is evidence that a moderate leukocytosis and thrombocytosis is seen postprandially (Garrey and Bryan, 1935; Priest et al., 1982).

Physical activity is known to be a source of test variability. Significant changes in the red cell count and in hemoglobin and haptoglobin levels following strenuous exercise have been described (Horder and Klorder, 1970; Refsum, Meen and Stromme, 1973; Refsum et al., 1973). The increased values are most likely caused by a loss of circulating plasma and by re-entry into the circulation of red cells that had been sequestered in the marginal capillaries; increased red cell counts of up to $0.5 \times 10^{12}/1$ and of hemoglobin up to 15 g/l have been reported (Eklund, Eklund and Kauser, 1971).

Brief severe exercise produces a mild lymphocytosis; prolonged exercise can cause leukocytosis, principally derived from a neutrophilia of up to $30 \times 10^9/1$ (Sturgis and Bethell, 1943). The leukocytosis is believed to result from cellular release from the marginal pools into the circulation. Heavy manual labour has been reported to be accompanied by neutrophilia, lymphopenia and eosinopenia (Karvonen and Kunnas, 1952, 1953; Hurkat and Jain, 1973).

Leukocytosis has also been reported following

emotional stress (Milhorat, Small and Dietheim, 1942). Stress as well as exercise is believed to influence coagulation by increasing fibrinolysis (Astrup, 1973).

The effect of patient posture on routine test results is well established (Statland, Bokelund and Winkel, 1974). Hemoglobin and packed cell volume (PCV) levels average 5% less when the patient is in a recumbent position rather than upright. These changes occur rapidly, usually within 20 min, after which the values stabilize at the lower level (Lange, 1946; Eisenberg, 1963; Eklund, Eklund and Kauser, 1971; Tombridge, 1978). Similarly, PCV values are 4–6% higher after prolonged standing (Mollison, Engelfriet and Contreras, 1987).

The position of the arm during phlebotomy also influences test results. When the arm is held at the atrial level, the PCV is 2–4% lower than when it is held in a vertical position (Eisenberg, 1963). The changes are likely related to a shift of body water from the vascular to the interstitial compartment.

Increased erythropoiesis is seen following cigarette smoking; an increase in hemoglobin and PCV has been reported (Isager and Hagerup, 1971; Helman and Rubinstein, 1975; Smith and Landaw, 1978) as well as leukocytosis and eosinopenia (Winkel and Statland, 1981). Platelet hyperaggregatability and decreased platelet survival have also been found (Hawkins, 1972).

Many hematological test result variations are difficult to document accurately (Statland and Winkel, 1977a). Substantial physiological day-to-day and within-day variability has been reported for serum iron (Bowie et al., 1963; Statland, Winkel and Bokelund, 1976; Statland and Winkel, 1977b) and for the total iron-binding capacity (Statland and Winkel, 1977b). Diurnal variation of serum iron up to 30% has been noted (Hamilton et al., 1950) with maximum values found in the morning and lowest values in the late evening. Compared to the inter-individual variation, intra-individual variations of haptoglobin and transferrin are relatively small (Statland, Winkel and Killingsworth, 1976). A day-to-day variation of 10% has been reported for plasma fibrinogen (Grannis, 1970); a diurnal fibrinolytic rhythm has also been reported (Fearnley, Balmforth and Fearnley, 1957; Buckell and Elliot, 1959). Numerous reports have appeared (McCarthy and Van Slyke, 1939; Mole, 1945; Stengle and Schade, 1957; Elwood, 1962) indicating a diurnal variation for hemoglobin and PCV: compared with morning levels, hemoglobin levels as much as 3 g/l lower in the afternoon have been reported (Statland et al., 1978). Significant diurnal variation has also been found for the total white cell count (Kennon, Shipp and Hetherington, 1937) and for differential white cell counts (Statland and Winkel, 1977a; Statland et al., 1978; Winkel et al., 1981); only eosinophilic and basophilic granulocytes appear to show a more consistent pattern of lower

values in the afternoon and higher values in the morning (Rorsman, 1962). These variations appear to parallel diurnal glucocorticoid changes (Statland et al., 1978).

Other documented causes of test result fluctuations are altitude and pregnancy. Increased altitude results in increased hemoglobin levels and an increase in the number of circulating red cells. The magnitude of the increase depends on the degree of anoxia; at an altitude of 6500 feet (c 2000 m) for example, the hemoglobin level is approximately 10 g/l higher than at sea level (Myhre et al., 1970). Hemoglobin levels decrease during pregnancy because of the increased nutritional demands and hemodilution; leukocyte counts as high as $15 \times 10^9/l$ have also been reported. The white cell count peaks about 8 weeks before parturition and returns to normal about one week after delivery (Cruikshank, 1970).

12.3 Specimen collection

Specimens for the hematology laboratory may be whole blood, collected by venepuncture or skin puncture, peripheral blood smears or bone marrow obtained by aspiration or biopsy. Specimen collection by arterial puncture is generally reserved for blood gas tension and blood pH measurement (NCCLS, 1992a).

12.3.1 Test requisition

Organization is essential in areas where blood specimens are collected so that patient records may be accurately maintained. Each request for a blood specimen should be recorded. This accessioning provides a means of identifying all paperwork and supplies associated with each patient. Use a unique accession number on all specimens taken from a patient at one time; record on labels the information given on the specimen request form; include: (1) patient's full name; (2) identification number; (3) accessioning number; (4) date and (5) time of collection. Other information may be added, e.g. the physician, room number, name of test, initials of person drawing the specimen and relevant patient information. Labels should be printed in ink, indelible pencil or by computer print-out.

12.3.2 Patient identification

Before any blood specimen is drawn, the patient must be positively identified. The patient should be asked to give her or his full name, and outpatients should also give their home address. When dealing with hospitalized patients, it is important to verify the accuracy of the wrist or ankle bracelet issued on admission. When the patient is unable to speak, a

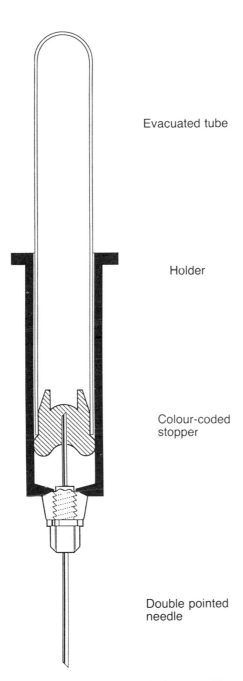

Evacuated tube

Holder

Colour-coded stopper

Double pointed needle

Figure 12.1 Components of an evacuated tube system (From NCCLS, 1991b, with permission)

family member, the doctor, or the nurse should be asked to positively identify the patient. When identifying a patient, it is important to always ask the patient to state his or her full name and not, for example, to ask the patient 'your name Smith?'

Immediately after collection and before drawing specimens from any other patient, all blood speci-

mens must be fully labelled with patient's first and last names, patient location, and date.

12.3.3 Blood collection: venous blood

Two systems are used in drawing venous blood specimens: the syringe and needle or the evacuated tube system. A syringe and needle is preferred when difficulty in drawing the specimen is anticipated, e.g. patients with fragile or hardened vein walls. In general, the evacuated tube system is a popular method for specimen collection. Evacuated tube systems are composed of three basic elements: a sterile needle, a holder securing both the needle and the tube, and an evacuated tube containing a pre-measured vacuum and with or without a pre-measured additive (Fig. 12.1).

Although the principal problems involving evacuated tubes for collecting blood affect biochemical and toxicological testing (Missen and Dixon, 1974; Pragay et al., 1979), poor specimen collection can influence hematological test results no matter how well the laboratory carries out the analyses. It is therefore wise to establish a specific quality assurance procedure for checking evacuated tubes. Parameters to check include the volume of blood drawn, stopper removal, and a visual check for anticoagulant as well as the presence of foreign material in the tube. Anticoagulated specimens should also be carefully inspected for the presence of clots.

The actual venepuncture procedure should be evaluated (ECCLS, 1987). In obtaining a venous specimen, it is standard procedure to apply a tourniquet to make the veins more prominent so as to facilitate needle entry and the rapid withdrawal of specimens. Venous flow is occluded and localized stasis may occur, especially if the tourniquet remains in place longer than one minute or if it is too tight. Stasis results in hemoconcentrated specimens and in erroneously high hematological test results. Because it is often difficult to draw blood without the aid of a tourniquet, it is important to limit the time the tourniquet remains in use and to determine the order of draw for the tests requested. The recommended (NCCLS, 1990b, 1991c) order of draw is blood culture tubes first, then tubes without additives, next tubes with additives for coagulation testing, and, finally, tubes with other additives. Non-additive tubes are drawn before tubes with additives to avoid contamination of non-additives tubes. Cross-contamination between different additives has also been reported (Jones, 1980). It is therefore recommended (Calam and Cooper, 1982; NCCLS, 1991c) to draw citrate-containing tubes first, followed by heparin-containing tubes, then EDTA-containing tubes, and finally any others, e.g. oxalate/fluoride-containing tubes.

When collecting multiple tubes, it is most important to mix the anticoagulant and the blood immediately by gently inverting the tube five to ten times before additional blood samples are collected. This helps minimize the formation of microclots.

The effect of hemolysis on hematological test results is not well documented. Most laboratories reject the blood specimen if any sign of hemolysis is detected. There is, however, evidence that minimal hemolysis, i.e. slightly pink plasma, does not effect the prothrombin time test, provided the hemolysis is not the result of a traumatic venepuncture (Engstrom, 1968). Complete blood counts should not be performed on hemolysed specimens, although hemoglobin assays can be done.

Hemolysis may occur during phlebotomy or during transport or processing of the specimens. During collection, blood may hemolyse from a variety of factors, including the expulsion of the blood through a small-bore needle with resultant froth formation, and from shaking the tube too vigorously when mixing. Technically difficult venepunctures may also result in hemolysed specimens. Sharp 19–22 gauge needles should be used to collect blood from adults: hemolysis occurs more frequently with smaller bore needles. Excessive negative pressure from either the syringe or the evacuated tube not only damages the red cells but may also fragment both leukocytes and platelets. Thus, blood specimens should be routinely examined and rejected, not only for the presence of microclots, but also for hemolysis.

Evacuated tubes should be allowed to fill to capacity to ensure a correct final concentration of anticoagulant. Excessive amounts of anticoagulant, resulting from incomplete filling of the tube, can result in falsely decreasing the PCV by up to 0.04, as well as producing a false leukopenia (Koepke et al., 1978).

When transferring blood from a syringe to an evacuated tube, do not remove the rubber stopper from the tube. Blood must be transferred from the syringe by the action of the vacuum in the tube; it must not be injected into the tube. This technique is extremely important if the tube contains an anticoagulant or other additive. The vacuum ensures that the proportion of blood to additive is correct.

12.3.4 Blood collection in special circumstances

For venous specimens, some hematological parameters will vary in response to changes in the physiological state of the patient. Apprehensive infants and children may have cyanotic extremities resulting from dilated capillaries. This, in turn, can result in falsely elevated hemoglobin values and red cell counts. Transient leukocytosis may also occur in frightened children in response to the liberation of sequestered cells from the marginal pool.

The collection of blood specimens from patients in special situations requires extra care and attention. Obtaining blood from indwelling lines or catheters may be a potential source of error. It is common practice to flush these lines with heparin to reduce the risk of thrombosis. Consequently, they must be flushed free from heparin before any blood is collected and used for testing. It has been recommended that at least three times the volume of the line be removed and the blood discarded before a specimen is obtained for analysis (NCCLS, 1986). If intravenous fluids are being administered in an arm, blood should not be collected from that side to avoid acquiring a hemodiluted specimen. The phlebotomist should obtain blood from the opposite arm or, if that is not possible, from a site below the intravenous infusion. In such situations the physician should be notified and, if possible, the intravenous infusion should be stopped for a few minutes prior to venepuncture. A vein other then the vein used for the infusion should be selected, and the first 5 ml of blood obtained discarded.

12.3.5 Complications in venepuncture

The use of evacuated tubes will occasionally cause collapsed veins, especially in patients with small veins, particularly hand or ankle veins. In these situations the syringe method is preferred to obtain a specimen because the phlebotomist can more easily control the negative pressure applied to the blood vessel.

On rare occasions, the vessel wall will be flattened against the needle lumen, occluding the needle with resultant inadequate collection. A remedy in such cases is to gently disengage the needle from the vein wall by slowly withdrawing and rotating the needle about one-half turn, taking care not to remove the needle completely from the vein. When evacuated tubes are used, this procedure is more easily accomplished by removing the tube from the tube holder, manipulating the needle, then reinserting a fresh evacuated tube into the holder.

12.3.6 Prevention of hematoma and/or hemolysis

Fully penetrating, yet only puncturing, the uppermost wall of the vein will prevent hematoma formation while performing a venepuncture. Partial penetration may allow blood to leak into the soft tissues surrounding the vein by way of the needle bevel. Only major veins should be used for a venepuncture and the tourniquet should be released before removing the needle.

Care must be taken to avoid drawing blood from a hematoma and to avoid using a needle with too small a bore size. When using needle and syringe, make sure the needle is fitted securely on the syringe to avoid frothing; avoid drawing back the plunger too forcefully. Anticoagulated specimens should be mixed gently but thoroughly; blood must not be injected from a syringe into an evacuated tube.

Bleeding from the venepuncture site will occasionally be seen, especially following phlebotomy on a patient with bleeding tendencies. Hematomas can be avoided even in such extreme situations by applying firm, constant pressure to the puncture site for at least 5 min. It is essential that the patient's arm is not bent upwards as this opens the wound site with resultant further bleeding. Pressure should be applied with the arm held high and straight in a vertical position, and a pressure bandage should be applied after overt bleeding has ceased.

12.3.7 Blood collection: capillary blood

For small quantities of blood required for hematological procedures or some chemical tests, adequate specimens can be collected by performing a skin puncture. Especially in premature infants, drawing large quantities of venous blood may result in anemia. Skinpuncture specimens from adults may be desirable from severely burned patients, extremely obese patients, patients with thrombotic tendencies, patients with malignancies where venepuncture is reserved for or limited to therapeutic purposes and geriatric patients.

Some studies have shown no significant difference between an individual's capillary and venous blood values for PCV, red and white cell counts, mean cell volume (MCV) and platelet counts (Stuart, Barrett and Prangnell, 1974); others have reported significant discrepancies in PCV (Nelson, 1976; Oski and Naiman, 1982); these discrepancies may, however, have been exaggerated by cold with resulting slow capillary blood flow (Oh and Lind, 1966).

12.3.8 Puncture sites

The most commonly used sites for skin puncture are: (1) the lateral or posterolateral portion of the heel; (2) the big toe and (3) the palmar or dorsal surface of the last digit of the finger. The heel is used most often prior to 1 year of age. Care must be taken to prevent the point of the lancet from penetrating the bone in newborns. Puncturing deeper than 2.4 mm on the plantar surface of the heel of infants may risk bone damage (NCCLS, 1991d). Puncturing the calcaneus can increase the risk of osteomyelitis. The puncture site must be non-edematous since tissue fluids can cause abnormal results, and preferably warm; the skin puncture must bleed freely.

Several types of containers are used to collect capillary blood (NCCLS, 1990a):

1. Capillary pipettes, most often used for collecting routine blood test specimens. The specimen is collected into several tubes and can be distributed easily. However, the pipettes are hard to label and must be broken after centrifugation to obtain serum or plasma.

2. Microcontainers composed of small polypropylene tubes with a capillary tube in the lid. The specimen is collected by capillary action and then flows into the tube. Little hemolysis results with the use of these microcontainers (Hicks, Rowland and Buffone, 1976).
3. 'Unopettes', disposable diluting pipettes consisting of a capillary tube and a reservoir containing a pre-measured volume of diluent.
4. Small conical glass or plastic tubes. To move blood to the bottom of the tube, the technologist must flick her or his wrist after each drop is collected. This drop-by-drop collection increases the chance of hemolysis of the specimen. Special precautions are required when collecting capillary blood for coagulation tests (Hathaway and Bonnar, 1978).

Hemolysis may also occur when blood is collected by skin puncture if excess alcohol is left on the skin puncture site or if the heel or finger is squeezed excessively. Massaging the site prior to puncture may reduce cell counts up to 5%; squeezing blood through an inadequate puncture wound may elevate cell counts by as much as 25%. Clotting from liberated tissue fluids and local alterations in the marginal leukocyte pool may account for these discrepancies. Hemolysis of blood collected from newborns and infants is more common, and particular attention should be paid to obtaining a free flow of blood from the puncture without the necessity of making multiple wounds.

Many neonatal screening programmes (e.g. hemoglobinopathy screening) use capillary blood collected on filter paper. Specimens may be collected directly from the puncture site, or the preprinted circles on the filter paper may be saturated with blood previously collected into sterile, heparinized capillary tubes. The following instructions must be observed: (1) Apply blood to one side of the filter paper only: (2) Examine both sides to make sure that the specimen has penetrated and saturated the paper. Avoid touching or smearing the blood spots; (3) Allow the specimen to air-dry in a suspended horizontal position for at least 3 h at ambient (15–22°C) temperature. Do not heat, stack or allow the blood spots on the filter paper to touch other surfaces during the drying process; (4) After the spot has dried, place each filter paper card into a separate mailing envelope, and mail to the laboratory within 24 h of collection.

Suitable filter paper should conform to specifications and the absorption capacity, homogeneity and retention volume of the 3 mm blood spot punch should be measured for each lot (Jensen et al., 1984; NCCLS, 1992d).

12.3.9 Phlebotomists

Reducing errors during the blood collection phase

Table 12.1 Dimensional guide for evacuated tubes

Nominal size (mm)	Nominal draw (ml of blood)	Outside tube diameter (mm)
10 × 65	3	10 –11
13 × 75	5	11.5–13
13 × 100	7	11.5–13
16 × 100	10	15 –16
16 × 127	15	15 –16

will result in biologically representative specimens, comparable from one institute to another. A standard procedure has been published by the European Committee for Clinical Laboratory Standards (ECCLS, 1987). Without question, a sound training programme is needed to develop efficient, well-trained phlebotomists. The National Committee for Clinical Laboratory Standards (NCCLS) has published guidelines for such a training programme (NCCLS, 1991c).

12.3.10 Evacuated tubes

The containers that form part of the evacuated tube system (see Fig. 12.1) are available in different sizes (Table 12.1) with or without additives. Colour-coding of the stoppers indicates the type of additive (Table 12.2).

The degree of vacuum in evacuated tubes is such that the tube generally will fill to within ± 10% of the stated draw volume, thus ensuring a correct final blood/additive ratio. However, the tube vacuum may diminish with time, resulting in 'incomplete draws'. Laboratories may determine the degree of vacuum draw of an evacuated tube using a calibrated buret (ISO, 1987; NCCLS, 1991b).

Evacuated tube systems are quite adequate for collecting blood specimens for routine coagulation testing, e.g. prothrombin time, partial thromboplastin time, fibrinogen. Activation of the coagulation factors is circumvented with the use of siliconized evacuated tubes. However, some studies showed inconsistent test results when tubes of different brands, or different lots of the same brand, were used (Heyns et al., 1981; Palmer and Gralnick, 1981; van den Besselaar and Loeliger, 1982; Thomson, 1984). Laboratories that use these tubes for coagulation testing specimens should validate the brand being used in the laboratory. More sophisticated coagulation studies may require more elaborate evaluation of collection systems before use.

Needles for evacuated tube holders are available in different sizes. Generally, #19 to #22-gauge needles (20–23 SWG; 1.06–0.71 mm outside diameter) are preferred. The choice of a needle is usually a compromise between optimal flow rate for blood collection and minimal size to reduce tissue/vessel wall damage and pain. Small-bore needles require considerable suction pressure through the needle resulting in a strong possibility of red cell damage in the needle (Nevaril et al., 1968). If a sufficient blood-flow rate through the needle is not obtained, the time required for collecting the specimen may be unduly prolonged, coagulation is liable to occur, and the normal plasma/cell ratio may be upset.

12.3.11 Additives

Heparin

Heparin is specifically recommended as anticoagulant when determining carboxyhemoglobin (Rodkey and O'Neal, 1974) and zinc (Dawson and Walker, 1969). It is also valuable as anticoagulant when unhemolysed, unaltered red cells are required for fragility studies and red cell enzyme determinations. The lithium salt of heparin has been particularly recommended (NCCLS, 1988). Heparin anticoagulation is not recommended for blood cell counting because it causes clumping of platelets and leukocytes. Blood films made from heparin-anticoagulated blood are difficult to stain clearly and show a blue background when stained with standard Romanowsky dyes.

To determine an upper limit of heparin as anticoagulant without increase in erythrocyte size, micro-hematocrit capillaries (NCCLS, 1993b) containing increasing amounts of heparin were tested at the Centers for Disease Control and Prevention (CDC). The packed cell volume (PCV) remained constant in capillary tubes containing from 4 to 7.5 IU per tube and increased by 1.5% with 9.75 IU per tube. Thus, 7.5 IU of heparin per capillary tube may be considered a 'safe' upper limit for PCV determination. An amount of 7.5 IU heparin per capillary tube is equal to 125 IU per ml of blood.

Trisodium citrate

Trisodium citrate, $Na_3C_6H_5O_7$, is the usual anticoagulant for coagulation investigations. For coagulation studies either a 109 or a 129 mmol/l (32 g/l or 38 g/l of the dihydrate form) solution in a 1:9 anticoagulant/blood ratio has been acceptable (NCCLS, 1991e). However, only the 109 mmol/l solution has been recommended by the International Committee on Thrombosis and Haemostasis, ICTH (Ingram and Hills, 1976a,b). If a patient's PCV is very high or very low, the results of the prothrombin time may be inaccurate when a 1:9 anticoagulant/blood ratio is used (Hardisty and Ingram, 1965). Different anticoagulant/blood ratios have been advocated for specimens with PCV ≤ 0.20 and ≥ 0.60 (Koepke, Rodgers and Ollivier, 1974; Ingram and Hills, 1976a; NCCLS, 1986).

For determining the erythrocyte sedimentation rate (ESR), a 109 mmol/l solution is recommended in a 1:4 anticoagulant/blood ratio (ICSH, 1977).

Table 12.2 Letter and colour codes for specimen tubes

Additive	Use	Letter code*		Stopper colour	
		ISO	NCCLS	ISO	NCCLS
None	Serum	Z		Red	Red
EDTA K_2, K_3	Plasma or whole blood	KE	K3E$^+$	Lavender	Lavender
Na_2		NE	N2E	Lavender	Lavender
Heparin (Na,Li)	Plasma or whole blood	NH	NAH	Green	Green
		LH	LIH	Green	Green
Trisodium citrate	Coagulation studies	9NC	NC9	Light blue	Blue
1:9					
1:4	ESR (Westergren)	4NC	NC4	Black	Blue
Acid citrate dextrose		ACD		Yellow	
Sterile interior of tube					Yellow
Fluoride/oxalate	Glycolysis inhibition	FX	NFX	Grey	Grey
Serum separation material	Serum	S		Red/black	
		S		Red/grey	

*Manufacturers of evacuated tubes are currently not using letter coding on the tube labels to indicate the type of additive.
$^+$ For EDTA K_2

Table 12.3 pH of aqueous EDTA-salt solutions and required amounts for adequate anticoagulation

Compound	pH	Required amount per ml of blood	
		μmol	mg
Na_2-EDTA.$2H_2O$	4.5 – 5.3	3.7 – 5.4	1.4 – 2.0
K_2-EDTA.$2H_2O$	⩽ 4.5	3.7 5.4	1.5 – 2.2
K_3-EDTA (anhydrous)	7 – 8	3.7 – 5.4	1.5 – 2.2

EDTA

The most frequently used anticoagulant in the hematology laboratory is ethylenediaminetetraacetic acid (EDTA), $C_{10}H_{16}N_2O_8$. EDTA acts as a sequestering or chelating agent and effectively chelates the calcium in blood. Because of its chelating properties, EDTA is unsuitable for specimens for calcium and iron analyses using colorimetric or titrimetric techniques. The lack of solubility of the free acid in aqueous solution makes using sodium and potassium salts preferable. The disodium and dipotassium salts are generally used in the dry form, the tripotassium salt usually in the liquid form.

The recommended range for adequate anticoagulation is 3.7–5.4 μmol/ml of blood of the free acid. Table 12.3 gives the amount and the pH of aqueous solutions of the sodium and potassium salts of EDTA. Na_3-EDTA is not recommended because of its high pH; in liquid form it may adversely affect glass and plasma proteins. EDTA is particularly useful in the hematology laboratory because it preserves the cellular components of blood, and ICSH has recommended the dipotassium salt as the anticoagulant of choice for blood cell counting and sizing (ICSH, 1993).

Acid citrate dextrose (ACD) and citrate phosphate dextrose (CPD)

Although acid citrate dextrose (ACD) is still widely used because of its anticoagulant and preservative properties, it has been largely supplanted by citrate phosphate dextrose with adenine (CPDA). The storage life of red cells in ACD is 21 days; in CPDA up to 35 days. CPDA-1 contains 26.3 g trisodium citrate (dihydrate), 3.27 g citric acid (monohydrate), 2.22 g sodium dihydrogen phosphate (monohydrate), 31.8 g dextrose (monohydrate), and 0.275 g adenine per litre; 14 ml are used per 100 ml of blood. In CPDA-2, the amount of dextrose is increased to 44.6 g and the amount of adenine to 0.55 g. The additional adenine hastens the loss of 2,3-DPG from the red cells (Mollison, Engelfriet and Contreras, 1987).

Oxalate

Combined ammonium/potassium oxalate was extensively used in the hematology laboratory before the introduction of EDTA, but is no longer recommended.

12.4 Specimen stability

In general, anticoagulated blood specimens for

hematological testing are less stable than the serum samples used in chemistry and serology testing.

When blood is anticoagulated with tripotassium EDTA and is stored, undisturbed, at room temperature (18–25°C), the hemoglobin concentration, PCV, red and white cell counts and the red cell indices (MCH, MCHC, MCV) are stable for up to 8 h and are within Tonks' 'allowable limits of error' (Tonks, 1968) for up to 24 h. Tests performed on blood stored at 4°C have produced conflicting data. It has been suggested that EDTA-anticoagulated blood remains within 5% of the initial values of the 'hemogram' when kept at 4°C for up to 24 h (Brittin et al., 1969) and at an acceptable level when kept for 48 h in a refrigerator (Lampasso, 1968).

Two problem parameters appear to be the white cell count and the mean cell volume, MCV. The leukocyte count is stable for 24 h if the specimen is stored at ambient temperature and for up to 48 h if stored at 4°C. However, individual differences are found, especially when an impedance-based method is used for counting.

Absolute lymphocyte counts are integral to the determination of the absolute number of CD4+ lymphocytes which is a very important laboratory parameter for the diagnosis and monitoring of treatment in patients infected with Human Immunodeficiency Virus (HIV). Studies have shown that there can be a progressive decline over time in the accuracy of absolute lymphocyte counts with up to 50% after 72 h of collection (Koepke and Landay, 1989; Koepke and Smith-Jones, 1992). Ideally these critical counts should be done within a few hours after the collection of the blood specimen. If delays are encountered, each laboratory doing such studies should evaluate the acceptability of their particular hematology analyser if specimen analysis is delayed for more than a few hours. Such validation studies are endorsed by the Centers for Disease Control and Prevention (CDC) in their guidelines for CD4+ testing (CDC, 1992).

After 8 h of storage at ambient temperature the MCV increases at a progressive rate of 3 to 4 fl every 24 h. In blood stored at 4°C the MCV is stable for 24 h and then progressively increases at the same rate as if it is stored at ambient temperature (Simmons, Wiseman and Fay, 1978; Simmons, 1982). If the blood is stored at 4°C and is mixed intermittently, the hemoglobin concentration, red and white cell counts, red cell indices and the platelet count are stable for up to 72 h (Cohle, Saleem and Makhaoui, 1981). Results of storage up to 48 h are summarized in Table 12.4. At the CDC, K$_3$-EDTA anticoagulated blood, stored at 4°C and 22°C, was followed for 24 h using a microhematocrit centrifuge and an automated hematology analyzer (Coulter S-880). The MCV of specimens stored at 22°C demonstrated a gradual increase over the 24 h period (+1.5%) but no change in the PCV. The platelet count of the speci-

mens stored at 4°C, however, showed a continuous decrease (−34° in 24 h; Table 12.5).

Reticulocyte counts have been reported to be reliable up to 48 h in blood stored at either 4°C or 23°C (Lampasso, 1968). However, the manufacturer's stability recommendations for their reticulocyte method should be confirmed.

Extended storage (24 h) is generally not recommended because stability can vary to a considerable degree. Stability depends on reagents, system, instrumentation, etc. and it is recommended that EDTA-preserved blood be processed not more than 6 h after being drawn (NCCLS, 1992c).

One variable frequently overlooked is the importance of the use of the correct EDTA concentration. For optimal storage conditions, a full-drawn tube of blood anticoagulated with K$_3$-EDTA, 1.25–1.75 mg/ml, should be used (Sacker, 1975). NCCLS (1992c) recommends that EDTA salts be used at a concentration of 3.7–5.4 μmol/ml blood, equivalent to 1.4–2.0 mg/ml Na$_2$-EDTA.2H$_2$O and 1.5–2.2 mg/ml K$_2$-EDTA.2H$_2$O or K$_3$-EDTA (anhydrous). When 2-ml pediatric evacuated tubes are used, specimens less than 0.5 ml demonstrate significant decreases in the leukocyte count and an increased MCHC due to the hypertonic action of the anticoagulant, causing cell shrinkage and a decreased MCV (Doyle, 1967).

Manual/visual differential leukocyte counts are stable for a long time, provided the blood film is made and fixed within 3 h of collection although the quality of staining may be impaired after 2–3 weeks. Blood films are best made directly from the venepuncture needle or from a direct skin puncture rather than from EDTA-anticoagulated blood. Films made from anticoagulated specimens may show morphological cellular changes even after a brief storage period. The first changes have been reported to occur within 30 min in the neutrophilic and other granulocytes and consist of swelling and the loss of nuclear lobe structure (Sacker, 1975). This is followed by stretching of the interlobular bridges, loss of cytoplasmic granulation, and vacuolization. These changes progress with more marked nuclear swelling and crossover of nuclear chromatin, resulting in typical cloverleaf patterns in the more extreme cases. Ultimately these changes progress to a more complete morphological disintegration of the cell, leaving a bare nucleus (Sacker, 1975). An absence of significant changes in cell morphology for up to 5 h (Kennedy, Machora and Baker, 1981) and up to 6 h (Lloyd, 1982) has, however, also been reported. At CDC, slight vacuolization of monocytes was found after 1 h, progressing to moderate after 4 h, and slight vacuolization of neutrophilic granulocytes at 3–4 h, progressing to moderate after 6 h. If an automated cytochemical flow method is used to determine the differential count, cell stability is acceptable up to 48 h.

Table 12.4 Effect of storage on hematological test stability

| | 21.5°C | | | | |
	O	4 h	8 h	24 h	48 h
Hemoglobin (g/l)	147	146	147	145	149
RBX (× 10^{12}/l)	4.81	4.83	4.87	4.78	4.78
WBC (× 10^9/l)	6.8	6.4	6.6	6.6	6.5
MCV (fl)	89.3	89.3	88.0	93.5	98.7
	4°C				
Hemoglobin (g/l)	147	148	145	146	148
RBC (× 10^{12}/l)	4.81	4.89	4.85	4.85	4.88
WBC (× 10^9/l)	6.8	6.3	6.4	6.6	6.1
MCV (fl)	89.3	89.3	90.4	89.0	92.6

Table 12.5 Effect of storage at 4 and 22°C of a K_3-EDTA–anticoagulated blood specimen on MCV and platelet count

| Time (h) | MCV (fl) | | Platelet count (× 10^9 per litre) | |
	4°C	22°C	4°C	22°C
0	93.8	93.8	294	294
3	94.1	94.4	268	285
6	93.7	94.7	243	286
12	94.6	95.3	246	292
24	93.9	95.2	195	280

MCV and cell counts determined with a Coulter S–880.

Platelets appear to swell, producing giant forms, then disintegrate over 48 h. Because the fragments are large enough to be counted as morphologically normal platelets, artificially high platelet counts are obtained.

Red cells also undergo changes in shape, leading to both macrocytosis and spherocytosis.

The erythrocyte sedimentation rate test ESR remains stable for 4–6 h when the specimen is stored at room temperature (Lugton, 1987) and for 24 h when refrigerated (Gambino et al., 1965). ICSH, however, recommends that the ESR test be set up within 4 h if the blood is left at room temperature (18–25°C) and within 6 h when the specimen is kept at 4°C (ICSH, 1977; NCCLS, 1993a). A pre-storage normal sedimentation rate is most likely to remain normal after storage; any grossly abnormal test result is likely to decrease after storage and will become either less abnormal or even normal.

Coagulation test stability is critical both for diagnosis and for maintenance of anticoagulant therapy. Depending on the temperature maintained during transport and storage of the specimen, various time intervals between obtaining the specimen and testing the sample have been recommended: 2 h when stored at 22–24°C, 4 h when stored at 4°C, 2 weeks when stored at −20°C, and 6 months when stored at −70°C (NCCLS, 1991c). Stability studies have, however, shown that, in an unopened vacuum-collected tube, samples for the prothrombin time test do not deteriorate for at least 6 and up to 12 h, even when stored at room temperature (Fig 12.2); the partial thromboplastin time meanwhile, increased 10–15% after 24 h of storage (Koepke, Rodgers and Ollivier, 1974).

Studies have been performed to document differences between the effect of Na_2-EDTA, K_2-EDTA, and K_3-EDTA on the apparent PCV using the microhematocrit method (NCCLS, 1993b; ICSH, 1993) and several automated hematology analysers (Koepke et al., 1988/89). K_3-EDTA causes the largest degree of red cell shrinkage with increasing EDTA concentration (11% at 7.5 mg/ml blood), the largest change in cell volume on standing (+1.6% after 4 h), and results in lower MCV values (−0.16–1.3%, depending on the type of analyser used). Similar findings were recently published by Broden (1992). A decreased white cell count has also been reported with K_3-EDTA in high concentration (Goosens, van Duppen and Verwilghen, 1991). Additionally, K_3-

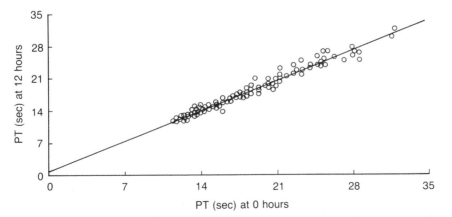

Figure 12.2 Correlation of prothrombin time (PT) determined immediately after drawing the speciment (0 hours) and after storage at room temperature (18–24°C) for 12 hours; n = 230, r = 0.986

EDTA is dispensed as a liquid, causing all directly measured values (hemoglobin concentration, red cell, white cell and platelet counts) to be 1–2% lower than the values in circulating blood. For this reason, and because K_2-EDTA is widely used in Europe and Japan, ICSH recommends K_2-EDTA as anticoagulant in specimen collection for blood cell counting and sizing, especially when PCV values are required for the calibration of automated hematology analysers (ICSH, 1993). When a laboratory switches from K_3-EDTA to the K_2 salt, the population (target) means will have to be modified: the MCV mean will increase about 2%; the MCHC mean will decrease by a similar amount (NCCLS, 1993b). Since K_2-EDTA is dispensed as a powder, special attention must be paid to adequate mixing of the specimen.

12.5 Blood films

The reliability of information obtained from blood films depends on the quality of the films. Properly spread films are essential for accurate work. Slides and cover glasses must be scrupulously clean and free of grease and dust so that they will allow uniform spreading of the blood. Two methods of preparing adequate films are used:

(1) The two-slide method. Place a small drop of blood about 2 mm in diameter on a slide 2 cm from the end. Place the edge of another slide, from which a small corner has been broken off, on the surface of the first at an angle of 30–40°. Draw this slide back against the drop of blood until the specimen runs across the end of this slide. Push the slide forward at a moderate speed to spread the blood evenly on the first slide into a thin film. Airdry the film rapidly by waving the slide or by using a fan.

(2) The coverslip method. Using 2 × 2 cm coverslips, place a small drop of blood on one coverslip. Place a second coverslip diagonally over the first and allow the blood to spread out evenly. Smoothly slide the coverslips apart, parallel to their surfaces, and airdry the smears.

Expert morphological evaluation of peripheral blood cells is one of the most vital procedures in hematology laboratory diagnosis. It is essential, therefore, that blood films be of ideal thickness. An acceptable wedge blood film (Method 1) has the following characteristics (NCCLS, 1992b): (1) A gradual transition in thickness from the thick to thin areas, ending in a squared, straight edge; (2) At minimum 2.5 cm long, terminating at least 1 cm from the end of the slide; (3) Narrower than the slide on which the film is spread, with smooth, continuous side margins that are accessible for oil immersion examination; (4) No artefacts introduced by technique; (5) A far end that becomes gradually thinner,

without streaks, troughs or ridges; (6) Granulocytes, monocytes and lymphocytes that appear evenly distributed in the 'usable' fields of the film; (7) When the white cell count is within the normal range, the number of leukocytes per field at the tail area should not exceed 2–3 times the number per field in the body of the film; the film edges should contain less than 2–3 times the number of cells per field in the body of the smear and (8) Less than 2% of cells should be disrupted or non-identifiable (except in certain pathological states, e.g. chronic lymphocytic leukemia).

12.6 Bone marrow aspiration and biopsy

In addition to taking a careful and complete patient history, conducting a thorough physical examination and reviewing a patient's peripheral blood film, collecting and studying a bone marrow specimen is of prime importance in clinical and laboratory hematology. The routine site for marrow sampling was formerly the sternum where the marrow is easily aspirated. The sternum has, however, been almost completely abandoned in favour of other sites. With the increasing need for marrow tissue biopsies, the posterior iliac crest has become the location of choice for both aspiration and biopsy. The anterior iliac crest in adult patients is also sometimes biopsied.

Other sites, such as the spinous process of a vertebra or a focal lesion localized by X-ray examination, are occasionally aspirated or biopsied. In infants up to 8 months old, the proximal anterior aspect of the tibia, 1–2 cm below the greater tuberosity, provides a convenient site for marrow sampling.

Aspirated marrow specimens are used to prepare films of marrow cells on glass slides. Cover glass 'squash' preparations have been very popular. Place a small particle of marrow on an acid-cleaned, alcohol-rinsed, 2.5 × 2.5 cm coverslip and place a second coverslip obliquely on top of the particle. Gently squeeze the coverslips together, then grasp the opposing corners of the two coverslips and quickly pull them apart, being careful to keep them parallel to each other. Make several preparations and fix them with water-free ($\leq$ 3%) methanol (Diggs and Bell, 1980).

Two 2.5 × 7.5 cm microscope slides can be used instead of coverslips. A marrow particle is placed in the centre of the slide and a second slide is placed lengthwise covering about two-thirds of the lower slide.

The slides or coverslip preparations can be stained in the usual way, manually or with a slide stainer. The resulting films characteristically contain marrow cells in the central portions and sinusoidal blood at the periphery. Thus, the morphology of circulating blood cells can be evaluated along with the morphology of marrow cells.

Bone marrow biopsy specimens should be fixed according to methods suggested by the surgical pathology department.

12.7 Specimen handling and processing

12.7.1 Specimen transport

Handling and transport of diagnostic specimens must adhere to procedures that maintain the viability and integrity of the specimen from the point of origin to the laboratory. Although delays of blood specimens in transit from a patient to the laboratory are usually short, the time elapsing from separation of cells and serum or plasma until analysis may be considerable. For some tests (e.g. ammonia, blood gas determinations), specimens must be kept at approximately 4°C from the time the blood is drawn until the specimens are analysed or until serum or plasma is separated from the cells. Such specimens must be transferred to the laboratory by placing the specimen container in ice water. For all analytes that are thermally labile, serum or plasma should be separated from the cells in a refrigerated centrifuge.

Due to the phenomenon of cold activation of certain procoagulants, specimens for coagulation studies should not be chilled, especially when evacuated tubes are used for specimen collection (Thomson, 1984). ECAT (the European Concerted Action on Thrombosis) has recommended that blood samples to be used for the partial prothrombin time test should remain at room temperature to avoid cold activation, and should be tested within 60 min (D'Angelo, 1993). The prothrombin time (PT) of a series of 230 specimens collected in buffered trisodium citrate (NCCLS, 1991b; Thomson, 1991) was measured shortly after the specimens were drawn and remeasured after 12 h of storage at room temperature. An initial mean PT of 16.05 s was found, standard deviation 4.2 s; after 12 h of storage a mean PT of 15.90 s was measured, standard deviation 3.9 s (Simmons, 1993). The measurement results are presented in Fig. 12.2. The addition of buffer to the anticoagulant has been reported to prolong the PT (Thomson, 1991), and control plasmas should thus be collected into the same anticoagulant that is used to collect the patient samples (NCCLS, 1991e).

Transferring specimens from the patient to the laboratory is usually done by messenger. In some institutions, however, pneumatic tube systems may be used to move specimens more rapidly over longer distances. In such systems, hemolysis may occur unless the tubes are completely filled and prevented from moving inside the carrier (Steige and Jones, 1971; Pragay and Edwards, 1974; Greendyke and Banzhaf, 1977; Lapidus and MacIndoe, 1978; Poznanski, Smith and Bodley, 1978; Weaver and Miller, 1978; Bruner and Kissling, 1980). Pneumatic tube systems should be designed to eliminate sharp curves and sudden stops.

Occasionally specimens are sent to a referral laboratory. Before a referral laboratory is used, the quality of its work should be verified by the referring laboratory (NCCLS, 1991a), and licensing and proficiency testing results should be reviewed. All specimens collected and sent to a referral laboratory should be stored at 4–8°C, or the plasma should be separated and frozen if the analyte is labile. The courier service picking up the specimens should transport them in an insulated container with cold packs to maintain a temperature less than 10°C. Such specimens should take no longer than 3 h to reach the testing laboratory for most hematological tests. If the required test is temperature-labile, the courier service should transport the specimens in the frozen state using a separate, insulated container with dry ice.

12.7.2 Specimen shipping

When shipping specimens over long distances, care has to be taken in both packing and in controlling the temperature of the specimens. All biological fluids, including blood specimens, should be packaged in sealed containers wrapped in absorbent material. The specimen containers should be protected from breakage by placing them in a screw-capped metal tube and by inserting extra absorbent material around and between the tubes so that they are tightly packed.

In general, whole blood for hematological testing is unsuitable for long distance shipping, and every effort should be made to locate a local laboratory that can test the specimen. If a plasma or serum sample is sent, the specimen is best shipped in a plastic container, fully labelled, accompanied by a clear test request form, packaged and placed in an insulated container surrounded by several blocks of dry ice.

Shipping containers must be capable of withstanding the weight and shock commonly associated with handling and shipment. Corrugated fibreboard, paperboard, polystyrene boxes or other materials with similar rigid characteristics are suitable if they securely enclose the specimen containers. Polystyrene or other materials with similar insulating qualities are suitable for shipping frozen and refrigerated specimens. The size and shape of the shipping container are critical. The container must permit the release of CO_2 gas and prevent the build-up of pressure that could rupture the package. Dry ice is the most convenient substance for maintaining a temperature of −70°C. The amount of dry ice needed depends on the insulating qualities of the shipping container and the length of time the specimen must be kept frozen. Excess air space or packaging material (e.g. newspaper, polystyrene chips) in the shipping container will cause dry ice to dissipate at a faster rate. A polystyrene container with a wall thickness of 2.5 cm and an interior capacity of 2 litres filled with a 5-lb block of dry ice will keep a specimen frozen for 48 h when the container is stored at room temperature (NCCLS, 1985).

Various laws and national postal regulations apply to the shipment of biological specimens. Airlines have rigid regulations covering the transport of specimens and deem dry ice to be a hazardous material. Thus, transporting most clinical specimens is affected by regulations (NCCLS, 1985; CDC, 1993). In the USA, the Department of Health and Human Services approved proposed Federal Regulations on Interstate Shipment of Etiologic Agents in 1992. Similar regulations are proposed by a Technical Committee of CEN on a European Standard for mailing packages for medical and biological specimens.

12.7.3 Specimen processing

Multiple factors associated with handling and processing blood specimens can introduce test result imprecision or a systematic bias after the specimen has been collected but before the test is done. Several potential problem areas in handling and processing of blood specimens have been documented (Martinek, 1966; Mathies, 1974; Laessig et al., 1976a,b,c; Spencer, Nelson and Konicke, 1976; Calam, 1977). Specific concerns are related to prolonged contact of cells with serum or plasma, concentration changes due to evaporation or cell lysis, the use of serum separation devices, analyte deterioration because of improper storage, and the use of certain anticoagulants. Recognizing and controlling these variables will reduce error and contribute to the medical usefulness of patient test results.

In general, blood specimens should be centrifuged within 60 min after collection. However, to obtain serum, the tube should be left to stand for a minimum of 30 min to allow clot formation. This minimum time should be extended to 60 min if the collected specimen has been chilled (2–8°C). When the collection device contains a clotting activator, the minimum waiting time before centrifuging the specimen can be as short as 5 min (thrombin) or 15 min (glass or silica particles) (Calam, 1977); anticoagulated specimens can be centrifuged within minutes after they are collected. If adequate time for clotting to occur is not allowed, latent fibrin formation may be

a problem for many of the instrument systems used by laboratories.

Tubes of blood should be kept in a vertical position with the stopper up. This promotes complete clot formation and reduces agitation of the tube contents, which in turn reduces the potential for haemolysis. The stopper is also less likely to come off the tube by accident.

Chilling specimens inhibits the metabolism of blood cells and stabilizes some labile constituents. Thus whole-blood specimens must not be chilled unless there are documented recommendations for doing so. To chill specimens adequately, they should be in either crushed ice or a mixture of ice and water. Good contact between the cooling medium and the specimen is essential. Large cubes of ice instead of water are not acceptable because of inadequate contact between coolant and specimen. The specimen must be completely immersed in the cooling medium.

Blood contact with tube stoppers may be a source of contamination. Current manufacturing practices are helping to eliminate problems of this type. Thus, for example, special tubes have been designed for trace element determinations to eliminate stopper interference for these assays (Helman, Wallick and Reingold, 1971; Hughes, Wease and Troxler, 1976). Vigorous handling of collected specimens must be avoided to minimize hemolysis.

Specimens from patients with hepatitis and other potentially transmissible diseases should be explicitly labelled and the label attached to the specimen container and the requisition to give high visibility to these particular specimens. It is essential to ensure that this identification also accompanies the specimen through successive handling and processing steps.

Exposure to light, which causes breakdown of certain analytes, in particular bilirubin must be avoided. This is especially important when the specimen is from an icteric newborn who is being monitored to decide on the necessity of an exchange transfusion. Specimens must be protected from light with, for example, aluminum foil wrap.

Under the following conditions blood specimens are not acceptable for testing purposes and should be rejected. Professional judgement at the laboratory supervisory level must be exercised in applying these criteria:

1. Inadequate specimen identification, e.g. a tube is not labelled or is mislabelled.
2. An inadequate volume of blood collected into an additive tube. The amount of additive placed in a tube is intended for a certain volume of blood; if the quantity of blood is less than is required, the excess amount of additive could negate the accuracy of the test result, e.g. pro-

thrombin time (Humphreys and McPhedran, 1970) and MCV.

3. Using the wromg collection tube when method-specific specimens are required. The wrong order of draw during multiple blood specimen collection can invalidate test results because of contamination by the additive (Calam and Cooper, 1982). When drawing several specimens during a venepuncture, draw blood culture tubes first, non-additive tubes second, EDTA-containing tubes third and oxalate/fluoride-containing tubes last (NCCLS, 1990b).

4. Excessive hemolysis can result from a difficult venepuncture or from improper handling of the collected blood. A complete blood count, or plasma hemoglobin determination should not be carried out on visibly haemolysed specimens, unless the clinical history suggests hemolysis may be present, e.g. hemolytic anemia, transfusion reaction.

5. Improper transportation, e.g. a specimen that should have been chilled is received by the laboratory unchilled.

All tubes should be kept closed until after centrifugation, either by leaving the tube stopper in place or by using a suitable tube closure.

Separating serum or plasma from cells is based on a time-honoured practice of empirical observation. The recommended time is 10 ± 5 min at 1000–1200 × g (NCCLS, 1990b). However, the manufacturer's literature should be consulted to check specific recommendations for separating devices integrated into collection tubes or inserted into the blood before centrifugation. Relative centrifugal force (rcf) ('g-force') is a more meaningful term than revolutions per minute (rpm). The rpm is of limited use without an indication of the centrifuge model and its specific rotor, head, or effective radius: $rcf = 1.118 \times 10^{-5} \times r \times N^2$ where r = rotating radius in cm, and N = speed of rotation (rpm).

Certain analytes require chilled conditions. Laboratories should have access to temperature-controlled centrifuges. Centrifuges often generate more internal heat than is appropriate for analyte stability. Unless documentation supports a specific temperature for a specific analyte, a centrifuge temperature setting of 20–25°C is adequate.

All tubes of blood must be kept closed until after centrifugation. Leave the tube stopper in place, or place a suitable tube closure on the tube. Inaccuracies in test results can occur when the tube stopper is removed because of a change in specimen pH. Keeping tubes closed also prevents evaporation and aerosol formation during centrifugation.

The multiplicity of laboratory tests makes it mandatory that the laboratory staff consult specific references to determine the exact handling and storage conditions necessary to ensure the stability of specific analytes (Juul, 1967; Gianpietro et al., 1980; Rossing and Foster, 1980).

Many analytes are stable for up to 48 h when serum is left in contact with the cell mass; many are not (e.g. glucose, chloride, potassium, iron). As a general rule, carefully separate serum or plasma from the clot or cells within 2 h after collecting the specimen. Pipetting is recommended to remove the sample. Separated plasma or serum should be visually free of erythrocytes.

If a test cannot be carried out within 5 h after the plasma or serum has been separated from the cells or the clot, storing plasma or serum at 2–8°C is acceptable for most analytes. For storage beyond 24 h, freeze the specimen at −20°C. For certain labile analytes, e.g. folate, vitamin B_{12}, it may be necessary to refrigerate or freeze the specimen immediately after centrifugation.

Plasma or serum specimens must be kept covered at all times to eliminate possible exogenous contamination and to prevent evaporation.

12.7.4 Serum separation devices

Serum separation devices are used extensively in the clinical chemistry laboratory (Laessig et al., 1976d) but have not been generally accepted in the hematology and immunohematology laboratory. Interference of gel barrier devices with the direct and indirect antiglobulin test and with compatibility testing has been described (Renton and Handcock, 1957; Geisland and Milam, 1980). A density gradient system (SIMWASH™) has recently been described that does not cause false-positive antiglobulin tests and will, on some occasions, allow demonstration of the cell-bound IgG that may otherwise escape detection (Treacy and Marsh, 1987).

12.8 Storage of specimens

In recent years it has become apparent that well-characterized, properly stored biological fluid and tissue collections are valuable as databases for epidemiologic studies of newly recognized or emerging diseases, e.g. Legionnaire's disease, acquired immunodeficiency syndrome. Such collections can effectively be stored in a 'specimen bank'. This section is limited to intermediate- and long-term storage of serum; cryopreservation of cells and other biological materials has been extensively documented by Hurn (1968) and Ashwood-Smith and Farrant (1980).

The eutectic point of human serum lies between −18 and −22°C. Therefore, to ensure a solid core of frozen material and to prevent cyclical freezing/ thawing of core material, which is damaging to protiens, serum collections should be stored at temperatures well below $-20°C$. Although storage at $-35°C$ $-45°C$ would be adequate, storage at $-70°C$ has become popular (Cowley, Timson and Sawdye, 1961).

12.8.1 Short- and intermediate-term storage

Specimens intended for testing and that are not part of an organized study specimen subset should be stored at temperatures dictated by the stability of the specific analyte, e.g. $4-8°C$ or $-20°C$. Refrigerators and freezers must have continuous temperature monitoring and an alarm system. Temperature recorder sensors or the sensing end of thermometers should be placed in no more than 250 ml of liquid (refrigerators) so that the heat transfer characteristics are similar to blood and blood component containers (NCCLS, 1987), or in a container of ice or antifreeze in water (freezers). The use of at least two temperature sensors is recommended for large refrigerators, freezers and walk-in cold rooms.

12.8.2 Long-term storage

If specimens are part of a study for which long-term storage is desirable or required, particular attention must be paid to sterile collection and processing techniques. Specimens should be divided into several separate aliquots of $0.25-1.0$ ml to avoid repeated freezing and thawing when small amounts are retrieved for testing. Under no circumstances should storage take place in a so-called 'frost-free' environment. 'Frost-free' freezers are characterized by intermittent defrost cycles. These will cause specimens to become desiccated with resultant denaturation of protein material.

Specimen aliquots should be placed in suitable plastic cryovials equipped with a seal and an externally threaded cap. When $-70°C$ storage is not available, lyophilization and storage at $-20°C$ is an acceptable alternative.

12.9　Laboratory infection precautions

The increasing prevalence of infections such as hepatitis and human immunodeficiency virus (HIV) increases the risk that laboratory workers, phlebotomists and other health-care workers will be exposed to blood from patients infected with such agents. Health care workers should, therefore, consider that all patients may be infected with HIV and/or other blood-borne pathogens and adhere rigorously to infection-control precautions minimizing the risk of exposure to blood and body fluids of all patients (CDC, 1987; NCCLS, 1991f).

HIV has been isolated from blood, semen, vaginal secretions, saliva, tears, breast milk, cerebrospinal fluid, amniotic fluid and urine. Epidemiologic evidence has implicated only blood, semen, vaginal secretions and possibly breast milk in transmission. Standard sterilization and disinfection procedures for patient-care equipment currently recommended in a variety of health care settings are adequate to sterilize or disinfect items contaminated with blood or other body fluids from persons infected with blood-borne pathogens, including HIV (Garner and Favero, 1985). Studies have shown that HIV is inactivated rapidly after being exposed to commonly used chemical germicides at concentrations that are much lower than used in practice (Spire *et al.*, 1984, 1985; Martin, McDougal and Loskoski, 1985; McDougal *et al.*, 1985). In addition to commercially available germicides, a solution of sodium hypochlorite (household bleach) prepared daily is an inexpensive and effective germicide. Concentrations ranging from 1:100 to 1:10 of household bleach are effective, depending on the amount of organic material (e.g. blood, mucus) present on the surfaces to be cleaned and disinfected.

Since medical history and examination cannot reliably identify all patients infected with HIV or other blood-borne pathogens, precautions should be consistently used when collecting and handling material from all patients.

References

AABB (1987) Standards for Blood Banks and Transfusion Services (12th edn) pp. 8–14; 17–20. Washington, D. C.: American Association of Blood Banks.

AABB (1990) Quality assurance. In Technical Manual (10th edn), pp. 469–484. Washington, D. C.: American Association of Blood Banks.

Ashwood-Smith, M. J. and Farrant, J. (eds) (1980) *Low Temperature Preservation in Medicine and Biology*. Baltimore, MD: University Park Press; Tunbridge Wells, Kent, UK: Pitman Medical Ltd.

Astrup, T. (1973) The effect of physical activity on blood coagulation and fibrinolysis. In: Naughton, J. P., Hellerstein, H. K. and Mohler, I. C. (eds) *Exercise Testing and Exercise Training in Coronary Heart Disease*, P. 169. New York: Academic Press.

Bowie, E. J. W., Tauxe, W. N., Sjoberg, W. E. *et al.* (1963) Daily variation in the concentration of iron in serum. *Am. J. Clin. Pathol.*, **40**, 491–494.

Brittin, G. M., Brecher, G., Johnson, C. A. *et al.* (1969) Stability of blood in commonly used anticoagulants. *Am. J. Clin. Pathol.*, **52**, 690–694.

Broden, P. N. (1992) Anticoagulant and tube effect on selected blood cell parameters using Sysmex NE-Series™ instruments. Sysmex Journal International, **2**, 112–119.

Bruner, K. W. and Kissling, C. W. (1980). Evaluation of a pneumatic-tube system for delivery of blood specimens to the blood bank. *Am. J. Clin. Pathol.*, **73**, 593–596.

Buckell, M. and Elliott, F. A. (1959) Effect of butter lipaemia on the rate of clot lysis in normal males. *Lancet*, **1**, 662–663.

Calam, R. R. (1977) Reviewing the importance of specimen collection. *J. Am. Med. Technol.*, **39**, 297–302.

Calam, R. R. and Cooper, M. H. (1982) Recommended

Bruner, K. W. and Kissling, C. W. (1980). Evaluation of a pneumatic-tube system for delivery of blood specimens to the blood bank. *Am. J. Clin. Pathol.*, **73**, 593–596.

Buckell, M. and Elliott, F. A. (1959) Effect of butter lipaemia on the rate of clot lysis in normal males. *Lancet*, **1**, 662–663.

Calam, R. R. (1977) Reviewing the importance of specimen collection. *J. Am. Med. Technol.*, **39**, 297–302.

Calam, R. R. and Cooper, M. H. (1982) Recommended 'order of draw' for collecting blood specimens into additive-containing tubes. *Clin. Chem.*, **28**, 1399.

Centers for Disease Control (1987) Recommendations for prevention of HIV transmission in healthcare settings. *Morbidity and Mortality Weekly Report* **36** (Suppl. 2S): 3S–18S.

Centers for Disease Control (1992) Guidelines for the performance of CD4+ T-cell determinations in persons with human immunodeficiency virus infection. *Morbidity and Mortality Weekly* Report 41 (Suppl. RR-8): 1–17.

Centers for Disease Control and Prevention (1993) *Reference and Disease Surveillance.* U.S. Department of Health and Human Services, Public Health Service, Centers for Disease Control and Prevention, National Center for Infectious Diseases, Atlanta, Georgia, 30333.

Cohle, S. D., Saleem, A. and Makhaoui, D. E. (1981) Effects of storage of blood on stability of hematologic parameters. *Am. J. Clin. Pathol.* **76**: 67–69.

Cowley, C. W., Timson, W. J. and Sawdye, J. A. (1961) Ultra rapid cooling techniques in the freezing of biological materials. *Biodynamics* **8**, 317–329.

Cruikshank, J. M. (1970) The effect of parity on the leucocyte count in pregnant and non-pregnant women. *Br. J. of Haematol.* **18**: 531–540.

D'Angelo, A. (1993) Coagulation testing in the clinical chemistry laboratory. *IFCC, Journal of the International Federation of Clinical Chemistry*, **5**, 62–73.

Dawson, J. B. and Walker, B. E. (1969). Direct determination of zinc in whole blood, plasma and urine by atomic absorption spectroscopy. *Clin. Chim. Acta*, **26**, 465–475.

Diggs, L. W. and Bell, A. (1980). Bone marrow and morphology of bone marrow cells. In: Schmidt, R. M. (ed.) *CRC Handbook Series in Clinical Laboratory Science, Section I: Hematology. Volume II*, pp.3–61. Boca Raton, FL: CRC Press.

Doyle, C. T. (1967) The effect of blood volume and choice of anticoagulant on the PCV, MCHC, and total white cell count. *J. Med. Sci.*, **6**, 429–433.

ECCLS (1987) Standard for Specimen Collection. Part 2: Blood Specimen by Venepuncture. ECCLS Document, Vol.4, No.1. Berlin: Beuth Verlag.

Eisenberg, S. (1963) The effect of posture and position of the venous sampling site on the hematocrit and serum protein concentration. *J. Lab. Clin. Med.* **61**, 755–760.

Eklund, L. G., Eklund, B. and Kauser, L. (1971) Time course for the change in hemoglobin concentration with change in posture. *Acta Med. Scand.*, **190**, 335–336.

Elking, M. P. and Kabat, H. F. (1968) Drug induced modifications of laboratory test values. *Am. J. Hosp. Pharmacy*, **25**, 484–519.

Elwood, P. D. (1962) Diurnal hemoglobin variation in normal male subjects. *Clin. Sci.* **23**, 379–382.

Engstrom, A. W. (1968) Effect of hemolysis on the one-stage prothrombin time. *Am. J. Clin. Pathol.*, **49**: 742–745.

Fearnley, G. R., Balmforth, G. and Fearnley, E. (1957) Evidence of a diurnal fibrinolytic rhythm, with a simple method of measuring natural fibrinolysis. *Clin. Sci.*, **16**, 645–650.

Gambino, S. R., Dire, J. J., Monteleone, M. *et al.* (1965) The Westergren sedimentation rate using K_3EDTA. *Am. J. Clin. Pathol.* **43**, 173–175.

Garner, J. S. and Favero, M. S. (1985) Guideline for handwashing and hospital environmental control, 1985. Atlanta: Public Health Service, Centers for Disease Control, HHS Publication No. 99–1117.

Garrey, W. E. and Bryan, W. R. (1935) Variations in white blood cell counts. *Physiol. Rev.*, **15**, 597–638.

Geisland, J. R. and Milam, J. D. (1980) Spuriously positive direct antiglobulin test caused by use of silicone gel. *Transfusion* **20**, 711–713.

Gianpictro, O., Navalesi, R., Buzzigoll *et al.* (1980) Decrease in plasma glucose concentration during storage at −20 °C. *Clin. Chem.* **26**, 1710–1712.

Goossens, W., van Duppen, V. and Verwilghen, R. L. (1991) K_2- or K_3-EDTA: the anticoagulant of choice in routine haematology? *Clin. Lab. Haematol.*, **13**, 291–295.

Grannis, G. F. (1970) Plasma fibrinogen: determination, normal values, physiopathologic shifts, and fluctuations. *Clin. Chem.*, **16**, 486–494.

Greendyke, R. M. and Banzhaf, J. C. (1977) Immunologic studies of blood samples transported by a pneumatic tube system. *Am. J. Clin. Pathol.* **68**, 508–510.

Hamilton, L. D., Gubler, C. J., Cartwright, G. E. *et al.*, (1950) Diurnal variation in plasma iron level of man. Proc. Soc. Exp. Biol. Med. **75**, 65–8.

Hardisty, R. M. and Ingram, G. I. C. (1965) *Bleeding Disorders, Investigation and Management*, Oxford: Blackwell Scientific Publications p.162.

Hathaway, W. E. and Bonnar, J. (1978) Technical aspects of blood coagulation. In: Hathaway, W. E. and Bonnar, J. (eds), *Perinatal Coagulation*, New York: Grune & Stratton, p.15.

Hawkins, R. I. (1972) Smoking, platelets and thrombosis. *Nature* **236**, 450–452.

Helman, E. Z., Wallick, D. K. and Reingold, I. M. (1971) Vacutainer contamination in trace element studies. *Clin. Chem.* **17**, 61–62.

Helman, N. and Rubenstein, L. S. (1975) The effects of age, sex, and smoking on erythrocytes and leukocytes. *Am. J. Clin. Pathol.* **63**, 35–44.

Heyns, A. du P., Berg, D. J. van der, Kleynhans, P. H. T. *et al.* (1981) Unsuitability of evacuated tubes for monitoring heparin therapy by activated partial thromboplastin time. *J. Clin. Pathol.* **34**, 63–68.

Hicks, J. R., Rowland, G. L. and Buffone, G. J. (1976) Evaluation on a new blood collection device (microtainer) that is suited for pediatric use. *Clin. Chem.* **22**, 2034–2036.

Horder, K. and Klorder, M. (1970) Plasma haptoglobin and physical exercise: changes in healthy individuals concomitant with strenuous march. *Clin. Chim. Acta*, **30**, 369–372.

Hughes, R. O., Wease, D. F. and Troxler, R. G. (1976) Collection of blood uncontaminated with Ca, Cu, Mg, or Zn, for trace metal analysis. *Clin. Chem.*, **22**, 691–692.

Humphreys, R. E. and McPhedran, P. (1970) False evaluation of partial thromboplastin time and prothrombin time. *JAMA*, **214**, 1702–1704.

Hurkat, P. C. and Jain, M. (1973) Some haematological changes during exercise. *Ind. J. Physiol. Pharmacol.* **17**, 71–74.

Hurn, B. A. L. (1968) *Storage of Blood.* London: Academic Press.

ICSH (1977) Recommendation for measurement of erythrocyte sedimentation rate of human blood. *Am. J. Clin. Pathol.* **66**, 505–507.

ICSH (1982) Standardization of blood specimen collection procedure for reference values. *Clin. Lab. Haematol.* **4**, 83–86.

ICSH (1993) Recommendations of the International Council for Standardization in Haematology for ethylenediaminetetraacetic acid anticoagulation of blood for blood cell counting and sizing. *Am. J. Clin. Pathol.*, **100**, 371–372.

Ingram, G.I.C. and Hills, M. (1976a) Reference method for the one-stage prothrombin time test on human blood. *Thromb. Haemost.*, **36**, 237–238.

Ingram, G.I.C., and Hills, M. (1976b) The prothrombin time test. Effect of varying citrate concentration. *Thromb. Haemost.*, **36**, 230–236.

Isager, H. and Hagerup, L. (1971) Relationship between smoking and high packed cell volume and haemoglobin levels. *Scand. J. Haematol.* **8**, 241–244.

ISO (1987) Evacuated tubes for blood specimen collection. Draft International Standard ISO/DIS 6710. Geneva: ISO.

Jensen, R. J., Adam, B., Turner, W. E. *et al.* (1984) An evaluation of different filter paper lots used for blood spot collection during the last five years. In: Ming, S. Chan (ed.) *National Newborn Screening Symposium.* Jacksonville, FL: Florida Department of Health and Rehabilitation Services.

Jones, J. D. (1980) Factors that affect clinical laboratory values. *J. Occup. Med.* **22**, 316–320.

Juul, P. (1967) Stability of plasma enzymes during storage. *Clin. Chem.*, **13**, 416–422.

Karvonen, M. J. and Kunnas, M. (1952) Erythrocyte and haemoglobin changes during protracted heavy muscular work. *Ann. Med. Exp. Biol. Fenn.* **30**, 180–185.

Karvonen, M. J. and Kunnas, M. (1953) Factor analysis of haematological changes in heavy manual work. *Acta Physiol. Scand.* **29**, 220–231.

Kennedy, J. B., Machara, K. T. and Baker, A. M. (1981) Cell and platelet stability in disodium and trisodium EDTA. *Am. J. Med. Technol.*, **47**, 89–93.

Kennon, B., Shipp, M. E. and Hetherington, D. C. (1937) A study of the white blood cell picture in six young men. *Am. J. Physiol.* **118**, 690–696.

Koepke, J. A. and Landay, A. L. (1989) Precision and accuracy of absolute lymphocyte counts. *Clin. Immunol. Immunopathol.*, **52**, 1927.

Koepke, J. A. and Smith-Jones, M. (1992) Lymphocyte counting in HIV-positive individuals. *Sysmex J. Int.*, **2**, 71–74.

Koepke, J. A., Bull, B. S., Gilmer, P. R., Jr *et al.* (1978) Hematology: essentials of quality assurance. In: S. L. Inhorn (ed.). *Quality Assurance Practices for Health Laboratories.* American Public Health Association, Washington, DC, p. 695.

Koepke, J. A., Rodgers, J. L. and Ollivier, M. J. (1974) Pre-instrumental variables in coagulation testing. *Am. J. Clin. Pathol.*, **64**, 591–596.

Koepke, J. A., van Assendelft, O. W., Bull, B. S. *et al.* (1988/89) Standardization of EDTA anticoagulation for Blood counting procedures. *Labmedica*, **5** (Dec/Jan), 15–17.

Laessig, R. H., Hassemer, D. J., Paskey, T. A. *et al.* (1976a) The effect of 0.1 and 1.0 percent erythrocytes and hemolysis on serum chemistry values. *Am. J. Clin. Pathol.*, **66**, 639–644.

Laessig, R. H., Hassemer, D. G., Westgard, J. O. *et al.* (1976b) Assessment of the serum separator tube as an intermediate storage device within the laboratory. *Am. J. Clin. Pathol.*, **66**, 653–657.

Laessig, R. H., Indrikson, A. A., Hassemer, D. J. *et al.* (1976c) Changes in serum values as a result of prolonged contact with the clot. *Am. J. Clin. Pathol.*, **66**, 598–604.

Laessig, R. H., Westgard, J. O., Carey, R. N. *et al.* (1976d) Assessment of serum separator devices for obtaining serum specimens suitable for clinical analysis. *Clin. Chem.*, **22**, 235–239.

Lampasso, J. A. (1968) Changes in hematologic values induced by storage of ethylenediaminetetraacetate human blood for varying periods of time. *Am. J. Clin. Pathol.*, **49**, 443–447.

Lange, H. F. (1946) The normal plasma protein values and their relative variations. *Acta Med. Scand.*, Suppl. 176: 1–202.

Lapidus, B. M. and MacIndoe, R. C. (1978) A multi-station gravity delivery system. *Am. J. Clin. Pathol.*, **69**, 73–76.

Lloyd, E. (1982) The determination of leukocyte morphology with time – its effect on the differential count. *Lab. Perspect.*, **1**, 13–16.

Lugton, R. A. (1987) The ESR reexamined. *Med. Lab. Sci.*, **44**, 207–214.

Martin, L. S., McDougal, J. S. and Loskoski, S. L. (1985) Disinfection and inactivation of the human T lymphotropic virus type III/lymphadenopathy-associated virus. *J. Infect. Dis.*, **152**, 400–403.

Martinek, R. G. (1966) Specimens for clinical laboratory analysis: collection and preservation. *Postgrad. Med.*, **39**, A46–56.

Mathies, J. C. (1974) Evaluation of a new device for rapidly separating serum or plasma from blood. *Clin. Chem.* **20**, 1573–1576.

McCarthy, E. F. and Van Slyke, D. D. (1939) Diurnal variations of hemoglobin in the blood of normal men. *J. Biol. Chem.* **128**, 567–572.

McDougal, J. S., Martin, L. S., Cort, S. P. *et al.* (1985) Thermal inactivation of the acquired immunodeficiency syndrome virus-III/lymphadenopathy-associated virus, with special reference to antihemophilic factor. *J. Clin. Invest.* **76**, 875–877.

Milhorat, A. T., Small, S. M. and Dietheim, O. (1942) Leukocytosis during various emotional states. *Arch. Neurol. Psychiatr.*, **47**, 779–792.

Missen, A. W. and Dixon, S. J. (1974) Contamination of blood samples by plasticizer in evacuated tubes. *Clin. Chem.* **20**, 1247–1249.

Mole, R. H. (1945) Diurnal and sampling variations in the determination of haemoglobin. *J. Physiol. (London)*, **104**, 1–5.

Mollison, P. L., Engelfriet, C. P. and Contreras, M. (1987) *Blood Transfusion in Clinical Medicine*, 8th ed. Oxford: Blackwell Scientific Publications, pp.79, 147.

Myhre, L. G., Dill, D. B., Hall, F. G. *et al.* (1970) Blood volume changes during a three-week residence at high altitude. *Clin. Chem.* **16**, 7–14.

NCCLS (1985) H5-A2. Procedures for the Domestic Handling and Transport of Diagnostic Specimens and Etiologic Agents. Approved Standard. Villanova, PA: NCCLS (ISBN 1–56238–037–0).

NCCLS (1986) H21-A. Collection, Transport, and Preparation of Blood Specimens for Coagulation Testing and Performance of Coagulation Assays. Approved Guideline. Villanova, PA: NCCLS.

NCCLS (1987) I16-T. Temperature Monitoring and Recording in Blood Banks. Tentative Guideline. Villanova, PA: NCCLS (ISBN 1–56238–077.X).

NCCLS (1988) H24-T. Additives to Blood Collection Devices: Heparin. Tentative Standard. Villanova, PA: NCCLS (ISBN 1–56238–053–2)

NCCLS (1990a) H14-A2. Use of Devices for Collection of Skin Puncture Blood Specimens. Approved Guideline. Villanova, PA: NCCLS (ISBN 1-56238-109-1).

NCCLS (1990b) H18-A. Procedures for the Handling and Processing of Blood Specimens. Approved Standard. Villanova, PA: NCCLS (ISBN 1-56238-110-5).

NCCLS (1991a) GP9-T. Selecting and Evaluating a Referral Laboratory. Tentative Guideline. Villanova, P: NCCLS (ISBN 1-56238-139-3).

NCCLS (1991b) H1-A3. Standard for Evacuated Tubes for Blood Specimen Collection. Approved Standard. Villanova, PA: NCCLS (ISBN 1-56238-107-5). American National Standard.

NCCLS (1991c) H3-A3. Procedures for the Collection of Diagnostic Blood Specimens by Venipuncture. Approved Standard. Villanova, PA: NCCLS (ISBN 1-56238-108-3).

NCCLS (1991d) H4-A3. Procedures for the Collection of Diagnostic Blood Specimens by Skin Puncture. Approved Standard. Villanova, PA: NCCLS (ISBN 1-56238-111-3).

NCCLS (1991e) H21-A2. Collection, Transport, and Processing of Blood Specimens for Coagulation Testing and Performance of Coagulation Assays. Approved Guideline. Villanova, PA: NCCLS (ISBN 1-56238-129-6).

NCCLS (1991f) M29-T2. Protection of Laboratory Workers from Infectious Disease Transmitted by Blood, Body Fluids, and Tissue. Tentative Guideline. Villanova, PA: NCCLS (ISBN 1-56238-023-7).

NCCLS (1992a) H11-A2. Percutaneous Collection of Arterial Blood for Laboratory Analysis. Approved Standard. Villanova, PA: NCCLS (ISBN 1-56238-043-5).

NCCLS (1992b) H20-A. Reference Leukocyte Differential Count (Proportional) and Evaluation of Instrumental Methods. Approved Standard. Villanova, PA: NCCLS (ISBN 1-56238-131-8).

NCCLS (1992c) H35-T. Additives to Blood Collection Devices: EDTA. Tentative Standard. Villanova, PA: NCCLS (ISBN 1-56238--162-8).

NCCLS (1992d) LA4-A2. Blood Collection on Filter Paper for Neonatal Screening Programs. Approved Standard. Villanova, PA: NCCLS (ISBN 1-56238-157-1).

NCCLS (1993a) H2-A3. Methods for the Erythrocyte Sedimentation Rate (ESR) Test. Approved Standard. Villanova, PA: NCCLS (ISBN 1–56238–198–9).

NCCLS (1993b) H7-A2. Procedure for Determining Packed Cell Volume by the Microhematocrit Method. Approved Standard. Villanova, PA: NCCLS (ISBN 1–56238–199-7).

Nelson, N. M. (1976) Respiration and circulation after birth. In: Smith, C. A. and Nelson, N. M. (eds). *The Physiology of the Newborn Infant*, 4th edn, Springfield, ILL.: Charles C. Thomas. p. 158.

Nevaril, C. G., Lynch, E. C., Alfrey, C. P. *et al.* (1968) Erythrocyte damage and destruction induced by shearing stress. *J. Lab. Clin. Med.*, **71**, 784–790.

Oh, W. and Lind, J. (1976) Venous and capillary hematocrit in newborn infants and placental transfusion. *Acta Paediatr. Scand.*, **55**, 38–48.

Oski, F. A. and Naiman, J. L. (eds) (1982) *Hematologic Problems in the Newborn*, 3rd edn, Philadelphia: W. B. Saunders. pp. 6–7.

Palmer, R. N. and Gralnick, H. R. (1981) Cold-induced contact surface activation of the prothrombin time in whole blood. *Blood* **59**, 38–42.

Poznanski, W., Smith, F. and Bodley, F. (1978) Implementation of a pneumatic tube system for transport of blood specimens. *Am. J. Clin. Pathol.*, **70**, 291–295.

Pragay, D. A., Brinkley, S., Rejent, T. *et al.* (1979) Vacutainer contamination revisited. *Clin. Chem.*, **25**, 2058.

Pragay, D. A. and Edwards, L. (1974) Evaluation of an

improved pneumatic tube system suitable for transportation of blood specimens. *Clin. Chem.*, **20**, 57–60.

Priest, J. B., Tjien, D. D. *et al.* (1982) Exercise-induced changes in common laboratory tests, *Am. J. Clin. Pathol.*, **77**, 285–289.

Refsum, H. E., Meen, H. D. and Stromme, S. B. (1973) Whole blood, serum and erythrocyte magnesium concentration after repeated heavy exercise of long duration. *Scand. J. Clin. Lab. Invest.* **32**, 123–127.

Refsum, H. E., Treit, B., Meen, H. D. *et al.* (1973) Serum electrolyte fluid and acid-base balance after prolonged heavy exercise and low environmental temperature. *Scand. J. Clin. Lab. Invest.*, **32** 117–122.

Renton, P.H. and Handcock, J. A. (1957), Antibody-like effects of colloidal silica. *Vox Sang.*, 117–124.

Rodkey, F. L. and O'Neal, J. D. (1974) Effects of carboxyhemoglobin on determination of methemoglobin in blood. *Biochem. Med.* **9**, 261–270.

Rorsman, H. (1962) Normal variation in the count of circulating basophil leukocytes in man. *Acta Allergol.* (Kbh), **17**, 49–65.

Rossing, R. H. and Foster, D. M. (1980) The stability of clinical chemistry specimens during refrigerated storage for 24 hours. *Am. J. Clin. Pathol.*, **73**, 91–95.

Sacker, L. S. (1975) Specimen collection. In Lewis, S. M. and Coster, J. F. (eds) *Quality Control in Haematology.* London: Academic Press, pp. 211–229.

Simmons, A. (1982) Blood Storage. *Am. J. Clin. Pathol.* **77**, 116–119.

Simmons, A. (1993) Prothrombin time stability and precision using buffered sodium citrate. *Labmedica*, **10** (Nov/Dec), 22–26.

Simmons, A., Wiseman, J. D. and Fay, R. (1978) The stability of hematological parameters when tested by the Coulter model S. *Int. Soc. Haematol. Meet.*, Paris, FPS 371:56.

Smith, J. R. and Landaw, S. R. (1978) Smoker's polycythemia. *N. Eng. J. Med.* **298**, 6–10.

Spencer, W. W., Nelson, G. H. and Konicke, K. (1976) Evaluation of a new system ('Corvac') for separating serum from blood for routine laboratory procedures. *Clin. Chem.* **22**, 1012–1016.

Spire, B., Montagnier, L., Barre-Sinoussi, F. and Chermann, J. C. (1984) Inactivation of lymphadenopathy-associated virus by chemical disinfectants. *Lancet*, **2**, 899–901.

Spire, B., Barre-Sinoussi, F., Dormont, D. *et al.* (1985). Inactivation of lymphadenopathy-associated virus by heat, gamma rays, and ultraviolet light. *Lancet*, **1**, 188–189.

Statland, B. E., Bokelund, H. and Winkel, P. (1974) Factors contributing to intra-individual variation of serum constituents. IV. Effects of posture and tourniquet application on variation of serum constituents in healthy subjects. *Clin. Chem.*, **20**, 1513–1519.

Statland, B. E. and Winkel, P. (1977a) Effects of preanalytical factors on the intra-individual variation of analytes in the blood of healthy subjects: consideration of preparation of subject and time of venipuncture: *CRC Crit. Rev. Clin. Lab. Sci.* **8**, 105–144.

Statland, B. E. and Winkel, P. (1977b) The relationship of the day-to-day variation of serum iron concentration values to the iron binding capacity values in a group of healthy young women. *Am. J. Clin. Pathol.* **67**, 84–90.

Statland, B. E., Winkel, P. and Bokelund, H. (1976) Variations of serum iron concentration in young healthy men: within-day and day-to-day changes. *Clin. Biochem.* **9**, 26–29.

Statland, B. E., Winkel, P. and Killingsworth, L. M. (1976) Factors contributing to intra-individual variation of serum constituents. VI. Physiologic day-to-day variation of concentration values of ten specific proteins in the sera of healthy subjects. *Clin. Chem.* **22**, 1635–1638.

Statland, B. E., Winkel, P., Harris, S. C. *et al.* (1978) Evaluation of biological sources of variation of leukocyte counts and other hematological quantities using very precise automated analyzers. *Am. J. Clin. Pathol.*, **69**, 48–54.

Steige, H. and Jones, J. D. (1971) Evaluation of pneumatic tube system for delivery of blood specimens. *Clin. Chem.*, **17**, 1160–1164.

Stengle, J. M. and Schade, A. L. (1957) Diurnal-nocturnal variations of certain blood constituents in normal human subjects. *Br. J. Haematol.*, **3**, 117–124.

Stuart, J., Barrett, B. A. and Prangnell, D. R. (1974) Capillary blood collection in haematology. *J. Clin. Pathol.*, **27**, 869–874.

Sturgis, C. C. and Bethell, F. H. (1943) Quantitative and qualitative variations in normal leukocytes. *Physiol. Rev.*, **23**, 279–303.

Sunderman, F. W. (1972) Effects of drugs on hematological tests. *Ann. Clin. Lab. Sci.*, **2**, 2–11.

Taswell, F. H., Smith, A. M., Sweatt, M. A. *et al.* (1974) Quality control in the blood bank – a new approach. *Am. J. Clin. Pathol.*, **62**, 491–495.

Thomson, J. M. (1984) Specimen collection for blood coagulation testing. In: Koepke, J. A. (ed.) *Practical Laboratory Hematology*, Vol. 2, New York: Churchill Livingstone: pp. 833–863.

Thomson, J. M. (1991) In: Koepke, J. A. (ed.) *Practical Laboratory Hematology*. New York: Churchill Livingstone, pp. 313–328.

Tombridge, T. L. (1978) Effect of posture on hematology results. *Am. J. Clin. Pathol.*, **49**, 491–493.

Tonks, D. B. (1968) A quality control program for quantitative clinical chemistry estimations. *Can. J. Med. Technol.*, **30**, 38–54.

Treacy, M. and Marsh, W. L. (1987) Enhancement of the sensitivity of the antiglobulin test. *Am. Clin. Products Rev.*, **6**, 24–27.

van den Besselaar, A. M. P. H. and Loeliger, E. A. (1982) The effect of contact activation on the prothrombin time with special reference to insufficiently siliconised vacutainers and venoject devices. In: Triplett, D. A. (ed.) *Standardization of Coagulation Assays*, Skokie, ILL: College of American Pathologists. p. 95.

Weaver, D. K. and Miller, D. (1978) Evaluation of a computer-directed pneumatic tube system for pneumatic transport of blood specimens. *Am. J. Clin. Pathol.*, **70**, 400–405.

Winkel, P. and Statland, B. E. (1981) The acute effect of smoking on the concentrations of blood leukocyte types in healthy young women. *Am. J. Clin. Pathol.*, **75**, 781–785.

Winkel, P., Statland, B. E., and Saunders, R. M. *et al.* (1981) Within-day physiologic variation of leukocyte types in healthy subjects as assayed by two automated leukocyte differential analyzers. *Am. J. Clin. Pathol.* **75**, 693–700.

13

Standards, reference materials and reference methods

International Council for Standardization in Haematology*

Standards have an essential role in the laboratory to ensure test reliability and interlaboratory harmonization. A standard may be a process for measurement of accuracy or it may be a degree of excellence. The former may be a material of known value or a defined chemical or physical characteristic or a written specification. Various terms have been used in this context and this has led to considerable confusion. It is thus necessary to explain the concepts which are encompassed in standardization.

Reference Standard has been identified by ICSH as a substance or device, one or more properties of which are sufficiently well established to be used for the calibration of an instrument, for checking a measurement method or for assigning values to a material. This is also known as a material standard or a reference preparation. Three categories are recognized, namely, primary (International), secondary (National or regional) and tertiary (commercial or local).

The method for assigning values to standards is based on one or more of the following requirements:

1. Traceable to a primary reference standard (see below)
2. A collaborative exercise by a number of expert laboratories
3. A certification procedure (Sizaret, 1988; WHO, 1987)

13.1 Traceability

The science of measurement is known as metrology. There are certain measurements which have such well defined physical properties that any other material measured against these metrological standards will be equally well defined. The fundamental measurements in this context include length, mass and molar concentration. If a ruler is calibrated directly

and precisely against the defined reference standard metre this will give a measure of its true length. If a second ruler is calibrated against the first ruler this will give a measure of its true length (within limits of precision), and similarly with a third, fourth and many more rulers, all of which will have been calibrated indirectly against the original metre. Thus, these successive measurements are **traceable** to the metrological standard of length. There are similar examples of standards based on weight and traceable to the kilogram. Included in this group are chemical standards which can be defined in terms of their relative molecular mass. Hemoglobin belongs to this category (ICSH, 1987).

When a biological substance cannot be expressed directly in terms of either chemical or physical quantities, it may be defined in terms of international units. These are arbitrary units based on some type of reaction which relates to its biological activity. The unit concentration of any other preparation which reacts in the same way can be determined by comparing their reactions, thus making the second preparation traceable to the primary standard. Thromboplastin provides an example of this.

As described above, metrological standards ensure accuracy (truth); on the other hand, biological standards are arbitrary, and thus cannot be claimed to be 'accurate' but at least they ensure consistency.

In biomedical science the authority for international standards is the World Health Organization. WHO standards have, in the past, been mainly intended for controlling the potency, activity and specificity of preparations that are used in prophylaxis and therapy. More recently diagnostic standards have come to the forefront. In this work ICSH and IFCC advise WHO; in some instances ICSH has carried out collaborative studies and has provided the preparations which have been adopted by WHO as international standards. A number of primary standards are also produced by National Standards bodies such as the UK National Institute for Biological Standards and Control (NIBSC) and the USA National Institute for Standards and Technology

* Draft prepared by S. M. Lewis.

(NIST). These organizations are also responsible for producing secondary standards which are required to conform to the criteria described above; however, by relating such a standard to an international standard it indirectly fulfils traceability and allows a value to be assigned without the need for an extensive collaborative study. The European Community Bureau of Reference (BCR) is in a special category as a regional international body; it has a formal protocol for assigning values by a collaborative exercise by expert laboratories in the EC states, together with an authoritative certification Board.

Tertiary standards are the equivalent of calibrators which are used to calibrate, graduate or adjust a measurement. These preparations are usually manufactured by a commercial firm, often for use with a specific instrument.

In summary, **primary international standards** and **reference materials** are only available in restricted amounts. **Secondary standards** are established by direct comparison with a primary standard, usually by a national authority. They are more freely available and are intended for assigning values to **testing standards** or **calibrators,** which are commercial (or privately) manufactured products. Some calibrators are clearly seen to be traceable to the relevant primary standard; with other materials labelled as calibrators the link is tenuous and unfortunately sometimes non-existent.

Material standards may be complemented by written standards. These are specifications from which an instrument can be calibrated or a value assigned to a preparation. Thus, for example, the concentration of a hemoglobincyanide preparation (in mg/l) can be calculated from its spectrophotometric absorbance by a formula:

$$c \ (mg/l) = \frac{A^{540} \ (of \ HiCNPreparation) \times 64\,458}{44 \times d}$$

where 64 458 is the relative molecular mass of the Hb tetramer, 44 is the absorptivity* and d is the length of the lightpath in cm.

This assumes that the spectrophotometer is correctly calibrated and functioning; the certified hemoglobin standard serves this function and thus continues to have an important practical role in standardization for hemoglobinometry even if, in theory it can be replaced by a written specification.

Written standards are, in general, guidelines for laboratory practice, and for product manufacture. They are, thus, more akin to method standards which are described below.

A control is a substance, a device or procedure for checking that the performance of an analytic instrument is constant.

Calibrators and controls both have a place in

internal quality control; they have interrelated but different functions. A control must be stable and homogeneous; the exact analytic value is not important although the approximate value should be known in order to select a preparation at the upper or lower limit of the normal reference range or at other clinically important levels. By contrast, a calibrator must have an assigned value as close to the true value as can be established. The essential difference is that a calibrator is used for accuracy and inter-laboratory harmonization, whilst a control is used for precision.

The materials used as calibrators and controls are, in general, interchangeable but establishing an assigned value is an expensive, time-consuming procedure which makes it sensible to use it sparingly, whereas a control should be used with each batch of tests. Some controls are provided with stated values but this information should be treated with caution unless their accuracy can be confirmed independently by reference methods in expert laboratories. Material used in an external quality assessment scheme will usually have a value or values obtained as consensus mean or median value when the result from all participants are analysed (see Chapter 19). However, it is not good practice to regard the material with that assigned value retrospectively as a calibrator, and it should never be used to readjust an instrument.

A control is included alongside patients' samples in a batch of tests. It is subjected to the same reactions and the end-point of the reaction is read in the same way as in the adjacent samples. Thus, it must closely resemble test specimens in its behaviour. This is not always easy to achieve and for the blood count, especially, there is an inverse relationship between specimen-like behaviour and stability: blood in EDTA is unstable within a few hours of collection, and preservation that is necessary to prolong the stability may seriously affect its physical properties. On the other hand a reference standard need not behave in the same way as natural blood, but it is important to ensure that the instrument that is to be calibrated is not adversely affected by the material, e.g. by blocking the system's pathway or by giving an inconsistent reaction with its reagents or diluent. It may also be necessary to convert the measurement obtained with the standard to the measurement which would have been obtained on the same instrument with a fresh blood with equivalent dimensions.

13.2 Method Standards

The next group of standards are Method Standards. ICSH defines several categories as follows:

Reference Method: A clearly and exactly described technique for a particular determination which, in

---

* Or 'extinction coefficient'; now termed 'molar area (decadic) absorbance', expressed as L mmol^{-1} cm^{-1}.

the opinion of a defined authority, provides sufficiently accurate and precise laboratory data for it to be used to assess the validity of other laboratory methods for this determination. The accuracy of the reference method must be established by comparison with a definitive method where one exists. A reference method should be traceable to a primary metrological standard, and the degree of inaccuracy and imprecision must be stated.

An *International Reference Method* is one that has been established by a defined international authority.

A *Reference Reagent* is one which has defined and clearly described properties; it is used with a reference method or procedure, or when appropriate, in conjunction with an international reference material.

Standardized Method: A procedure whose reliability has been verified by a defined authority following a study based on a reference method where it exists and which is suitable for routine use, taking account of its limits of accuracy and precision in the context of its intended purpose, economy of labour and materials, ease of operation and safety.

ICSH Selected Method: A method which has been recommended for routine use by ICSH on the basis of advice by an ICSH expert panel or another defined authority, after verification of its comparability with a standardized method.

As an example, for hemoglobinometry, the ICSH *reference method* is by spectrophotometric measurement as hemiglobincyanide (ICSH, 1987). Both hemiglobincyanide and oxyhemoglobin measured by calibrated photometers are acceptable as *standardized methods*, whilst simple photometry of hemiglobin azide, hemiglobincyanide or oxyhemoglobin and several types of direct reading hemoglobinometers are recommended as *selected methods* (Evatt *et al.*, 1992), whereas the Tallquist, Sahli and Copper Sulphate methods do not warrant recognition as being acceptable in any category.

13.3 Preparation of material standards and calibrators

Certified reference materials for a number of hematological analytes are available as described below.

WHO has published guidelines for the preparation and establishment of reference materials and reference reagents (WHO, 1978). These include information on international collaborative studies on candidate preparations and collaborative assays for assigning values.

Calibrators and controls are now available commercially for a number of hematological tests and details can be found in various manufacturers' catalogues. Where possible, the user should ensure that these have a record of traceability to an appropriate primary standard.

When biological activity is the essential factor it may be more appropriate to express values in terms of international units (IU) of activity. A model for this is thromboplastin for use in the prothrombin time test in oral anticoagulant control (Lewis, 1987; WHO, 1983).

In essence WHO, following extensive collaborative studies in expert laboratories, established a primary international reference preparation (IRP 67/40) consisting of a human brain extract with added calcium chloride, fibrinogen and factor V. Subsequently WHO accepted as primary IRPs batches of bovine, rabbit and human (plain) thromboplastins which had been calibrated against IRP 67/40. Following extensive studies by an expert panel of ICSH jointly with the (then) International Committee on Thrombosis and Hemostasis (now the Standardization Committee of ISTH), a method was developed to express the relationship of different batches of thromboplastin as International Sensitivity Index, based on an ISI of 1.00 allocated to IRP 67/40. The panel also recommended standardization of method and expression of results as an international normalized ratio (INR) with the aim of harmonizing therapeutic control of oral anticoagulation. The majority of manufacturers now specify the ISI of their products and there are international recommendations on the appropriate levels of INR for patients on oral anticoagulant therapy for different clinical conditions.

Blood count calibration has proved to be more difficult; blood anticoagulated with EDTA is unstable; blood preserved in acid citrate dextrose (ACD) or citrate phosphate dextrose (CPD) is stable for only a few weeks and moreover is unsuitable as it behaves differently in each combination of automated counter and diluent. Stabilization of cells (by partial or total fixation) inhibits osmotic shifts which occur when fresh blood is exposed to the diluent, and thus there are differences in behaviour of fresh blood and stabilized cell suspensions, resulting in different MCV/Hct on different instruments (England, 1990). A similar situation occurs with artificial materials such as latex particles. The discrepancies between these materials and fresh cells are reflected in what is described as the 'shape factor'. Shape factor is defined as the apparent volume of the cell divided by the true value.

In essence the instruments are designed to analyse fresh blood and not stabilized cell suspensions which may not undergo the same shape change when diluted in the manufacturer's specified diluent. Conversely, calibration by fresh blood is impractical except under special circumstances. A procedure is necessary to provide a link between fresh blood and stabilized blood or artificial material (Lewis, England and Rowan, 1991).

13.4 Artificial materials as standards

Materials that have been suggested as surrogate blood cells fall into two main groups: artificial materials and natural blood cells that have been modified by fixative treatment. Artificial materials have included pollens, mould spores, yeasts and plastic polymers. None of these seem to have been suitable. This is partly because they do not have the relevant physical properties, but also by their nature or method of preparation, they lack homogeneity. Monosized, spherical, polystyrene latex particles are now available in a series of defined sizes, with a CV of 2–3%. Apart from their homogeneity they have the major advantages that they are perfect spheres and they spontaneously form two-dimensional arrays with no gaps between the particles when a suspension is placed on a glass slide and covered by a coverglass. This allows their diameters to be measured directly using a calibrated stage micrometer, and their volumes to be calculated from:

$$V = \lambda d^3/6$$
$$\text{where } V = \text{volume}$$
$$d = \text{diameter}$$

Two sets of latex particles have been established by the Community Bureau of Reference (BCR) of the Commission of the European Communities as Certified Reference Materials (CRM), with mean diameter (and volume) of 2.2 μm (5.7 fl) as a platelet equivalent, and 4.9 μm (60.0 fl) as a red cell equivalent, respectively (Thom, Marchandise and Colinet, 1985). Other sizes have been prepared as working standards. These have mean diameter (volume) of 3.9 μm (31.3 fl) and 6.9 μm (172 fl), respectively. The last is a leukocyte equivalent.

Specification of the CRMs include an approximate concentration. An accurate particle concentration has not yet been established for the BCR material, but preliminary studies indicate that there should be no major problem in establishing counting standards in parallel to the size standards.

When measured on instruments calibrated with fresh blood cells the latices give a different volume from that obtained by calculation from diameter. The different sized latex particles should show linearity when their true volumes are plotted against instrument results, although this may require recalibration of the counter (either by the laboratory or service engineer). The relation of true-volume:counter-volume ratio of the latex will then provide the relative shape factor, the latex:red cell ratio, for that particular instrument. The set of lattices would provide a means to check that the counter remains correctly calibrated and linear. In this way it would be a useful control, readily available, and easy to use in the individual routine laboratory on a regular basis. Latex has an added advantage of remaining stable for several years.

When the relative shape factor has been established the counter can be used to obtain volume measurements of subsequent batches of latex particles. These measurements are thus directly traceable to the primary standard.

13.5 Standards setting organizations

13.5.1 Written standards

The two main international authorities concerned with written standards are the International Organization for Standardization (ISO) and the International Electrotechnical Organization (IEC). Their responsibilities are roughly divided into the 'nonelectrical' and the 'electrical and electronic engineering' fields with some joint activities. ISO is a federation of the national standards bodies (e.g. ANSI, AFNOR, BSI, DIN, JISC) (ISO, 1993). Its work is mainly done by about 200 technical committees (TCs) with a large number of working groups. Their draft documents are submitted for approval to all ISO members and published as 'International Standards'. In total about 7000 such standards have been published by ISO. Only a small minority of TCs are directly involved in medical standardization and some others have implications for clinical laboratory practice. These are listed in Table 13.1.

Whilst ISO standards have a high reputation there is no legal obligation to implement their specifications in national standards. In Europe coordination and unification of national standards bodies are being achieved by Comité Européen de Normalisation (CEN) and Comité Européen de Normalisation Electrotechnique (CENELEC). Their areas of interest are similar to those of ISO and IEC respectively. The membership consists of the national standards bodies of the 12 countries of the European Union (EU) and the 6 countries of the European Free Trade Association (EFTA).

The primary concern of CEN is related to 'product' standards and not to the use made; their priority is given to standards to be used by manufacturers. Different technical committees were created to prepare standards for medical devices in Europe. They are coordinated by the 'bureau technique sectoriel' health care (BTS 3). They include:

In vitro diagnostic medical services (TC 140)
Biotechnology (TC 236)
Biological safety and biocomparability (TC 206)
Sterilization procedures (TC 204)

TC 140 is of particular concern to the laboratory. Its scope is standardization in the production of reliable *in vitro* diagnostic systems. *In vivo* diagnostics which could be regarded as drugs are excluded, while associated equipment to *in vitro* diagnostic systems are included in the present scope.

Table 13.1 ISO Technical Committees

TC 12	Quantities, units, symbols, conversion factors
37	Terminology
46	Informatics
48	Laboratory glassware and related apparatus
76*	Transfusion, infusion and injection equipment
84	Medical devices for injection
130	Graphic technology
171	Micrographics and optical memories for document and image recording, storage and use
172	Optics and optical instruments
176†	Quality management and quality assurance
184	Industrial automation systems
194	Biological evaluation of medical devices
198	Sterilization of health care products
199‡	Safety of machinery

*Also includes a working group on blood-collecting tubes but excludes syringes which are dealt with by TC84.
† Responsible for ISO 9000 series.
‡ Liaison with IEC.

Table 13.2 ICSH Expert Panels and Standing Committees

Expert Panels
Cytometry
Cytochemistry
Hemoglobinometry
Vitamin B_{12} and Folate
Iron and Ferritin
Diagnostic tests and radionuclides
Serology (including a Working Party on Blood-grouping reagents)*
Abnormal hemoglobins
Red cell enzymes
Stains and staining methods
Hemostasis (including a task-force on quality control for coagulation tests)†
Platelet function tests
Leukemia and lymphoma immunophenotyping
Blood rheology

Standing Committees
Quantities and units
Quality assurance
Instrument evaluation
Specimen preparation
Training programmes‡

*Jointly with International Society of Blood Transfusion
† Jointly with International Society on Thrombosis and Hemostasis
‡ Jointly with World Health Organization and International Society of Hematology.

When CEN standards which are known as 'European Norm' are accepted in a weighted vote by their members, they have the status of national standards in each of the 18 member countries and any conflicting national standard must be withdrawn. Directives on any of these harmonized standards by the European Commission may result in their mandatory adoption by all the member states, thus ensuring free circulation of devices which conform to the specifications in all EU and EFTA countries. Of particular concern to the laboratory practice is the Directive on *in vitro* diagnostic medical devices (CEC, 1993).

Professional voluntary organizations are also concerned with written standards. These include international groups such as ICSH, IFCC, COWS-WASP and also inter-regional and national bodies such as NCCLS, JCCLS and formerly ECCLS. These organizations prepare guidelines and recommendations both for specific test procedures and for good laboratory practice including quality system and quality management. The main activities of ICSH are reflected in the expert panels and standing committees which are listed in Table 13.2, and examples of various ICSH recommendations have been published in professional journals.

Although the recommendations of these organizations are voluntary they are likely to be adopted, to a greater or lesser extent, by the professions who are represented on the associations involved in their preparation. Moreover there is close cooperation between ICSH and ISO and between ICSH and WHO, thus ensuring not only harmonization of recommendations but also that they are realistic in meeting the needs of the users and are within their capability taking account of the facilities that may be available in different countries and for different aspects of laboratory practice.

13.5.2 Material Standards

As already indicated the main organization involved with primary reference (diagnostic) standards for hematology tests are WHO, BCR and ICSH, but there are also regional standardizing organizations such as BCR and national bodies such as NIBSC and NIST (see above). These have different status, authority and administrative procedures. WHO provides standards to national authorities whereas regional and national bodies are more concerned with the needs of commercial manufacturers of calibrators and reagents whose products require standardization whilst ICSH is especially concerned with educating the profession in the use of standards in their laboratories, although it has been responsible for developing primary material standards, carrying out collaborative exercises for assigning values and establishing international standards that have been adopted by WHO.

Standards are also often available from national authorities; these should be traceable to the international one.

The following lists the international standards that are currently available (Community Bureau of Reference, 1992; WHO, 1990).

General

Hemoglobin (HiCN) (ICSH/WHO, BCR)

HbA$_2$; HbF (ICSH/WHO)
Ferritin (ICSH/WHO)
Vitamin B$_{12}$ (ICSH/WHO)
Erythropoietin (WHO)
Monosized latex particles for cell sizing (BCR)

Cytopoiesis

Interleukins 1α, 1β, 2, 3, 4, 5, 7, 8 (WHO)
Granulocyte–macrophage colony stimulating factor (WHO)
Macrophage colony stimulating factor (WHO)
Tumour necrosis factor (WHO)

Immunohematology

Blood typing sera: anti-A; -B; -AB; -R° (D); -r' (C) (WHO)*
Anti-human globulin reagent (ICSH)
Antinuclear factor (WHO)
Human serum complement components (WHO)*

Coagulation

Thromboplastins: Rabbit, Bovine, Human (ICSH/WHO*, BCR)
Factors II, VII, X, VIII:Ag, VIII:C (WHO)
von Willebrand factor (WHO)
Antithrombin III (WHO)
Thrombin (WHO)
Plasmin (WHO)
Human tissue plasminogen activator (t-PA) (WHO)
Urokinase (WHO)
Streptokinase (WHO)
Protein C (WHO)
Alpha-thrombin (WHO)
Heparin (WHO)
Platelet factor 4 (WHO)
Prekallikrein activator (WHO)
β-thromboglobulin (WHO)
Immunoglobulins: IgG; IgA; IgM; IgE (WHO)

Details of the various products and the conditions under which they are supplied may be obtained as follows:

(1) WHO – World Health Organization, Biological Standards Division, CH-1211 Geneva 27, Switzerland. FAX: 22791 07 46
(2) ICSH – c/o Dr R. M. Rowan, Department of Haematology, Western Infirmary, Dumbarton Road, Glasgow G11 6NT. FAX: 041 339 7327
(3) BCR – Community Bureau of Reference, rue de la Loi 200, B-1049 Brussels, Belgium. FAX: 322 295 8072
(4) NIBSC – National Institute for Biological Stand-

ards & Control, Blanche Lane, South Mimms, Potters Bar, Hertfordshire EN6 3QG, UK. FAX: 0707 646730
(5) CLB – Central Laboratory of the Netherlands Red Cross Blood Transfusion Service, Plesmanlaan 125, 1066CX Amsterdam, The Netherlands.

13.6 Appendix

In this appendix methods are given for preparation of control materials. They may also be used as calibrators provided that values can be assigned reliably to the analytes.

13.6.1 Hemoglobin (as hemiglobincyanide)

For calibrating a hemoglobinometer or a photometer for measuring hemoglobin the ICSH hemiglobincyanide reference preparation, or a solution derived from it, should be used (van Assendelft, Holtz and Lewis, 1991). The standard is an aqueous solution of hemiglobincyanide with a concentration in the range 550–850 mg/l.

The following method which is based on that of Holtz (Holtz, 1965) is suitable for preparing a working standard for use in an individual laboratory.

1. Blood (human or bovine) in any anticoagulant is suitable. Centrifuge blood in bottles of appropriate size (e.g. 30 ml screw-cap glass containers). Remove the plasma and buffy coat aseptically.
2. Add to each red cell deposit and excess of physiological saline (9 g/l NaCl), mix well and recentrifuge. Discard the supernatant and any remaining 'buffy coat'.
3. Repeat saline wash two times to ensure complete removal of plasma, white cells and platelets, each time removing the top layer of packed red cells.
4. Add to the washed cells half their volume of carbon tetrachloride (or an equal volume of water and 0.4 vol of toluene), cap the containers and then shake vigorously on a mechanical shaker or vibrator for one hour. Refrigerate overnight to allow the lipid/cell debris to form a semi-solid interface between carbon tetrachloride and lysate.
5. On the following day centrifuge at about 2500 g or more for 20 min. Remove the upper lysate layers and pool them in a clean bottle.
6. Filter through ash-free filter paper or sintered glass filter to remove remaining cellular debris.
7. To each 70 ml of lysate add 30 ml of glycerol. Optionally, in order to help prevent infection of the material add antibiotics (e.g. 5–10 mg of penicillin and 5–10 mg of gentamycin per 100 ml). This stock may then be stored at 4°C until required for dispensing.

---

* The majority of the WHO standards are held and distributed by the International laboratory for Biological Standards at the UK National Institute for Biological Standards and Control (NIBSC); some (indicated by an asterisk) by the Central Laboratory of the Netherlands Red Cross Blood Transfusion Service (CLB).

8. Measure the Hb concentration approximately in the lysate. Then add sufficient cyanide-ferricyanide (modified Drabkin) reagent to the lysate to obtain a concentration of ca 700 mg/l. Allow to stand at room temperature for about 1h.

9. Filter through a micropore filter at 0.2 μm, and dispense 10 ml volumes aseptically into sterile containers, preferably glass ampoules. Heat-seal the ampoules or if vials are used cap and seal them. The material will be satisfactory for several years if kept at 4°C, provided that it is sterile.

10. Measure absorbance in a spectrophotometer against reagent blank at 540 nm and also at 504 nm and 750 nm. The ratio of A^{540}/A^{504} should be 1.59–1.63 and A^{750} should be <0.003 per 1.000 cm lightpath. The spectrophotometer should be checked by means of the ICSH hemiglobincyanide standard (van Assendelft, Holtz and Lewis, 1991).

11. Calculate Hb concentration (mg/l) =

$$\frac{(A^{540} \times 16114.5)}{(11.0 \times 1.000)}, \text{ where } 11.0 = \text{absorption in}$$

Lmmol^{-1} cm^{-1} (see page 129) and 16114.5 = monomeric mol. wt of hemoglobin.

13.6.2 Hemoglobin (lysate)

This is intended for use when hemoglobin is one of the tests in an automated blood counting system with a preset diluter. The method of preparation of a lysate is described above. To assign a value for hemoglobin concentration use the ICSH reference method (page 130) with a spectrophotometer, the calibration of which has been checked against the ICSH hemiglobincyanide standard or a secondary standard derived from it. Establish the coefficient of variation (CV) by ten replicate tests, sampling from several tubes taken at random from the batch. The CV should not exceed 2%.

When the instrument to be calibrated is an automated counting system in which hemoglobin is one of a set of interrelated parameters, whole-blood preparations should be used (see next section). The value of hemoglobin concentration is assigned to this material in the same way as for lysate.

13.6.3 Preparation of stabilized whole blood control (Reardon et al., 1991)

Reagent

Formaldehyde 37–40%	6.75 ml
Glutaraldehyde 50%	0.75 ml
Trisodium citrate	26 g
Distilled water to	100 ml

Method

1. Obtain preserved whole blood in CPD or ACD. This should be as fresh as possible and not more than 48 hours old. Filter through a 40 μm blood filter and measure the volume.

2. Add 1 volume reagent to 50 volumes blood.

3. Add antibiotics (see 13.6.1 7).

4. Mix continuously with a magnetic stirrer for one hour at room temperature. Then leave to stand overnight at 4°C.

5. To obtain different values remove 50 ml of supernatant plasma, and keep in reserve.

6. Remix the remainder and then with continuous mixing dispense part of the stock in 2 ml volumes into sterile containers.

7. Return the plasma (see 5) to the remaining stock, remix and dispense the rest of the stock in the same manner in 2 ml volumes into sterile containers.

8. Cap and seal; refrigerate at 4°C until needed.

9. For analysis the sample should be gently mixed on a roller mix or by hand before opening. Unopened vials keep in good condition for all blood count parameters for 2–3 years.

10. Methods for assigning values: ICSH recommended methods for Hb (ICSH, 1987), RBC (ICSH, 1994), WBC (ICSH, 1994) and Platelets (ICSH, 1988).

Other reference and selected methods for various hematological measurements are included in the ICSH bibliography in the Preface.

References

Commission of the European Communities (1993) Proposal for a Council Directive on *in vitro* diagnostic medical devices. Document III/0/4181/93-EN. EC, Brussels.

Community Bureau of Reference (1992) BCR Reference Materials. Commission of the European Communities, Brussels.

England, J. M. (1990) Recommended methods for the assignment of assay values to stabilized cell suspensions. *Clin. Lab. Haematol.*, **12** (Suppl.), 13–21.

Evatt, B. L., Gibbs, W. N., Lewis, S. M. *et al.* (1992) *Fundamental Diagnostic Haematology: Anaemia.* 2nd edn. US Department of Health and Human Services, Atlanta; Geneva: WHO. pp. 68.

Holtz, A. H. (1965) Some experience with a cyanhaemiglobin solution. *Bibl. Haematol.*, **21**, 75–78.

International Committee for Standardization in Haematology (1987) Recommendation for reference method for haemiglobinometry in human blood (ICSH Standard 1986) and specifications for international haemiglobincyanide reference preparation (3rd edn). *Clin. Lab. Haematol.*, **9**, 73–79.

International Council for Standardization in Haematology (1988). Recommended methods for the visual determination of white cell and platelet counts. WHO/LAB/88.3.

International Council for Standardization in Haematology (1994a) Rules and operating procedures Glasgow: ICSH Secretariat.

International Council for Standardization in Haematology (1994b) Reference method for the enumeration of erythrocytes and leucocytes. *Clin. lab. Haemat.* **16**, 131–138.

International Organization for Standardization (1993) ISO Memento. Geneva: ISO.

Lewis, S. M. (1987) Thromboplastin and oral anticoagulant control. *Br. J. Haematol.*, **66**, 1–4.

Lewis, S. M., England, J. M. and Rowan, R. M. (1991) Current concerns in haematology 3: Blood count calibration. *J. Clin. Pathol.*, **44**, 881–884.

Reardon, D. M., Mack, D., Warner, B. *et al.* (1991) A whole blood control for blood count analysers, and source of material for an external quality assessment scheme. *Med. Lab. Sci.*, **48**, 19–26.

Sizaret, P. (1988) The preparation of international reference materials for biological substances. *J. Biol. Standard.*, **16**, 129–137.

Thom, R., Marchandise, H. and Colinet, E. (1985) The certification of monodisperse latex spheres in aqueous suspensions with nominal diameter 0.2 μm, 4.8 μm and 9.6 μm. BCR Report EUR 9662 EN. Brussels: Commission of the European Community.

van Assendelft, O. W., Holtz, A. H. and Lewis, S. M., (1991) Recommended method for the determination of the haemoglobin concentration of blood. Document LAB/84/0 Rev 1. Geneva: WHO.

World Health Organization (1978) WHO Expert Committee on Biological Standardization, 29th Report, Technical Report Series, **626**, 101–141

World Health Organization (1983) WHO Expert Committee on Biological Standardization. 33rd report. WHO *Tech. Rep. Ser.* 687, 81–105.

World Health Organization (1987) WHO Expert Committee on Biological Standardization. 37th Report. WHO *Tech. Rep. Ser* 760, 39–81.

World Health Organization (1990) Biological Substances: International Standards and Reference Reagents, Geneva: WHO

14

Harmonization, concordance and truth of measurement

J. M. England

14.1 Introduction

Harmonization is the process of 'bringing into harmony, agreement or concordance', and the word *harmony* brings to mind the idea of music. However, this is a poor analogy; in music, harmony is subjectively assessed, listeners can select which harmony they find truly the best and many still prefer music from the 18th and 19th centuries! Hematologists do not have this privilege as far as their work is concerned as they have to make late 20th-century measurements. For such measurements accuracy or 'truth in measurement' is required if possible, rather than harmonization. It may have been perfectly acceptable, even as late as the 1960s, to harmonize hemoglobin measurements on the Haldane percentage scale, but we now have standards, reference materials and reference methods by means of which hemoglobin concentrations can be accurately measured. Nevertheless there are still some areas in hematology, such as the measurement of mean cell volume, where harmonization and concordance are more readily achieved than truth, though even here accuracy is gradually becoming possible. The greater part of this chapter will therefore deal with accuracy but we will return briefly to harmonization at the end.

Chapter 13 describes the Standards, Reference Materials and Reference Methods which are the foundation on which accuracy in hematology is based. However, there are still many obstacles to be overcome if these principles are to be applied to achieve truth in routine hematological practice. This chapter examines the difficulties and suggests ways in which the problems may be solved. Particular emphasis will be given to blood counting since the most significant advances have been made in this area.

Standards and reference materials are difficult to prepare and it is expensive to assign values to them; they are therefore, made available in relatively small quantities. They are developed by international organizations such as the World Health Organization (WHO), International Council for Standardization in Haematology (ICSH) and European Union/Measurement and Testing Unit also known as Community Bureau of Reference (EU/BCR) (see Chapter 13). Table 14.1 summarizes the types of International Standards available for the measurements which form part of the blood count. It can be seen from this table that standards suffer from the serious disadvantage that they differ from the fresh blood used in diagnostic tests.

The ICSH/WHO hemoglobin standard, for example, is an aqueous solution of hemiglobincyanide (HiCN) with a concentration in the range 550–850 mg/l dispensed as a sterile solution in individual doses in sealed ampoules (ICSH, 1987). It differs from natural hemoglobin which is found in red cells since the standard is prepared from a hemolysate. During the preparation the normally occurring forms of hemoglobin are also converted to HiCN by the addition of a modified Drabkin reagent recommended by van Kampen and Zijlstra (1961).

Similarly, the monosized latex particles available from EU/BCR, serve as volume standards for red cells, white cells and platelets (Community Bureau of Reference, 1992), but the latex particles differ in

Table 14.1 International Standards available for measurements which form part of the blood count

International organization	Standard	Details
WHO/ICSH	Hemoglobin (HiCN)	An aqueous solution of HiCN with a concentration in the range 550–850 mg/l dispensed as a sterile solution in sealed ampoules for single use
EU/BCR	Monosized latex particles, nominal diameter RM165 2.0μm RM166 4.8μm RM167 9.4μm	Vials of calibration material are available in suspensions with about 10% solids

shape from naturally occurring cells, especially the red cells and platelets. They are also more rigid than blood cells so that they resist the shape changes which are induced when natural cells pass through the sensing zone of modern blood counting instruments.

National Standards can also be prepared and their values assigned in a way which is traceable to the International Standards. However, even National Standards are produced in relatively small quantities and cannot be supplied to the routine diagnostic laboratories which might wish to include them with each batch of specimens. Ways must therefore be found to *transfer the values* from the Standards and Reference Materials to the instruments used in routine tests. This chapter will describe some of the ways in which values are transferred, and other ways in which they might be transferred in future.

Reference Methods also have serious limitations against their *direct* application to routine practice. The objective of a reference method is to provide: 'Sufficiently accurate and precise laboratory data for it to be used to assess the validity of other laboratory methods for (a particular) determination' (ICSH).

The degree of inaccuracy and imprecision must be stated and the method must also be traceable to a primary metrological standard. It follows from these strict requirements that reference methods are designed with requirements which are absolute and, as such, reference methods are free from the compromises which are often made when routine methods are devised. Consequently, they are usually too difficult to use in routine diagnostic laboratories because:

1. High levels of technical skills must be developed and maintained by continuous practice.
2. Specialized equipment may be required to ensure the traceability to the primary metrological standard
3. Time constraints in a busy service department would not permit staff to spend the necessary time since the reference methods usually require considerable periods – for example it can easily take most of a working day to make a few reference measurements on 2 or 3 blood samples
4. Relatively large volumes may be required, over and above those normally collected for a blood count.

Thus, in practice it is necessary to *transfer the values* obtained by the reference method to the instruments which will be used routinely. The next section describes the general principles involved.

14.2 The use of intermedia for the transfer of accuracy to the diagnostic laboratory

As indicated above, whilst standards, reference materials and reference methods provide the foundation for accuracy, they cannot be used directly in the diagnostic laboratory. The values inherent in the standards and reference materials, or the values obtained by the reference methods must be transferred via some sort of *intermedium* to the diagnostic laboratory (Figure 14.1). Because the diagnostic laboratory is required to assess accuracy on a regular basis the ideal 'intermedium' must possess the following characteristics:

1. *Stability* sufficient to allow time to assign values, distribute the material and provide a reasonable shelf-life, e.g. at least two weeks, in the diagnostic laboratory.
2. *Availability* in sufficient quantity for all the laboratories who might wish to use the material. Batches also have to be available at a relevant frequency; this will depend, inter alia, on the stability of the intermedium and the instrument.
3. *Reasonable cost*, taking account of the frequency with which the material has to be used and the quantity required by the instrument for each test.
4. *Ease of use* as assessed by whether the material can be treated in the same way as fresh blood, e.g. can it be readily suspended and is it suitable for aspiration into the instrument in the same way as blood samples from patients.
5. *Suitability* for all instruments performing the relevant determinations. This is desirable because, if the measured response is a function of the instrument, it may be difficult or impossible to use the same material to transfer accuracy to different types of instrument. In this context there are three possible options:
   a. the material is suitable for all instruments and transfers the same value regardless of instrument type;
   b. the material is suitable for all instruments but the value transferred is a function of the instrument type;
   c. different materials are used for different instruments.

Obviously these options can be inter-related. For instance, one material could have the same values transferred for a subset of instruments, but a different value for others (a and b combined). Alternatively, any material may be suitable for a certain subset of instruments but unsuitable for others (b and c combined).

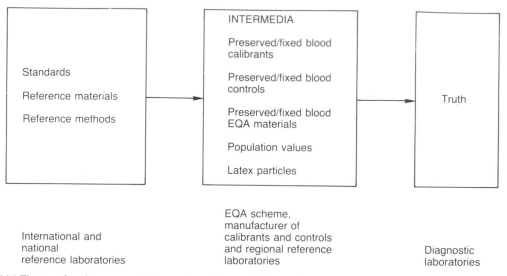

Figure 14.1 The transfer of accuracy via intermedia to diagnostic laboratories

14.3 The different types of intermedia

As explained in the previous section, the values inherent in the standards and reference methods must be transferred via an *intermedium* to the diagnostic laboratory. The intermedium will be a compromise between stability, availability, reasonable cost, ease of use and, as far as possible, suitability for many instrument types. It was recognized, however, that one intermedium may not be suitable for all instrument types.

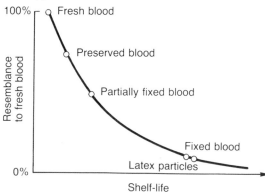

Figure 14.2 Shelf-life (see text) as a function of resemblance to fresh blood for various intermedia

14.3.1 Fresh blood

Fresh blood would, of course, be the perfect intermedium were it not for its short period of stability, i.e 2–4 h. As this time is barely sufficient to make any reference measurements the remaining shelf-life of a fresh blood intermedium is effectively zero!

Unfortunately, as illustrated in Figure 14.2, there is an inverse correlation between the shelf-life of an intermedium and its resemblance to fresh blood.

14.3.2 Preserved blood

Blood can be preserved in acid citrate dextrose (ACD), 'NIH-A', pH 5.4; Alsever's Solution, pH 6.1; citrate phosphate dextrose (CPD) or CPDA with the addition of adenine, pH 5.6–5.8.

With the addition of antibiotics, e.g. 5 μg/ml benzylpenicillin sodium and 50 μg/ml gentamycin this material should be stable for a minimum of three weeks at 4°C.

14.3.3 Partially fixed blood

A partially fixed whole blood preparation suitable for use as a stable control material for full blood count instruments was described by Reardon *et al.* (1991). When fresh CPDA-1 whole blood is partially fixed by the addition of both formaldehyde and glutaraldehyde it has a stability up to 175 days at 4°C. Such material can still be lysed for the measurement of hemoglobin.

14.3.4 Fixed blood

Red cells can be totally fixed using a greater concentration of glutaraldehyde (Lewis and Burgess, 1966). However, although this material has a long stability it suffers the disadvantage in blood cell counting that totally fixed cells cannot be lysed for the measurement of hemoglobin. Monosized latex particles are equally stable and are to be preferred since their volumes can be accurately determined by independent methods (see below). Though fixed red cells may have a shape more akin to a biconcave disc than a spherical latex particle this is irrelevant because blood counters never count or size red cells in their native biconcave disc shape. Some counters, especially those based on light scatter, isovolumetrically sphere the cells prior to analysis. Other instruments, particularly those based on aperture impedance, have such hydrodynamic forces in the sensing zone that the red cell is transformed into an elongated shape more akin to that of a cigar.

Fixed chicken red cells have been used as convenient substitutes for leukocytes, but, as described above, leukocytes stabilized by being *partially* fixed, are more suitable for use in blood cell counters, whilst platelets and red cells can be sized by reference to monosized latex particles.

14.3.5 Latex particles

Though these particles bear little or no resemblance to fresh blood they have a widely accepted role as a volume standard. Latex standards are readily available commercially with values traceable to the international standard. Traditionally platelets and leukocytes have been sized by reference to latex standards but not red cells. There are two reasons for this:

1. On most light-scatter systems the red cells are isovolumetrically sphered and therefore are the same shape as a latex particle. However, latex particles cannot be used as volume standards on these systems.
2. With aperture-impedance systems the fresh red cells remain flexible and are hydrodynamically forced into an elongated 'cigar like' shape whilst the latex particles are rigid and remain spherical. Studies with models have shown that the impedance change produced by a 'cigar-shaped' cell is 1.05 times that expected from the true volume whilst a sphere produces an impedance change 1.50 times that expected from the true volume. This means that the red cell measurements are totally incorrect if latex particles are used as volume standards. Incidentally, the same is probably true for platelets whose natural shape is discoidal, but the error with the platelet is of less significance: the platelet-crit (the product of mean platelet volume × platelet count) is hard to measure objectively by other methods and has yet to find a diagnostic, prognostic or therapeutic application which supersedes that of the platelet count. By contrast the hematocrit can easily be measured objectively by other methods and its value must conform to the product of mean (red) cell volume (MCV) and red cell count which it obviously would not do if red cells were sized relative to a latex standard.

14.3.6 Population values

In theory the fresh blood circulating in the veins of the local populace might be seen as an intermedium (Bull and Korpman, 1982). The possibility of using population values then follows from the fact that the blood count is fairly stable if a person is in good health. This is so even though there are minor variations on a diurnal basis and as a result of other factors such as exercise. Thus, if the reference methods were to be applied to a sufficiently large number of healthy subjects, the mean of their blood count parameters would be robust. Such a robust population mean could then be assumed if blood samples were taken from any other group of healthy subjects.

In practice population values cannot yet be used with complete certainty as an intermedium because:

1. Health is difficult to define and there are no agreed criteria for rejecting outliers, e.g. those beyond 2.0, 2.5 or 3.0 SD from the mean.
2. The initial sample would have to be large to reduce the standard of error of the mean (SEM) and reference methods would be virtually impossible to apply on such a scale.
3. The later samples would also have to be large to reduce their SEM.

However, population values may have some value as a check on instrument drift (see below).

14.4 The assignment of accurate values to intermedia

The values transferred to the intermedium must be accurate, i.e. derived from standards, reference materials or reference methods. But they must also be accurate for their intended application.

14.4.1 Latex particles

A consideration of latex particles as an MCV intermedium for aperture-impedance counters gives an idea of the underlying difficulties, i.e. that on such systems the absolute volume of latex particles is overestimated by approximately × 1.50 whilst red cell volume is only overestimated by approximately × 1.05 (typical values for an orifice of $100 \times 75 \ \mu m$). This means that if latex particles are to be used to size red cells it must be assumed that the latex particle is overestimated, relative to the red cell in the ratio:

$$\frac{1.50}{1.05} = 1.43$$

The factor of 1.43 can then be applied to 'correct' the true volume of the latex particle to the volume

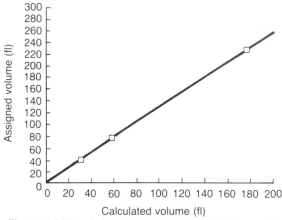

Figure 14.3 The relationship between calculated latex particle volume, based on diameter measurements and assigned volume on a Coulter Counter Model S Plus VI calibrated with fresh blood. The regression line has a slope of 1.285 and the intercept is 1.2 fl

which it is assumed to have when it is used as a standard for red cell measurement. But the real difficulty rests in the approximate nature of the 1.50 and 1.05 multipliers, and the resulting 1.43 multiplier. Regrettably these multipliers cannot be assumed because they vary according to the stated dimensions of the counter orifice. They also vary from orifice to orifice even for those stated to have the same dimensions. This is because the orifices are usually very small and the method used to drill them into gemstones will result in some variation between them.

If latex particles are to be used as an MCV intermedium the following procedure must be adopted at the manufacturer of the instrument or at a regional reference laboratory (England, 1990):

1. Obtain 3 sets of latex particles over a suitable volume range, whose certified volumes are traceable to a national or international reference preparation.
2. Calibrate the instrument with fresh blood as explained in the Appendix (page 144) and then estimate the volume of the latex particles.
3. Plot the results as shown in Figure 14.3. If the regression line does not have a zero intercept then the manufacturer must correct the fault in the instrument which has caused the zero offset. The slope of the regression line gives the relevant multiplier for the particular instrument and its orifices and this value is certified. It can be seen that the value on this instrument is lower than described above because the orifice dimensions are different. (It should also be noted that the exercise would have to be repeated if the orifices are changed).

The diagnostic laboratory can then use any one latex particle of suitable volume as a standard for

that particular blood counter provided, of course, that the volume of the latex particle is traceable to a national or international reference preparation. Under these circumstances the certified volume of the latex particle must be adjusted for the instrument/orifice factor certified by the instrument manufacturer or regional laboratory.

This procedure is summarized in Figure 14.4.

14.4.2 Preserved or partially fixed blood

Preserved or partially fixed blood may also be used as an intermedium for many or all of the blood count parameters. Values are normally assigned to the material for instruments of particular types (Figure 14.5); it is not practicable, though it would be desirable, to assign values for any particular instrument. To assign values the manufacturer of the blood intermedium must either have, or have access to, a sufficient number of instruments of the particular type(s) for which the intermedium is to be used. All of these instruments must be fresh-blood calibrated (ICSH, 1988) (Appendix). The manufacturer of the blood intermedium then tests this material on the instruments, averaging the results obtained from the instruments of each particular type. These then form the assigned or label values which are used by the diagnostic laboratory (England *et al.*, 1983) (Figure 14.6).

It is usually helpful if the manufacturer of the preserved blood has close working relationships with the instrument manufacturer since the instruments used to assign the values should be as typical as possible of that particular type.

14.5 The use of intermedia in the diagnostic laboratory

As explained in Figure 14.1, the intermedium is used as the final stage of the process to transfer accuracy to the diagnostic laboratory. The actual process itself will depend on how the instrument is calibrated.

1. If the instrument has been 'factory precalibrated' by the manufacturer, either in part or whole, then those aspects which are 'factory precalibrated' can only be checked by use of the intermedium. Assuming the values for the intermedium which are recorded by the instrument agree, within the predefined limits, with the values assigned to the intermedium then all is well and the instrument can be used for routine tests. On the other hand, should there be disagreement, the instrument cannot be used and a service engineer should be requested to correct the problem.
2. If the instrument or the parameter being checked can be adjusted by the user then the instrument

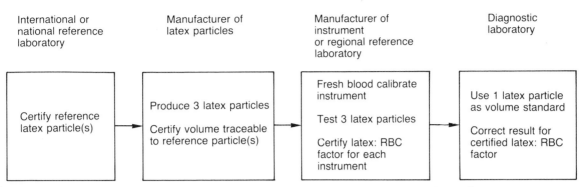

Figure 14.4 A schema for the use of latex particles as red-cell volume standards in diagnostic laboratories

PARAMETER	UNITS	DILUENT (1)	DILUENT (2)	DILUENT (3)
White Cell Count	$10^9/L$	9.0	9.0	9.0
Red Cell Count	$10^{12}/L$	4.22	4.22	4.22
Hemoglobin	g/dL	12.6	12.6	12.6
Packed Cell Volume	L/L	0.368	0.359	0.359
MCV	fl	87.1	85.1	85.1
MCH	pg	29.9	29.9	29.9
MCHC	g/dL	34.2	35.1	35.1

Figure 14.5 An example of a package insert from a commercial calibrant, showing that certain assigned values vary from diluent to diluent

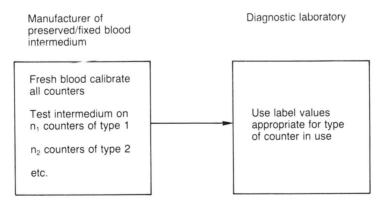

Figure 14.6 The assignment of label values to preserved/fixed blood intermedia by their manufacturer

must be *calibrated* when the values recorded for the intermedium differ beyond the predefined limits from the assigned values.

ICSH define the process of calibration as: Adjustment of instrument bias or assigning of a bias conversion factor in order to obtain accurate measurements. Accuracy over the operation range must be established by appropriate use of reference methods, reference materials and/or calibrators.

14.6 The choice of an intermedium for transfer of accuracy to the diagnostic laboratory

The possible intermedia have already been described, as have their desirable characteristics of stability, availability, reasonable cost, ease of use and suitability for use with all instruments. In this section the various possible intermedia will be assessed in

Table 14.2 The choice of intermedia for transfer of accuracy to the diagnostic laboratory

	Stability	Availability	Reasonable price	Ease of use	Suitability for all instruments
Fresh blood	No	Yes	Yes	Yes	Yes
Preserved blood	Yes	Yes	Yes	Yes	Yes
Partially-fixed blood	Yes	Yes	Yes	Yes	Yes
Fixed blood	Yes	Yes	Yes	Yes	Yes
Latex particles	Yes	Yes	Yes*	Yes*	Not†
Population values	Yes	No	No	No	Yes

*Assuming that the instrument can be modified to allow the latex particles to be introduced into the orifice baths.
†Aperture-impedance instruments only.

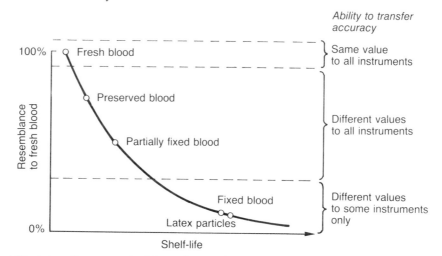

Figure 14.7 The ability to transfer accuracy by different intermedia

relation to these characteristics (Table 14.2); their ability to transfer accuracy is summarized in Figure 14.7.

14.6.1 Fresh blood

As already explained, fresh blood fails on the stability criterion, and its only use as an intermedium is for 'fresh-blood' calibrating instruments that are then used to assign values to more stable intermedia. Such instruments are usually located either in the facilities of manufacturers of instruments or intermedia or in regional reference laboratories.

14.6.2 Preserved blood

Blood preserved, other than by use of fixation, has a reasonable shelf-life but it is preferable to use partially-fixed blood.

14.6.3 Partially-fixed blood

This is probably the most satisfactory intermedium though it suffers from the disadvantage that the assigned values will be a function of instrument type.

14.6.4 Fixed blood

Fixed blood offers no advantages over latex particles in this context.

14.6.5 Latex particles

Latex particles are the ideal intermedium for aperture-impedance counters, though only volume reference standards are available (England *et al.*, 1990). However it is hoped that count standards may be developed.

The main shortcoming of latex particles is their relatively high cost which precludes their aspiration by the instrument through the blood sampling system. Instead, the particles have to be introduced directly into the baths which contain the orifices. In this way they can be introduced in a dilute, and hence relatively inexpensive, suspension with a similar particle concentration to the diluted blood which is aspirated through the orifices. Manufacturers may make such an option available on special request.

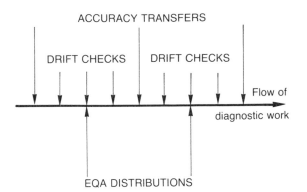

Figure 14.8 The use of accuracy transfers, drift checks and EQA distributions during the flow of diagnostic work

14.6.6 Population values

The logistical difficulties, outlined earlier, mean that this approach would be difficult and expensive although possibly useful in the future.

14.7 Ensuring that accuracy is maintained in the diagnostic laboratory

As explained, it is essential to use a suitable intermedium to transfer accuracy into the laboratory, either to check that a factory pre-set calibration is satisfactory, or to calibrate if the user is permitted to do so (Figure 14.8). However, this must not be seen as a once and for all phenomenon because every instrument has a degree of instability, albeit much less than they used to have, and faults can still occur. For this reason it is essential to check the instrument's accuracy at intervals specified by the manufacturer, whenever it appears to drift if a major component is changed or if unsatisfactory results are obtained in an external quality assessment (EQA) Scheme.

14.7.1 The assessment of drift

Materials used to assess drift are selected from the materials detailed in Table 14.2. One important criterion is stability and the other is as close a resemblance as possible to fresh blood (Figure 14.2). The second criterion follows from the fact that some instrument faults are so subtle that they are not detected using totally fixed blood or artificial particles such as latex.

It can be seen that only preserved or partially-fixed blood and population values can reasonably satisfy both criteria.

a. Controls

When preserved or partially fixed blood specimens are interposed into the flow of diagnostic work to check for drift the specimens are termed controls. Controls do not need to have values assigned to them by their manufacturer; if they do so the value should be taken merely as an indication as to whether the control has a high, intermediate or low value. Under no circumstances should any label values on controls be seen as part of the transfer of accuracy.

Regardless of whether or not the control has a label value it is the responsibility of the diagnostic laboratory to assign an initial value as the mean of however many replicate determinations are specified by the manufacturer of the control and the manufacturer of the instrument. In the same way there should also be a predefined band around the mean value within which the instrument is, by definition, in control and outside which the instrument has drifted. There should also be a stated frequency with which the control should be tested, i.e. after how many patient specimens.

The results from the controls should be plotted on a suitable graph. Most manufacturers use a Levy–Jennings plot which permits a graphical assessment of trends as well as formal definition of in and out of control.

However, it must be admitted that modern instruments may be more stable than preserved or partially-fixed blood and the cost-benefit trade off may be hard to define.

b. Population values

Here, again, the issue of instrument stability is crucial and in many instances the instrument may be more stable than the patient values derived from the flow of diagnostic work. Various algorithms can be used to calculate the patient values; all are types of moving average with systems designed to minimize or reduce the effect of outliers (Bull and Korpman, 1982).

The continuing debate between the proponents of population values and the proponents of controls suggest that the issue still has to be settled. Indeed, both techniques may become increasingly unnecessary now that instruments are much more stable.

14.7.2 EQA schemes

These schemes, which are described more fully in Chapter 19, occupy a central role in ensuring that accuracy exists and persists. They can do so largely because they are external and view the situation independently from outside the closed loop in which the diagnostic laboratory is held by the

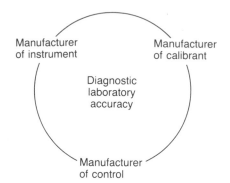

Figure 14.9 The accuracy of a diagnostic laboratory dependant on the manufacturer of instrument, calibrant and control

manufacturers of the instrument, calibrant and control (Figure 14.9). The loop is obviously tight when the same manufacturer supplies all three items, but even when manufacturers differ, their independence can sometimes be more apparent than real, e.g. different manufacturers may cross calibrate their calibrants.

14.8 Harmonization or accuracy?

Performance in EQA schemes has improved over the past 25 years, as evidenced by greater and greater harmonization. But has this meant improved accuracy? The answer is yes, but one cannot say how much because the process of transfer of accuracy (see Figure 14.1) is, in many respects, shielded from view.

The key activity in the transfer of accuracy is the fresh blood calibration of the blood counters and their behaviour when they are used to assign values to the calibrants. Consumer groups such as the British Committee for Standards in Haematology have checked the accuracy of blood calibrants and found generally satisfactory results, but this sort of activity should be more widespread and continuous (England *et al.*, 1983).

Quis custodiet ipse custodies?

Acknowledgements

Mrs V. J. Newman kindly prepared the chapter and Mr P. McTaggart the illustrations. Miss J. Wardle read the document and made numerous helpful comments.

APPENDIX
The assignment of values for fresh blood used for calibrating automated blood cell counters

THE FOLLOWING PROCEDURES ARE SUMMARIZED FROM ICSH (**1988**)

The instability of fresh blood restricts its use to short-term procedures over a few hours.

Materials
Blood Samples

1. Anticoagulant: K_2 EDTA or K_3 EDTA* in a final concentration of 1.4 – 1.6 mg/ml.

2. Donors: Healthy subjects fulfilling the following criteria:

   K_2 EDTA: Mean cell volume (MCV) 86–96 fl and mean cell hemoglobin concentration (MCHC) 33.0–34.5 g/dl. The PCV/RBC and Hb/PCV values for these calculations being obtained by the methods described below.

   *K_3 EDTA: MCV 84–94 fl and MCHC 33.7–35.2 g/dl obtained by the same methods.

3. Sampling: Either by syringe or evacuated containers. Samples should be rejected if they show any visible hemolysis or if microclots are present and should remain at room temperature (circa 20°C) being tested within 4 hours.

*ICSH has recommended K_2EDTA (*American Journal of Clinical Pathology*, 1993, **100**, 371–372); however some laboratories still use K_3EDTA.

Glassware

1. Pipettes: Officially certified Class A glassware which achieve an inaccuracy of pipetting of < 0.5%. They should be kept clean and dry but never heated above 50°C.

The following pipettes are required:
Maclean (white shell-back) blood pipettes (ml)
   0.05 ± 0.0005
   0.2 ± 0.002
   0.5 ± 0.005
Volumetric pipettes with controlled draining time and prescribed waiting time (ml)
   20   ± 0.03
   25   ± 0.03

2. Capillary tubes for haematocrit determination. Disposable capillary tubes satisfying the specifications of a national standards body (BSI 1968;

Table 14.3 Direct measurements in fresh blood

	No. of tests	Maximum permissible bias (%) (± 2 CV)
Hemoglobin	Two dilutions	1.0
Packed cell volume	Four tubes	1.0
Red cell count	Two dilutions each counted twice on each polarity,* i.e. four counts per dilution	3.5
White cell count	As for red cell count	4.0
Red cell/platelet count ratio	Four replicates	15.0

* If counter changes polarity.

American Society for Testing and Materials, 1980). A clay-like sealing compound should be used.
3. Volumetric flasks. Certified Grade A borosilicate glass volumetric flasks.
   Volumetric flask (ml) 100 $\pm$ 0.1
4. Counting vials. Clean plastic or glass vials with a minimum volume of 10 ml. It should be experimentally demonstrated that cells do not adhere to the vials.

Direct measurements

Considerable practice is needed to eliminate inter-technologist biases in the direct measurements which are summarized in Table 14.3

1. Hemoglobin: in accordance with the ICSH Reference Method (ICSH, 1987) using 100 ml of reagent in a volumetric flask and rinsing in 0.5 ml of blood to give a dilution of 1 in 201. This solution should be filtered through a low protein binding membrane filter, mean pore diameter of 0.20–0.25 μm to ensure the absence of turbidity and the hemoglobin estimated spectrophotometrically.
2. Packed cell volume: by the (ICSH, 1989) selected method for microhematocrit determination without correction for trapped plasma.
3. Red cell count: performed using a semi-automated single channel aperture-impedance counter without sheath flow working on a known displaced volume basis.
   The instrument design should incorporate the following points:
   a. Sterile, non-toxic buffered salt solution diluent.
   b. Cylindrical counting aperture having a nominal diameter of 80–100 μm and a length of 70–100% of diameter.

c. Minimum recirculation of cells inside the orifice tube.
d. Avoid turbulence and trapped bubbles.
e. The sample flow lines must not change volume in response to fluid pressure.
f. Cells should not adhere to the instrument.
g. The displaced volume should be accurate to within 1% and traceable to a recognized standard.
h. The detection electronics should be verified as conforming to ICSH (1987) with validated count thresholds.
i. Coincidence correction can be provided automatically or by means of a coincidence correction chart, but in either case it should be verified.

For counting, a primary dilution is prepared (0.05 ml blood plus 25 ml diluent), and from this a secondary dilution (0.2 ml primary dilution plus 20 ml diluent). Counting must be accomplished within 5 minutes of the last dilution step.

Potential sources of error in counting procedures are:

a. Sampling – including measurement and mixing.
b. Transport – caused by sedimentation, cell loss and/or recirculation, inaccuracy and imprecision of displaced volume.
c. Counting – arising from improper discrimination, spurious counts or inaccurate correction for coincidence loss.

4. Red cells indices: calculated from the measurement already described:
   MCV = PCV/RBC
   MCH = Hb/RBC
   MCHC = Hb/PCV
5. White cell count: instrument principle and specifications are as for red cell counting. The lytic agent must be capable of completely lysing red cells, leaving no residual material capable of contributing to the count. The red cell primary dilution is used incorporating the dilution effect of the lytic agent. The count should be stable for 15 minutes after preparation.
6. Platelet count: methods employing platelet-rich plasma produce biases and are therefore unacceptable, neither is there available an instrument, aspirating whole blood, and directly counting platelets in the presence of red cells. Thus it is only possible to use an instrument for determining the ratio of red cell to platelet count. The RBC is performed as detailed above and the platelet count can then be calculated. A sheath flow instrument is used, which has been validated as described by ICSH (1988).

For 95% of the specimens the value calculated must be within $\pm$ 10%.

References

Bull, B. S. and Korpman, R. A. (1982) Intralaboratory quality control using patient's data In *Quality Control* (I. Cavill, ed.), Edinburgh: Churchill Livingstone, pp. 121–150.

Community Bureau of Reference (1992) *BCR Reference Materials*. Brussels: Commission of the European Communities.

England J. M., Chetty M. C., Garvey B. *et al.* (1983) Testing of calibration and quality control material used with automatic blood counting apparatus: application of the protocol described by the British Committee for Standards in Haematology. *Clin. Lab. Haematol.*, **5**, 83–92.

England, J. M. (1990) Recommended methods for the assignment of assay values to stabilized suspensions. *Clin. Lab. Haematol.*, **12** (Suppl. 1) 13–21.

England J. M., Lewis S. M., Rowan R. M. *et al.* (1990) Surrogate materials for calibration and control: the use of latex particles as calibrants for red cell volume measurements. *Clin. Lab. Haematol.*, **12** (Suppl. 1), 55–63.

International Committee for Standardization in Haematology (1987) Recommendation for reference method for haemoglobinometry in human blood (ICSH Standard 1986) and specifications for international haemiglobincyanide reference preparation (3rd edition). *Clin. Lab. Haematol.*, **9**, 73–79.

International Committee for Standardization in Haematology (1988) The assignment of values to fresh blood used for calibrating automated blood cell counters. *Clin. Lab. Haematol.* **10**, 203–212.

International Committee for Standardization in Haematology (1989) Recommended methods for the determination of packed cell volume: prepared on behalf of WHO by ICSH Expert Panel in Cytometry. WHO document LAB 89.1.

Lewis S. M. (1975) Standards and reference preparations. *Quality Control in Haematology* (S. M. Lewis and B. J. Burgess eds) Symposium of the International Committee for Standardization in Haematology pp. 79–95.

Lewis S. M. and Burgess B. J. (1960) A stable standard suspension for red cell counts. *Lab. Practice*, **15**, 305.

Reardon D. M., Mack D., Warner B. *et al.* (1991) A whole blood control for blood count analysers, and a source of material for an external quality assessment scheme. *Med. Lab. Sciences*, **48**, 19–26.

Van Kampen E. J. and Zijlstra W. G. (1961) Standardization of hemoglobinometry. II. The hemiglobincyanide method. *Clin. Chim. Acta*, **6**, 538–544.

Ward P. G., Wardle J. and Lewis S. M. (1982) Standardization for routine blood counting – the role of interlaboratory trials. *Methods in Haem.*, **4**, 102.

15

Reference values, reference intervals, quantities and units

R. L. Verwilghen

15.1 Reference values, reference intervals

An isolated result of a laboratory measurement has no practical value. It becomes useful only when it can be compared to another result obtained for the same parameter. Thus, for example, by comparison with a previous similar measurement on the same patient, one can conclude that the new value has increased/decreased or has remained constant. By far the best reference value for a given patient is thus the result from a previous similar measurement. Most biological parameters, if measured in similar conditions, remain remarkably constant in healthy adults. Minor changes in the measured parameter can thus be relevant and be an early sign of disease. Mainly for parameters that show major inter-individual variations, a previous measurement of the same person is even the only valable comparison. Thus for example if we wish to know if our patient gained or lost weight a previous measurement of his weight is essential.

When the measurement is a first one on an individual person, the only possible comparison is with a result obtained for the same test in other people. From such comparison one can conclude if the result is 'higher', 'lower' or 'similar' to that of other persons. The significance of the observed value will be understood from this comparison with the result seen in 'normal conditions' in 'normal people', with 'normal values'.

The concept 'normal', however, gives rise to much confusion. Commonsense applies the word 'normal' to what is seen in a 'healthy' person. However, it can as well be used for the 'mean value' observed in 'not-ill' people, as for the optimum value, seen in individuals with potentially the longest survival. Many variables influence laboratory parameters, such as the age, sex, race, environment, social conditions of the concerned patient. Other factors are the diurnal variations of the measured parameter, exercise, feeding status, smoking, alcohol intake, etc.

Thus, it is not practicable to use 'normal values' as the yardstick for the interpretation of laboratory results seen in a patient. We use, instead, the more appropriate and better defined 'reference values', computed from an appropriate 'reference population'.

If no previous value is available for the patient, as is generally the case for a 'new' patient, we have to compare our result with that of other people. When the inter-individual variations are not too pronounced, reference values based on measurements in a comparable population can be used. For the establishment of such reference values, the selection of an appropriate 'reference population' is of utmost importance. It is also important to take the 'reference specimens' in conditions similar to those in which the patient's specimens are taken and to use a similar or at least comparable measurement's technique. Using such information, a 'reference interval' can be determined, containing the central 95% of the population (Gräsbeck and Alström, 1981).

Different recommendations have been published by IFCC (International Federation for Clinical Chemistry) and by ICSH on the theory and practical establishment of appropriate reference values in hematology and in clinical chemistry (ICSH, 1982; IFCC and ICSH, 1987 a,b,c).

These recommendations describe the rules to be followed for the selection of the reference sample from the whole reference population, for the measurement of the reference values and for the statistical treatment of the reference values.

It is useful to start with a clear definition of the terms used in this context (IFCC and ICSH, 1987a):

- A *reference individual* is an individual selected on the basis of defined criteria.
- A *reference population* consists of all possible reference individuals.
- A *reference sample group* is a statistically adequate number of reference individuals selected to represent the reference population.
- A *reference value* is the value obtained by observation of measurement of a particular type of

quantity in the reference individuals belonging to a reference sample group.

- A *reference limit* is derived from the distribution of reference values.
- A *reference interval* is the interval between, and including, two reference limits.

For practical purposes, the most frequently used reference interval or reference range includes the 95% central reference values, excluding the 2.5% highest and lowest values (respectively).

A first step in establishing reference values for a given test is the selection of an *appropriate reference sample from the reference population*. At first glance this may seem to be relatively easy, but it is, in fact, the most difficult step of the whole procedure.

This chapter will be limited to a discussion of the selection of a reference population to obtain reference values and reference ranges to be used in clinical medicine. It will not include the special problems met when reference values are used in epidemiological investigations, for public health purposes, etc. What will be discussed is the production of reference values obtained from a healthy (normal) population to be used in clinical medicine to judge if a patient's result is within or how far outside this reference range. For some purposes reference populations with a given disease or abnormality can be of use in the same way: for disease-specific clinics (e.g. monitoring of diabetic patients, or renal patients on dialysis or for the follow-up of bone marrow transplants) a reference population composed of diabetic or renal patients under control, or bone marrow transplanted patients 'doing well' might be useful.

It is very important to consider *all criteria used for inclusion and exclusion* of individuals from the reference population and to decide if these criteria are acceptable.

The reference population should, of course, be matched to the patient population for all characteristics known to influence the measured parameter. This is not only age and sex, but also many other factors such as race, socioeconomic factors, environmental conditions, etc.

The reference population should be as similar as possible to the patients for all factors known to influence the measured parameter: time of the day when the specimen is taken, pre- or post-prandial state, smoking, oral contraceptives and many other factors must be considered and standardized.

At first glance it might seem easy to obtain such a 'healthy' reference group. For tests done on blood samples, one often uses blood donors from transfusion collection centres. However, this is a highly selected population and it has been shown to be significantly different from the population as a whole. The same is true for another 'easy access' reference population composed of young doctors, nurses and technicians. Once again, this is a selected population significantly different from other similar aged groups.

When appropriate reference samples are obtained from an acceptable population, the next step will consist of the measurement of the specified parameter. If a reference method is available, it can be used for this purpose. One should, however, consider whether the routine method currently used gives result comparable to the former methods and if any bias exists in this routine method. It is often best to make the measurements with the currently used routine method in order to obtain the reference intervals to be used in the laboratory.

To compute the reference interval, different approaches may be followed. If the measured values follow a normal distribution, the 95% central values are situated between the mean $\pm$ 2 standard deviations. For most biological parameters the distribution will not be Gaussian. If the data show a skew or other forms of non-normal distribution, they can be subjected to different transformations, so that the distribution becomes normal and a parametric approach (calculation of mean and standard deviation) becomes possible.

A different approach, when the distribution is not Gaussian, is the non-parametric method. In the most commonly used procedure results are sorted according to increasing numerical values. The top and bottom 2.5% of results are excluded, and the new highest and lowest values constitute the reference interval containing the central 95% of all measurements.

The size needed for the reference sample, or the needed 'number of controls' from which the reference sample is taken, should be as large as conveniently possible. For a statistical, acceptable analysis, a minimum of 120 samples should be measured. If a non-parametric approach is followed, the sample should be larger to ensure reliability.

The introduction of automation in laboratory medicine, the use of complex systems and the availablity of 'kits' have increased the need to establish appropriate reference values.

When, for a given analyte, a well-established reference method exists and reference materials are available, kits and systems can be calibrated using such reference measurement system. Comparability of results obtained with different devices in different laboratories can thus be guaranteed by their manufacturer.

In many instances, the only method available to the manufacturer, will be to establish a 'reference interval' to be used with the new test. This will make it possible, using arbitrary units, to place the patient's result in the range of results measured in the 'healthy' population or in a population of patients with a similar pathology. In this way one can compare results obtained with different tests or kits, claiming to measure the same parameter, but both expressed in a different set of arbitrary units.

15.2 Quantities and units

In the Vocabulaire International de Métrologie (VIM) (1993) and in documents prepared by TC 140 of the 'Comité Europcén de Normalisation' (CEN) a quantity is defined as follows:

(measurable) quantity

attribute of a phenomenon, body or substance, that may be distinguished qualitatively and determined quantitatively

NOTES

1 The term quantity may refer to a quantity in a general sense (see example a) or to a *particular quantity* (see example b).

EXAMPLES

a) quantities in a general sense: length, time, mass, temperature, electrical resistance, amount-of-substance concentration:

b) particular quantities:

    – length of a given rod

    – electrical resistance of a given specimen of wire

    – amount-of-substance concentration of ethanol in a given sample of wine.

2 Quantities that can be placed in order of magnitude relative to one another are called *quantities of the same kind*

3 Quantities of the same kind may be grouped together into *categories of quantities* for example:

    – work, heat, energy

    – thickness, circumference, wavelength

unit (of measurement)

particular quantity, defined and adopted by convention, with which other quantities of the same kind are compared in order to express their magnitudes relative to that quantity.

From a practical point any measurement should be done using a set of units.

Originally units were used only locally: the mile of Brabant was different from the mile in Flanders, as were the pound and the yard. Until the French revolution many if not most units in Europe were still different from region to region, probably the only exception being the units for time (day, hour and minutes). In the 18th century the measurement of time remained extremely inaccurate, clocks were running fast or slow according to many factors, e.g. the ambient temperature, and they were corrected to measurements done with sophisticated albeit still very unreliable sundials. Only with the advent of the telegraph, did synchronization of time became possible at national and supranational level, when, the gun at noon or at sunset, or the church bells ringing the 'Angelus' as the method of time synchronization could be replaced.

In most countries of Europe, starting from the French revolution, integrated sets of units were adopted and progressively used, based on length (originally the metre defined as $1/4 \times 10^7$ part of the equator), mass (the kilogram, weight of 1 decimetre³ of distilled water) and time (the second). International resolutions were adopted by the Conférence générale des poids et mesures (CGPM) set up by the 'Convention du Mètre' signed in Paris in 1875. This system evolved progressively and was refined by CGPM between 1954 and 1960 to the 'système international d'Unités' (SI system), It was endorsed by the World Health Assembly in 1977 (WHO, 1977). The International Organization for Standardization (ISO) adopted an international standard (2955 of 15th May 1983) about the representation of SI and other units in systems with limited sets of characters.

The European Union considers that differences in 'units of measurement' between the member states could be a barrier to trade. For this reason the 'Council Directive' of 20 December 1979, last amended by the Council Directive of 27 November 1989 directs the member states to harmonize their legislation and to adopt the SI system.

The directives introduce the concept of 'legal units' to be used in the European Union for expressing quantities. These include the 7 SI base units (metre, kilogram, second, ampere, kelvin, mole and candela), supplementary (radian and steradian) and derived (e.g. hertz, newton, pascal, gray) SI units. They include further units defined on the basis of SI units but that are not decimal multiples or submultiples thereof (e.g. minute, hour and day), a few units defined independently of the seven SI base units (e.g. the electronvolt) and a few units permitted in specialized fields only (e.g. dioptre, carat).

For transitional periods and often limited to countries where they were previously used, or for specific applications, other specified units are legal units and can remain in use (e.g. the mile, yard, foot and inch for road traffic signs, distance and speed measurements, the gill for spirit drinks).

Use of SI units in the medical laboratory

The introduction of SI units for the expression of laboratory results has been of concern to the medical profession in general. Part of this concern was due to modifications in the way in which concentrations of different essential biological parameters are expressed. Inevitably each change will meet resistance from many physicians accustomed to the previous situation, and any change could give rise to confusion endangering a patient's life; moreover, some modifications, claimed as improvement, have subsequently been shown to be more influenced by 'fashion' than by real progress.

In the SI system there is a strong preference for using *substance concentration* (mol/l) for all substances whose molecular weight is known. *Mass concentration* (g/l) must be used for other substances and this group includes many proteins (e.g. the immunoglobulins). Of special concern to hematologists is the expression of the hemoglobin concentration. Both substance and mass concentration are compatible with the SI system. While organizations of clinical chemists strongly favour the use of substance concentration for hemoglobin, many hematologists prefer to use grams hemoglobin per litre. ICSH has recommended the use of grams per litre but accepts the expression of results for hemoglobin as substance concentration provided it is specified whether the monomer or tetramer is used.

References

Council Directive of 20 December 1979 (80/181/EEC) on the approximation of the laws of the Member States relating to units of measurement and on the repeal of Directive 71/354/EEC, *Official Journal of the European Communities*, No. L39, 15.2.1980, p. 40.

Council Directive of 27 November 1989 (89/617/EEC) amending Directive 80/181/EEC on the approximation of the laws of the Member States relating to units of measurement, *Official Journal of the European Communities*, No. L357, 7.12.89, p. 28.

Gräsbeck, R. and Alström T. (eds) (1981) '*Reference Values in Laboratory Medicine. The Current State of the Art*'. Chichester: John Wiley, p. 413.

International Committee for Standardization in Haemotology (ICSH) (1982) 'Standardization of Blood Specimen Collection Procedure for Reference Values'. *Clin. Lab. Haemat.*, **4**, 83–86.

International Federation of Clinical Chemistry (IFCC) and International Committee for Standardization in Haematology (ICSH) (1987a) 'Approved Recommendation (1986) on the Theory of Reference Values. Part 1: The Concept of Reference Values'. *J. Clin. Chem. Clin. Biochem.*, **25**, 337–342.

International Federation of Clinical Chemistry (IFCC) and International Committee for Standardization in Haematology (ICSH), (1987b) 'Approved Recommendation (1987) on the Theory of Reference Values. Part 5: Statistical Treatment of Collected Reference Values. Determination of Reference Limits'. *J. Clin. Chem. Clin. Biochem.*, **25**, 645–656.

International Federation of Clinical Chemistry (IFCC) and International Committee for Standardization in Haematology (ICSH) (1987c) 'Approved Recommendation (1987) on the Theory of Reference Values. Part 6: Presentation of Observed Values Related to Reference Values'. *J. Clin. Chem. Clin. Biochem.*, **25**, 657–662.

Vocabulaire International de Métrologie (1993) 'International Vocabulary of Basic and General Terms in Metrology' (2nd edn). Geneva: ISO

World Health Organization, (1977) 'The SI for the Health Professions'. Geneva: WHO.

16

Instrument and kit evaluation

A. Richardson-Jones

16.1 Introduction

Most clinical hematology laboratories rely on commercially produced instruments and kits for analytic tests. The evaluation of these instruments and kits is a useful first stage in establishing a performance base-line against which future performance of the analysis method may be compared as part of the routine quality control procedures. The need to establish this type of base-line is now embedded in the regulation that controls the practice of laboratory medicine in the USA. This regulation, 42 CFR 493, Sub-part K (1992), empowered by the Clinical Laboratory Improvement Amendments of 1988 (CLIA '88), requires the performance specifications of newly installed test methods to be verified before reporting the results on patients' specimens.

A further purpose of instrument and kit evaluation is to help buyers to choose among the wide selection of currently available commercial products. The consumer may make an unsuitable choice of test method if his selection is based only on printed (labelling) information or on published studies. The importance of this buying decision is recognized in the UK by an ongoing programme of instrument evaluation sponsored by the Department of Health (Lewis and England, 1992). Testing a candidate product under conditions of actual use may reveal undesirable characteristics and prevent the purchaser from becoming locked into an unhappy relationship with the product or its manufacturer or supplier. In addition to its use by consumers, it is hoped that this chapter will aid manufacturers in maintaining or improving standards of design and fabrication.

The methods described here have evolved in our laboratory over many years in the course of providing a major manufacturer of hematology instruments (Coulter Corporation) with a critical, independent analysis of product performance. The information produced by these evaluation procedures has been used for proof of safety and effectiveness required by US law and for independent design verification re-quired for conformance to the future European Communities Directive on *in vitro* medical devices and the anticipated pre-production quality assurance requirements of FDA.

16.2 Preliminary evaluation

The preliminary evaluation should include the following steps:

16.2.1 Examination of documents

These documents should include the product reference manual for instruments and package inserts for kits. In addition, the evaluator should review advertising material or other pertinent sales literature.

There are two purposes in scrutinizing these documents. One is to compare the claimed performance of the product against the laboratory's current and projected needs. Under-estimating workload growth or future interest in more recently available analytical capabilities such as reticulocyte and cell-surface marker assay can result in costly premature obsolescence of the contemplated investment. On the other hand there is little to be gained by paying for more capability in an instrument than is actually needed.

The second purpose is to ensure that the physical requirements (such as ambient temperature limits) are appropriate for the environment in which the evaluation will be carried out. Every item in these specifications should be checked against the ability of the laboratory to meet them. Often overlooked is the impact of added specimen testing on personnel and workflow patterns and whether there is a requirement for laboratory personnel to possess special skills or receive additional training.

The contents of the product reference manual or package insert should follow the requirements of the United States Code of Federal Regulations 21 CFR 809.10 (1992). Since this document is comprehensive, it is recommended that the evaluator obtains a copy of it for direct study. If the instrument or kit is manufactured in the United States, it can be assumed that the manual or insert will conform to this Standard. The *in vitro* diagnostic device Directive stemming from the International Standards Organization (ISO) standards will impose similar requirements on European Union manufacturers in the future. However, a product reference manual may conform in all respects to statutory requirements and yet be ineptly written. Because of the importance of communicating the complex world of the hematology instrument to ordinary people, readability of a manual can become a critical aspect of a decision to buy a product. This includes having the manual in the commonly used language of the country.

Quality control and calibration procedures should be provided by the supplier as a section of the product reference manual and must teach the steps of the calibration procedure, if one is required. Quality control instructions should describe methods for verifying the calibration set-point, detecting set-point change and detecting departure from the specified limits of precision, accuracy, clinical sensitivity and specificity. Of particular importance is the proper application of positive and negative control materials and procedures.

16.2.2 Review of Service and Warranty Provisions

Even the most robust product will eventually fail and require repair. Manufacturers are frequently reticent on these points but should be closely questioned about them. Consider the following:

Warranty. What is the duration of the warranty? For instruments, at least one year should be expected. Does it provide for full replacement, full refund or merely repair? Remember that the cost of the warranty has been built into the purchase price!

Service contracts. After the warranty has expired, what is the cost of service? Is there a comprehensive contract or separate charges for labour and materials? Can you chose between these arrangements?

Service calls. How far will your serviceman need to travel? Is service available 24 hours in the day and seven days in the week? Do you require such complete coverage? Determine the support available from the factory. Does the manufacturer offer a 'hot-line' trouble-shooting service?

Service history. What is the device's mean time between failures (MTBF)? How many changes have been made to this, or a similar product, during the time it has been in distribution? Are you entitled to have changes installed outside the warranty period at no cost? Has this, or a similar product ever been recalled?

User serviceability. How much preventive maintenance can the owner perform? Are certain types of repair forbidden to the owner? Will service training (and parts) be available to hospital engineers?

16.2.3 Review of emergency service ('stat') capability

This is an important and often overlooked situation. In addition to it being desirable for an instrument to require minimal preparation for the performance of emergency assays, consideration should be given to the calibre of personnel available at all hours of the day and night to do such work, and whether they can be expected to operate the instrument properly. This capability should be thoroughly tested by simulated stat tests under worst-case conditions.

16.2.4 Review of flagging capability

It is probably not reasonable to expect an instrument or kit to be capable of accurate assays on all specimens. Extremely high or low analyte values, the presence of interfering substances and the alteration of analyte properties by pathological conditions may induce deterioration of accuracy and/or precision. The manufacturer should have investigated the response of his product to such circumstances and should provide the user with due warning (flagging) of the conditions under which performance may deteriorate. In some cases the warning may be automatic and expressed by displayed or printed information. In other cases, particularly kits that do not use a dedicated instrument, the sole source of warning may be only in the product manual or package insert. The manufacturer should have addressed the question of whether to suppress a questionable result or whether to display it together with a warning. The evaluator should acquire an understanding of the flagging criteria and decide whether they are reasonable and safe. This is particularly important in the case of automated differential counters.

16.3 Verification of performance specifications

A few comments about terminology will be helpful. Note the use of the word 'verification'. This means that we have evaluated the performance specification, found it acceptable for our purpose and are now going to test its truth. It is also useful to use the term 'Performance Characteristic' to describe a sub-set of the specification such as *precision* or *clinical sensitivity*. The performance characteristics that are useful in describing a product are:

- Accuracy
- Precision
- Reportable or Dynamic Range

- Analytical or Clinical Sensitivity and Specificity
- Reference Ranges or Intervals

The alternative terminology, e.g. 'Reference Ranges' versus 'Reference Intervals' reflects alternative authorities. The former is preferred by 42 CFR 493 (1992). The latter is preferred by the NCCLS Proposed Guideline NRSCL8-P2 (1993). The reader should refer to the NCCLS document to resolve terminological ambiguities.

Accuracy means the degree to which the test method agrees (or disagrees) with a result accepted as 'true' by an alternative analysis system. An important component of the measurement of accuracy is the range of analyte values over which a given standard of accuracy holds true.

Imprecision, frequently expressed as precision, is a statement about the repeatability of the test method. It should give the user an understanding of the meaning of differences that might be observed when a specimen is re-tested to verify a result that does not seem to agree with clinical expectations. It is useful to include the measure of imprecision in statements of accuracy but low imprecision (high repeatability) must not be taken to imply high accuracy. Note that the usual indices such as standard deviation or coefficient of variation make a statement about error, not about the lack of it. For this reason the word 'imprecision' will be found in this text more frequently than its antonym.

Analytical or Clinical Sensitivity and Specificity are used in the sense defined by Galen and Gambino (1975) with particular emphasis on errors produced by pathological conditions and interfering substances. The definition is further refined for differential leukocyte counting in NCCLS document H20-A (1992).

Reportable or Dynamic Range is a relatively new term for hematologists. It means the range of analyte values over which patients' results are can be measured with accuracy and precision. We believe it to be a more useful term than linearity. Reportable Range may be affected by a variety of errors of which lack of linearity is one special case.

Reference Ranges or Intervals should be stated by the supplier in the performance specifications. This statement should include subcategories of the sample population from which this information was obtained together with a description of the statistical methods that were used. Gender distribution, age range, the effect of smoking, alcohol or drugs, demographics and race may be factors affecting reference ranges.

16.4 The evaluation process

The quality control procedure given in the manual or insert should be followed rigorously throughout the entire evaluation process and a comment on its effectiveness made a part of the final report. Any imperfections in the procedure should be noted and discussed with the manufacturer at the earliest moment. An ineffective quality control procedure or one that is not meticulously followed could invalidate the evaluation process. If used, the make or source of stabilized blood control material recommended by the manufacturer may be different from that currently used by the evaluator. Do not make a substitution without good reason.

Statistical methods useful for analysing the data from the various evaluation procedures are described in simple terms in this text and stated in more formal terms in a glossary at the end of the chapter. Additionally, the reader should consult standard reference books such as Geigy Scientific Tables (1982) for more details of statistical procedures.

16.5 Measurement of precision

Precision is estimated by performing a set of replicate tests within a stipulated time frame. The dispersion of these results is the measure of the imprecision of the system and is expressed as an index of dispersion.

Carefully performed estimates of imprecision are the best indicator of the integrity of an instrument or kit. Loss of precision does not provide information about the nature of a product defect but, when observed, should lead to a careful search for causative factors. Loss of precision may cause a systematic loss of accuracy (bias) if calibration is performed when the instrument response is momentarily offset as a result of some internal derangement. Therefore, verification of the precision specification should always be the first stage of the calibration procedure and must precede measurement of accuracy.

Every system of analysis contains variables. It is important to have an understanding of the 'error budget' of the total system when verifying precision and accuracy. Some of these variables may not be controllable since they lie outside the measuring device. For example, a blood cell counter may be temperature-sensitive. Even though the laboratory temperature may be equable, the analyser may have been installed close to a radiator. Reagents may not have equilibrated with room temperature or blood specimens or the control material may have been stored in the refrigerator and not adequately warmed before use.

After ensuring that external factors have been controlled or minimized (it is a good idea to have a checklist for them), two types of testing may be undertaken for both short-term and long-term precision studies.

16.5.1 Simple replication

This test uses both stabilized blood control material and fresh blood from a normal individual. The characteristics of the control material lie in the hands of its manufacturer. Ideally, it should provide different levels of each analyte, covering, as nearly as possible, the full reportable range and cover the normal ranges as well as values near the critical decision levels used by the clinicians. Fresh whole blood from a normal individual, rather than a patient is to be used in order to minimize the errors of analyte instability or other interferences that are possible in pathological specimens.

Usually, 31 replicate determinations are made. A lesser number may be used on the understanding that the statement of precision may be compromised thereby and the conventional descriptors of precision such as standard deviation (s) and coefficient of variation (CV) will not be robust. The results of lesser numbers of replications (n) should be more properly expressed as confidence limits. This is a term that evokes a more descriptive mental image than s or CV and we recommend its use regardless of whether the value of n is equal to or less than 31.

Some instruments provide automatic calculation of precision from a set of replicated control assays. Should this capability be used here? We think it should, providing it has been checked once against a hand calculator. But make sure that your method of rounding or truncating numbers is the same as that used by the instrument manufacturer.

1. *Replicate assays with n = 31*

Perform 31 consecutive assays of three levels of control material and 31 replicate assays of a normal whole blood specimen. For each analyte, calculate s and CV using formulas (1) and (2) from the Glossary (pp 163–165).

For instruments in proper working order, replicated results should differ randomly from the mean 66% of the time by amounts up to the specified value of s and will differ from the mean 95% of the time by amounts up to twice the specified value of s. An instrument giving results that deviate beyond these limits should be considered to be defective and cause should be sought for the disparity.

2. *Replicate assays with n < 31*

Replications less than 31 do not give the classical bell-shaped curve of data distribution. Instead there is a tendency for the data to occupy the tails of the curve rather than the centre, making simple calculation of s inaccurate. This problem was solved by Gosset (1908), writing under the *nom de plume* 'Student'. His work provides us with a factor, t (Student factor) by which s should be multiplied to give confidence limits appropriate for the degree of replication used in the test of precision.

Perform the calculation for s using the formula 1 from the Glossary. The divisors for calculating the means and s will now be the chosen n and (n − 1).

Look up, in Table 16.2, the value of t that is appropriate for (n − 1) and multiply s by this number to obtain the 95% confidence limits for the chosen degree of replication as shown in formula 3. Since t increases as n decreases, the 95% confidence limits given by this method will be greater than the simple 2s limits (based on n = 31) that are usually quoted in manufacturers' performance specifications. This can make it difficult to compare the test results with the specifications. A method of avoiding this difficulty is given later in this chapter.

3. *Pair Difference Analysis*

This test is performed on at least 31 clinical specimens. These specimens should be selected to give as broad as possible a spread of all analyte values and a 'smooth' dispersion of results. Analyse all specimens in duplicate. Label the data 'Run 1' and 'Run 2' and tabulate accordingly, taking care to match the rows in the table exactly. Inspect the values to determine whether there are cases in which adjacent tests have been affected by preceding high values or low values. If this is seen it indicates that the system is sensitive to carry-over. Make a note of such cases but do not delete them. The effect of carry-over on the repeatability of results is an inherent part of the real-life use of analysis systems. The usefulness of the pair-difference method for long-term precision measurement is discussed below.

Most, if not all, instruments provide a means of flagging results that exceed the capability of the method due to interfering substances, extreme high or low analyte levels or other causes of untrustworthy results. Whether on not to include such results in the pair difference table will depend on the flagging criteria given in the product reference manual. These criteria will differ from supplier to supplier so no firm rules for exclusion can be given here other than, 'if in doubt, leave it out'. Make sure that the record reflects this exclusion.

The table of results should have a third column headed 'Difference' (d). It will contain the difference between each row-member of the first and second columns, i.e. $d_1 \ldots d_n$. Calculate the Mean and s of the data in the difference column. The value of n will be the number of rows in the table.

The index of dispersion of the data in the difference column can be expressed as either s or confidence limits. Because the number of tests will be over 31, $\pm 2s$ will be very nearly equivalent to 95% confidence limits.

16.5.2 Within-run and between-run imprecision

It is customary to distinguish two types of imprecision, namely within-run or short-term, and between-
run or long-term. Any of the simple replication
methods can be used to verify the within-run imprecision specification. The meaning of within-run imprecision is that it teaches the limits of difference between
results of a test, on the same specimen, that is repeated within an interval short enough to exclude
analyte change as a cause of test-to-test disparity.

The implication of the between-run imprecision
specification is less clear for hematology measurements than for chemistry measurements because tests
on the same specimen performed on different shifts
or different days may be affected by the instability of
cellular analytes. Even labile biochemical analytes
can be preserved between runs by freezing. Cellular
analytes cannot be conveniently preserved in this
manner. In spite of these problems the between-run
test is important in providing evidence of instrument
stability and drift of calibration set-point

The lability of cellular analytes may obscure underlying instrument instability or may give a falsely
pessimistic impression of an analytic system. For this
reason, pair-difference measurement of imprecision,
if spread over several days, is a better method than
spaced sets of replicate tests for estimating the effect
of time-lapse on repeatability. If the instrument is
time-stable, the index of dispersion given by pair
difference will be only slightly greater than that
given by replication.

Between-run imprecision specifications should be
verified by sets of replicate tests of stabilized blood
control material at various analyte levels with n =
31. These tests should be performed on at least three
different shifts or days. On each occasion, the observed value of s should not exceed the specification
and the means of each set of 31 results should agree
with the mean of all sets within twice the Standard
Error of the Mean (SEM). SEM is calculated by
dividing the measured s by the square root of n as
shown in formula 4. If all values of s are the same,
or nearly so, but the means are in disagreement, it is
almost certain that the calibration set-point of the
instrument has drifted.

Measurement of the imprecision of the leukocyte
differential count presents a separate statistical problem since the variance of proportional differential
count data is concentration-dependent. If the
concentration of a cell type is expressed as p and the
concentration of the sum of all other cell types is q,
then the square root of $((p \times q) \div n)$ provides an
index of dispersion of p for any value of n where n is
the total number of cells classified. This index is the
Standard Error of p (SEp) and is found in the glossary
as formula 5. From this it is clear that the confidence
limits of the differential count can be improved by
increasing n. This rule is based on the work of Clopper

and Pearson (1934) and its importance was pointed
out by Rümke (1977). The method for deriving SEp
is given in NCCLS document H20-A and is further
discussed under Measurement of Accuracy, below.

16.5.3 Measurement of carry-over

Most, if not all, instruments suffer in some degree
from interaction between adjacent specimens. Typically, less than 1% of a sample will be contaminated
by the preceding one (or contaminate the subsequent
one). Since the analyte levels of juxtaposed specimens
are likely to be randomly related, the effect of carry-
over can be thought of as a contributing factor to the
repeatability of the test method and a component of
imprecision.

Although a variety of methods have been proposed
for this test, the underlying principle is the same for all.
1. Replication: Because the measured value of carry-
over is small, it challenges the limits of sensitivity of
most analysers. To minimize error due to imprecision, replicate testing is essential. At least ten replications should be used
2. Choice of material: In some laboratories there may
be problems in selecting blood specimens with major
differences in analyte concentration. Therefore manipulation of a single specimen can be carried out to
yield both high-valued and low-valued 'specimens'.
The cellular components of a normal whole blood
specimen may be concentrated by low-speed centrifugation. Remove only enough plasma to give a nominal cell concentration that approximates the upper
limit of the claimed Reportable Range. Add this
plasma back to an uncentrifuged portion of the
specimen to lower the cell concentration as close as
possible to the lower limit of the Reportable Range.
Occasional specimens may show platelet or neutrophil
clumping with this treatment. Examine all preparations, appropriately diluted, under the microscope
before use to exclude this potential source of error.

Rather than juxtaposing high- and low-valued
specimens, a normal-valued (or manipulated high-
valued) specimen may be partnered with cell-free
plasma or the system's own diluent reagent.

Artificially concentrated blood may be replaced by
high-valued stabilized blood control material. Take
care! Some commercial control material may have a
concentration/viscosity characteristic that could exag-
gerate an otherwise acceptable carry-over result.
3. Protocol: The instrument should have been verified
as meeting the within-run imprecision specification.
Perform three consecutive analyses of the high-
valued specimen (H_1, H_2, H_3) followed by three
consecutive analyses of the low-valued specimen
(L_1, L_2, L_3). Repeat this ritual 10 times. Tabulate the
data so that all 'first shot' results and all 'third shot'
results of both high and low specimens can be averaged. Carry-over percent is the ratio of the average
of 'first shots' to the average of 'third shots' times

100 minus 100. As shown in the following example of measurement of red cell carry-over where the H_1 average is 5.62 and the H_3 average is 5.65.

$$((5.62 \div 5.65) \times 100) - 100 = -0.531$$

Although this carry-over quantity is arithmetically negative, for descriptive purposes it is convenient to ignore the sign. True negative carry-over would cause H_1 to be greater than H_3 and would raise the suspicion that the manufacturer had over-corrected carry-over error in software.

Carry-over for all analytes should be calculated. It might seem unnecessary to do this for analytes that share the same fluidics pathway but the adhesive property of surfaces for various cell types may differ so that different cell types sharing the same pathway may have differences in carry-over.

16.6 Measurement of accuracy

Accuracy is estimated by a comparison test in which the instrument or kit assays specimens in parallel with an alternative method whose accuracy has been verified. The choice of the alternative or comparator method will depend on the availability of equipment, time, manpower and skills. It is reasonable to expect a manufacturer to use state-of-the-art devices and methods to ensure the accuracy of his product but it is unreasonable to expect the average buyer of his product to work to this standard.

The most elementary approach to verification of accuracy is the assay of stabilized blood calibrant (calibrator). Recovery of the labelled assigned values within the limits imposed by the imprecision of the system and the degree of replication provides a preliminary estimate of accuracy but does not predict the behaviour of the instrument or kit with actual blood specimens (Koepke, 1977). The span of results covered by the assigned values is usually less than the span of patient results. At best, this method of assessing accuracy is a screening test. If assigned values are not recovered, the test method (or the calibrant) must be suffering a grievous disorder. If assigned values are recovered it is worthwhile proceeding with a more definitive investigation.

The recommended use of calibrant rather than control material is based on the supposition that its manufacturer has assigned calibrant values by a closed-loop method using multiple fresh whole blood specimens to transfer assay instrument calibration set-points from reference method measurements (ICSH, 1988; Richardson-Jones, 1990; Bull *et al.,* 1992). The confidence limits of these values should be stated in the product labelling. The assigned values of control material may have been obtained from instruments that were calibrated with calibrant and thus might contain an additional order of error.

Verification of accuracy will be simplest in the case of the laboratory that already possesses an instrument or kit of a type equivalent to the device that is undergoing evaluation. Let us call the device under test the *propositus device* and the existing device to which it is equivalent the *predicate device*. The predicate device should have a carefully documented history and a clean record of performance in internal and external quality control programmes. Its conformance to precision specifications should be verified by one or more of the methods described above. The accuracy of the predicate device should be confirmed by re-calibration. Regardless of the number of replicated assays of calibrant recommended by the manufacturer, we think at least 16 should be used for this purpose. A data string of this length will have a SEM = 0.25s for each analyte. Therefore the mean recovered value of all calibration assays should be within 0.75s (t = 2.9467 for 2P = 0.01 and (n − 1) = 5). If the assigned values of the calibrant are not recovered within these limits, the accuracy of the predicate device may not be in conformance with the manufacturer's specifications or the calibrant may be defective, or both. The supplier's service organization should then be consulted.

Employing a currently used predicate device assumes that no new analytes will be assayed. Additional analytes will require additional testing capability. The most likely additions to the instrument repertoire will be reticulocyte, CD4 and CD8 counts. A reticulocyte reference method suitable for comparison testing is described in NCCLS Publication H44-P (1993). Comparison testing of cell surface markers presents a problem since no method has yet been agreed upon to provide an independent standard of accuracy. At the time of writing, stabilized cell preparations for use as calibrants or as quality control material for these special tests should be used with caution. The package inserts of monoclonal antibodies for CD4 and CD8 identification provide satisfactory descriptions of flow cytometric procedures that can be used as comparator methods. If the laboratory does not have a flow cytometer, the evaluator will have to generate predicate data in a remote institution or persuade his own institution to buy the necessary equipment.

Manufacturers of instruments and kits are presumed to have solved this problem and will be expected to hold themselves to higher standards of accuracy in cell counting, sizing and classification than can be achieved by institutions that are limited to the use of calibrated comparator instruments. Manufacturers will be expected to use true Reference Methods conforming to the definition in NCCLS document NRSCL8-P2 (1993) where these are available and establish an audit trail of accuracy to fundamental units of mass, length, etc. For instance, the manufacturer's reference hemoglobinometry method should use the extinction coefficient of hemiglobincyanide (ICSH, 1987; NCCLS, 1993) rather than a calibrant solution as the means of setting the spectrophotometer concentration/absorbance relationship. A reference cell counter should measure the volume of cell suspension presented to the particle sensing zone by a positive-displacement, gravimetrically calibrated system and the identification of cell type by size should be verified for every assay by size distribution analysis. A practical dissertation on the choice of reference methods is given by the ICSH Expert Panel on Cytometry (1984).

Reference leukocyte differential counts can be performed by virtually all institutions and certainly by all manufacturers. The method is described in NCCLS Publication H20-A (1992). Although two 200-cell counts are proposed in this document, consideration should be given to using an 800-cell count (4 observers, each counting 200 cells) when examining abnormal specimens. This will improve the probability of finding low-frequency abnormal cell types by a factor of 1.4.

Observer validation is an essential part of the method. The microscopists used for the reference differential count should be validated by a double-blind protocol that tests the dispersion of individual observer performance against the mean of all assays for each of four specimens covering the reference interval of each normal cell type. All observer values should fall within the 99% SEp. If they do not, the disparate results should be submitted to arbitration and a microscopist re-training programme should be considered.

16.6.1 Range of analyte values

This should be as broad as possible. The record of the results of the Accuracy Test will provide documentation of the range of test results which are valid, i.e. where there is agreement between the propositus and predicate methods. This will provide verification of reportable or dynamic range. It will be suggested that the reportable range defined in this way can be extended by experimentally defining the limits of linearity of the propositus method.

16.7 Analysis of comparison test data

There is no single 'best' method for analysing the data from tests for the measurement of accuracy. Choice is largely determined by the amount of information the evaluator needs to form a judgement about the product and the types of analyte under evaluation. The following methods of data analysis should be considered when making this choice. Bear in mind that this list is practical rather than exhaustive and that good practice calls for the use of more than one method.

16.7.1 Comparison of means

This is the simplest method. It looks for bias between the methods reflected by the difference, if any, between the average (formula 5) of all results from the predicate method and all results from the propositus method. Its sole merit is that it frequently can provide a quick answer. The dispersion of individual differences should be included in the table of results as s. However, this method does not permit analysis of whether analyte concentration affects differences.

16.7.2 Cumulative mean difference

This test tells whether the dispersion of differences is influenced by factors other than statistical variation and it provides a graphical expression of the adequacy of the data-base. Use the string of differences between propositus and predicate methods. Average the first four differences, five differences, six differences and so on according to formula 6. Plot each incremental average (mean) on the y-axis against its sequential number on the x-axis. An example is shown in Figure 16.1.

Note that the line connecting the points becomes progressively smoother and asymptotic. Combine the s for each method and plot the SEM of the cumulative mean differences over the data plot. If the variance (scatter) of the data plot tracks the SEM line, method differences are due to statistical factors. If the data plot violates the SEM line, additional causes of difference must be pursued.

16.7.3 Difference/concentration plot

When the means of propositus and predicate instruments differ, this method shows whether the difference is due to slope, offset or a combination of both. Plot the string of differences between the methods (y) as a function of analyte concentration (x). If the methods agree, the data points will lie along the zero difference coordinate as illustrated in Figure 16.2.

Other conditions such as slopes, shifts and curves require explanation. Remember that this and other difference or ratio plots speak only of difference, or lack of it, and are silent as to truth.

16.7.4 Regression analysis

This is probably the most abused and least understood method for comparing two data sets. It only works well when both x- and y- data have similar variance that is not concentration dependent and there are no isolated, non-linear data-points with very high or very low values (formula 7). The Correlation Coefficient (r) and the predictive value of x for y (r²) apply only to the data set as a *whole*. An individual value of x will predict y only within the limits

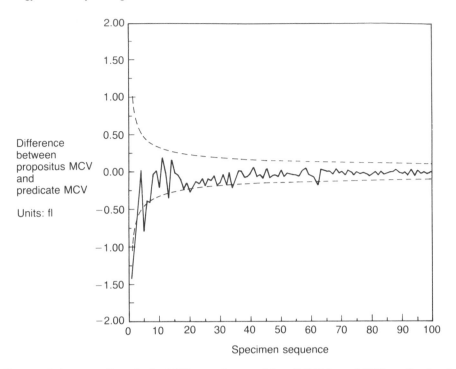

Figure 16.1 The cumulative mean (formula 6) of differences between Mean Cell Volume (MCV) results given by a predicate method and the results given by a propositus instrument. Predicate values are from NCCLS H7–A packed cell volume (PVC) method divided by the red cell count from a validated (see text) single-channel Coulter Counter®. The dotted line limits of the standard error of the mean (SEM, Formula 4) provide a guide to the progress of the experiment. The good fit between the data and the SEM is the result of selecting specimens having predicate Mean Cell Hemoglobin Concentration (MCHC) values of 33.7 ± 1.0 gm/dL (Arnfred, Christensen and Munck, 1982).

of imprecision. A low value of r may mean that the data sets correlate poorly but it may also suggest that regression analysis is an unsuitable method for analysing the case (formula 8).

16.7.5 Binomial envelope

The Standard Error of the Parameter (SEp) for 95% limits for both propositus and predicate methods are combined by taking the square root of the sum of their squares over the appropriate range of p (formula 4). This will give a composite binomial envelope that should be set at a slope of 1.00. No more than 5% of data points may escape the envelope if method agreement is to be assured. Bias or offset, if present, is easily seen. Morphologically abnormal specimens, whether flagged by the microscopist or by the instrument, should be excluded from an analysis of the accuracy of the distributional differential count.

It should be borne in mind that the binomial dispersion is not the only component of instrument error. All instruments contain sources of variance (process variation) that are independent of the concentration of analyte. The imprecision that results

from the combination of these errors can be measured by replication (see above) at an arbitrarily chosen concentration, subtracted from the calculated SEp for that value of p and added back to the SEp, as a constant, for each increment of concentration. This has the effect of making the fusiform binomial envelope wider at each end and provides a kinder statistical environment for assessing performance for low-concentration cell types such as basophil. An example of this adjusted binomial envelope is given in Figure 16.3. It illustrates performance that would be unacceptable without the addition of process variation but becomes acceptable with it.

Although the binomial envelope method has grown in popularity, it was not always thus. As recently as NCCLS Publication H20-T (1984), the double arc-sine transform was tentatively recommended as one way to define the relationship between the microscopic, neuro-optical (low precision) and instrument (better precision) differential count methods. The final approved standard H20-A (NCCLS, 1992) uses the binomial method. Publications on the performance of automated differential counters not uncommonly contain statements of correlation coefficient rather than fit to a binomial envelope. Inspection of the data in these publications often shows

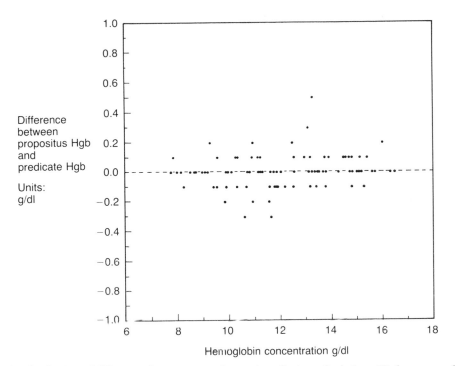

Figure 16.2 The distribution of differences between propositus and predicate methods (n = 98) for assays of hemoglobin (Hgb) as a function of analyte concentration. It demonstrates that agreement between the methods is independent of concentration over the range studied. The spread of differences should not exceed three times the standard deviation previously measured by pair-difference analysis. Data that slopes upward or downwards suggests calibration set-point error. Data that is grouped above or below zero difference but is not sloped cannot be corrected by re-calibration

that a low value of r is not inconsistent with a good binomial fit.

16.7.6 Comparison of confidence limits

There will be occasions when one must compare the means of two sets of data that are based on differing values of n. If n for each set differs but equals or exceeds 31, statistical variation as a contributor to an apparent difference between the methods can be ignored. If n for each set is less than 31, calculate s for each set and derive the 95% confidence limits for each, based on its unique n. Divide the larger value of t by the smaller to make a ratio. Multiply the confidence limits of the set with the larger n by this ratio to make the limits comparable.

16.8 Measurement of clinical sensitivity and specificity

For instruments that produce continuously variable data (as contrasted to a simple positive or negative result), sensitivity is defined as the smallest input

that will produce a measurable response. In practice this means the smallest response that can be differentiated from random variation, or the difference between a pair of results that exceeds the 99% confidence limits.

Specificity is the measure of the test method to differentiate accurately among the various cell types or analytes. Rightly or wrongly, the criteria for recognition of analytes will have been set by the predicate method or the reference method, if one is available. Therefore, specificity and accuracy are inter-related. As an example, Mean Cell Volume (MCV) reported by most automated blood cell counters differs in some degree from that reported by the reference method (Arnfred, Christensen and Munck, 1982). This difference cannot be entirely explained by random variation and must be ascribed to a difference of specificity between the methods. Therefore lack of specificity can be expressed as the residual bias in a comparison study after subtraction of statistical error limits.

For all estimates of sensitivity and specificity, there must be some form of reference measurement that is presumed to be true. Thus the ability of an instrument to detect abnormal cell types will be compared to the performance of human observers engaged in

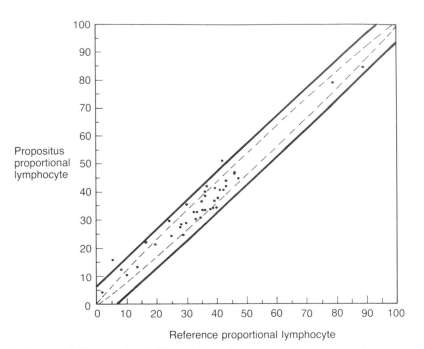

Figure 16.3 The distribution of 41 proportional differential lymphocyte counts from a propositus instrument compared to NCCLS H20–A reference counts. When only binomial limits, indicated by dotted lines, are used to judge method agreement, 24% of the results appear to be in error. When binomial distribution error (formula 5) and process variation (formula 1 and text) are combined to produce the solid line envelope, the error rate becomes 5%

the same task. We do not have to know whether the instrument is 'better' than the human observers, only whether it is similar or different.

For kits and for qualitative or discontinuous instrument parameters, the methods and definitions of Galen and Gambino (1975) are recommended. The ability of an instrument to detect or flag specimens containing morphologically abnormal leukocytes provides an example.

The first stage of the test is to define the criteria of abnormality. For instance, how many blasts must be seen in order to label the specimen 'abnormal'? NCCLS Publication H20-A (1992) provides a useful set of limits. Although that publication gives a choice of absolute or proportional counts, we now recommend using the absolute number. The ratio of normal to abnormal specimens has an important bearing. The effect of *prevalence* on the robustness of the information yielded by the study, should lead, if possible, to the use of approximately equal numbers of normal and abnormal specimens.

A minimum of two, and preferably four trained and validated microscopists will each classify 200 cells in blind coded specimens as 'normal' or 'abnormal' on the basis of these criteria. They must agree on the presence and type of abnormal cells. Disagreements that exceed the limits predicted by binomial analysis must be referred to an arbitrator.

When a specimen satisfies the criteria for abnormal-

ity, it is so labelled. The nature of the abnormality is also recorded. The terms 'normal' and 'abnormal' are preferred but 'reference positive' or 'reference negative' are often used. The latter designators, we believe, should be reserved for the instrument or kit results, the former for reference results. Note the use of the term 'reference' rather than 'predicate' in the case of differential counter analysis. This term is used because the method given in NCCLS H20-A (1992) has the formal status of a reference method. Classification of reference results and propositus results in this manner allows the construction of a table that uses the layout given in NCCLS H20-A (1992) (Table 16.1).

Beware of the self-serving manufacturer who expresses false negatives as (negatives minus abnormals) divided by the total number of tests. Even worse is the inclusion of distributional normals and abnormals in the table. Both of these manoeuvres artificially dilute the error frequency and make the performance picture rosier than it really is.

Evaluation of the types of pathology associated with false positives and false negatives is necessary to assess the gravity of these errors. Borderline abnormals should always be reassessed in the light of the Standard Error of the Parameter (SEp). The evaluator might thus find a basis for hardening or softening his decision level.

The following is a suggested method (formula 8)

Table 16.1 Analysis of clinical specificity and sensitivity of an automated differential counter by comparing its flagging rate for morphologically abnormal specimens (27/230 cases) with NCCLS H20-A reference method

	Instrument flagged or positive test result	Not flagged or negative test result
Reference Positive (abnormal)	TP (True positive) 24	FN (False negative) 3
Reference Negative. (normal)	FP (False positive) 26	TN (True negative) 177

$$\text{Agreement} = \frac{TP(24) + TN(177)}{TP(24) + FN(3) + FP(26) + TN(177)}$$
$$\times 100 = 88\%$$

$$\text{False positive ratio} = \frac{FP(26)}{FN(26) + TN(177)}$$
$$\times 100 = 14\%$$

$$\text{False negative ratio} = \frac{FN(3)}{FN(3) + TP(24)}$$
$$\times 100 = 11\%$$

for obtaining a numerical value for the specificity of propositus analysis systems such as cell counters that produce a continuum of data. Make sure propositus and predicate systems are exactly calibrated

1. Measure the variance (s squared) of propositus and predicate systems by the pair-difference method shown in formula 1. Add the two variances.
2. Take the square root of the sum of the variances to obtain the combined standard deviations of the precision tests. Label this $s_{\text{precision}}$.
3. Make a column of differences between predicate values and propositus values. Calculate s for this column. Label it s_{accuracy}.
4. Make a ratio of $s_{\text{precision}}$ to s_{accuracy}. If this ratio is unity, or nearly so, the two methods have equal specificity. If it is greater or less than unity, the methods have differing specificity. and an explanation should be sought.

As an example, consider the case of hemoglobin measurements made by the NCCLS H15-A (1993) reference method (predicate) compared to the results from the same set of specimens given by the propositus automated blood cell counter. The pair difference estimate of s for the reference method was ± 0.12. For the propositus method it was ± 0.16. The combined s for both methods ($s_{\text{precision}}$) was ± 0.20. The standard deviation of the differences between the methods (s_{accuracy}) was ± 0.31. Applying formula 7 gave an index of 1.55, suggesting that the propositus method was less specific than the predicate method. Inspection of the data showed that the disagreements between the methods were associated with predicate values having elevated absorbance at 750 nm caused by turbidity. The automated instrument, having no means to compensate for turbidity, gave slightly, but falsely, elevated hemoglobin values in these cases. The significance of this type of finding must be left to the judgement of the evaluator.

16.9 Assessment of linearity

The non-linear response is a special case of loss of sensitivity as a function of analyte concentration. The measurement of linearity is of importance to instrument designers because it can help define potential error sources. In addition to verifying specifications the institutional evaluator will find it useful for establishing extended reportable or dynamic range limits. Linearity measurement should not be the sole source of data for this purpose but if it is so used, the test should be modified to enable propositus and predicate methods to be assayed in parallel.

The cell count analytes will be expected to decrement proportionately with dilution. However, cell size analytes and ratios, e.g. MCV and differential count percentages, should not change with dilution unless the system is defective. For this reason the linearity test of a differential counter should use absolute counts in addition to proportional values.

If measurement of linear response is undertaken, several factors should be taken into account:

16.9.1 Material

It will be necessary to concentrate platelets, leukocytes and red cells in varying degree to provide a high-end specimen. This may be done by making, from the same specimen, separate preparations of re-spun platelet-rich plasma, re-suspended buffy coat and sedimented red cells. The concentrates are then re-combined to give the following approximate cell counts:

Red cells	$7.0 \times 10^{12}/l$
Leukocytes	$150 \times 10^{9}/l$
Platelets	$2000 \times 10^{9}/l$

Verify, by microscopy, that the suspensions are free of agglutinates. Make triplicate dilutions of the modified specimen in its own cell-free plasma in 20% steps from 100% to 0%. Use TC pipettes that are rinsed into each suspension. Do not over-fill and drain back to the mark. This leaves cells on the pipette wall that cause a significant error.

16.9.2 Protocol

Perform 4 replicate counts on each dilution, discarding the first result in order to obviate carry-over error.

16.9.3 Analysis

Average the remaining three results for each dilution and plot these means with 'min/max' error bar against the dilution percentage. Connect the graph points and assess linearity with a straight edge. The dilution factor at which the line connecting the points falls one half the length of an error bar from the mean is the limit of linearity. Use a near-normal reported value from which to extrapolate the expected count limits. More sophisticated methods of linearity analysis may be used but these do not necessarily shed light on the causes of unsatisfactory results.

16.10 Evaluating reference ranges

The reference range or reference interval is the span of 95% of assay values that may be expected in a 'normal' population. As a corollary, values falling outside this interval suggest the presence of pathological conditions.

Responsibility for developing the reference ranges for an instrument or kit lies, in the first place, with the manufacturer. A user of the product has the responsibility for confirming that the manufacturer's proposed ranges are consistent with those found in individuals likely to patronize his institution. Local socio-economic, ethnic and geographic factors need to be considered if the evaluator's findings differ from the product labelling. Consideration should also be given to changes in reference intervals associated with the installation of a different type of analyser, reagent or calibrant. Analytical systems for coagulation measurements may be sensitive to this effect.

Reference should be made to NCCLS Publication C28-P (1992) and to an IFCC/ICSH publication (1987) on the topic of reference intervals.

A minimum of 120 males and 120 females who meet the wellness criteria given in the NCCLS document should be assayed after the physical and performance specifications of the instrument have been verified.

Prepare a histogram of each data-set, inspect for the presence of outliers and reject cases that are clearly not a part of the continuum. Fractile (ranked order) analysis is a useful way to do this.

If the data for any analyte is skewed (i.e. mode and mean are not in close agreement) the reference range will be the results that fall between the 2.5 and 97.5 percentiles (formula 10). If the data is symmetrical, the reference range will be $\pm$ 2s above and below the mean (formula 3). For analytes that do not show any gender-linked difference, pool male and female results. Separation of data on the basis of other variables such as race, alcohol use, tobacco use, etc. will be at the discretion of the evaluator and local institutional standards.

As a practical matter, data for reference range evaluation can be built up over a period of time, providing the manufacturer's published ranges do not conflict with the laboratory's prior experience.

16.11 Record keeping

Little has been said on this topic until now because laboratorians are generally inveterate, if not compulsive, keepers of records. In addition to the obvious documentation of lot numbers and expiration date of reagents, control materials and cleansing agents it is recommended that the temperature, barometric pressure, humidity and, if possible, line voltage in the evaluation laboratory be continuously recorded. The relationship of untoward episodes to fluctuations of ambient conditions may suggest a causative relationship. Be reminded that information that is not legibly and accurately compiled does not, for practical purposes, exist. Some differences between routine laboratory records and the documentation of evaluation tests deserve discussion.

16.11.1 Separation of records

Evaluation data must be clearly separated from the data of tests performed for diagnostic purposes. Use an 'all in one place' rule for record storage. Third-party auditors of the work will be more kindly disposed towards evaluation programmes that have easily accessible documents laid out in a consistent format.

16.11.2 Confidentiality

An audit trail is necessary to track down the possible impact of diagnosis on anomalous results. This trail must be securely keyed through a senior person in order to preserve anonymity of data. The manufacturer of the product should be informed if a third party, other than a duly authorized government agent or agent of a voluntary compliance organization seeks access to the data for purposes other than proof of compliance with regulatory performance standards.

16.11.3 Diagnostic use

In general, the results of evaluation tests should not be used for diagnosis unless supported by information from an alternative source. This is particularly important in cases where the propositus device carries an 'Investigational Use' or 'Research Use' label. In the latter case, diagnostic use of the results will be absolutely forbidden in the US. The report of the work should show that these constraints have been observed.

16.11.4 Institutional Review Board

Evaluation tests that use specimens left over from diagnostic procedures will not require the informed consent of the patient but it is strongly recommended that the Human Research Committee or Institutional Review Board of the hospital be given the opportunity to approve the terms of the evaluation project and be satisfied that its rules are understood and followed.

16.11.5 Alterations

White-out must never be used to alter a record. Strike out the erroneous entry with a single line; write in the correct entry and have the change initialled by another person. If necessary, use a footnote to explain the action.

16.11.6 Storage

Records, both paper and magnetic, must always be kept secure from tampering and accidental damage. Consult the manufacturer of the product as to whether he has a preference for the duration of storage and check with management of the institution as to their policies in this matter.

16.12 Cost accounting

Analysis of the cost of an evaluation, and hence cost of ownership, can make an important contribution to the decision to buy or not to buy, should this be the purpose of the project. The manufacturer or the institution's accounting department will usually prove helpful in setting up a costing system but the laboratory must be prepared to keep accurate records of man hours spent in generating data, i.e. labour burden per test result, and the amounts of reagents and control materials consumed. When doing this, the time spent bringing the instrument from standby to fully operational state and performing quality control procedures must be added to the time spent testing specimens. The chapter on workload and performance indicators (Chapter 9) may provide useful information for these studies.

Cost of commercial calibrants, quality control material, reagents and cleaners should be negotiated with the supplier at rates based on the laboratory's estimate of future use.

An important but often overlooked item is the cost of down-time and repair. It may be difficult to estimate future down-time during the course of an evaluation since the tested product may be relatively immature and more fragile than later members of the production cycle. Evaluation may betray design weaknesses that should be frankly discussed with the manufacturer. His attitude may reveal much and may influence a buying decision.

16.13 Glossary of statistical terms

In the interest of readability, formal definition of statistical methods, prepared by Dean Twedt, has been gathered here in the sequence the formulae appear in the text. The use of these equations should be reinforced by readings from any of the many standard works on medical statistics such as Brown and Hollander (1977), Dowdy and Wearden (1983), Weisbrot (1985).

Formula 1 Arithmetic mean
The arithmetic mean is the sum of values in an array of data divided by the number of elements within the array.

$$\bar{x} = \left[\frac{x_1 + x_2 \ldots x_n}{n} \right]$$

Formula 2 Standard deviation and coefficient of variation
Variance is the sum of differences between the mean of an array of data and the individual elements of that array.

$$s^2 = \left[\frac{\Sigma [x_i - \bar{X}]^2}{n - 1} \right]$$

Standard deviation is the square root of variance

$$s = \sqrt{\left[\frac{\Sigma (x_i - \bar{x})^2}{n - 1} \right]}$$

Coefficient of variation (CV) expresses s as a percentage of the mean

$$CV = \frac{s}{\bar{x}} \times 100$$

Formula 3 Confidence limits
For most applications 95% confidence is used. This predicts the limits of dispersion of members of a population sample when event frequency is a major variable. It implies that only 5% of the members will exceed predicted limits and assumes the dispersion to be symmetrical

$$Confidence\ (95\%) = (s) \times (t)$$

s = standard deviation
t = Student factor (p. 0.05) for (n − 1)

Formula 4 Standard error of the mean
The standard error of the mean estimates the error of a mean of data array. This gives the probable difference between mean of the sample as a function

Table 16.2 Values of t used to convert standard deviation to 95% confidence limits when an imprecision test has employed less than 31 replications. Use 2 as the multiplier (s × t) for 31 or more replications

n^*	Student factor or t	n^*	Student factor or t
1	12.706	16	2.120
2	4.303	17	2.110
3	3.182	18	2.101
4	2.776	19	2.093
5	2.571	20	2.086
6	2.447	21	2.080
7	2.365	22	2.074
8	2.306	23	2.069
9	2.262	24	2.064
10	2.228	25	2.060
11	2.201	26	2.056
12	2.179	27	2.052
13	2.160	28	2.048
14	2.145	29	2.045
15	2.131	30	2.042

*For estimates of imprecision the degrees of freedom (the value of n) are usually one less than the number of replications or (n–1).

of the number of replications and the true mean of the population.

$$SEM = \frac{s}{\sqrt{n}}$$

Formula 5 Standard error of the binomial distribution
Binomial distribution and expansion are concerned with alternative possibilities and their probabilities. Thus:

$$(p + q)^2$$

where p = probability of success
q = 1 − p
n = number of events

The standard error of this binomial distribution is thus:

$$SEp = \sqrt{\left[\frac{(p) \times (q)}{n}\right]}$$

Example:
What is the error of a nominal 30% lymphocyte assay for a 100 cell differential?

p = 30/100 = 0.3
q = (1 − p) = (1 − 0.3) = 0.7
n = 100

$$SE_{30} = \sqrt{\left[\frac{[0.3] \times [0.7]}{100}\right]}$$

$$SE_{30} = 0.046$$

Since p was divided by 100, multiply SE_{30} by 100.

Therefore the error of a 30% assay is 4.6% or approximately + 9% at 95% confidence.

Formula 6 Cumulative (moving) mean
Cumulative mean is an incremental, sequential series of means for an array of data. The first mean of this series represents the average of the first four elements of the data array; mean, the average of the first five elements of the data array, etc. The final mean or cumulative mean of the series is the arithmetic mean of the total array.

Plotting this series of sequential means as a function of specimen sequence (n) provides an estimate of the efficiency.

$$\bar{x}_4 = \left[\frac{X_1 + x_2 + \ldots x_4}{4}\right]; \ldots \bar{x}_n = \left[\frac{x_1 + \ldots + x_n}{n}\right]$$

Formula 7 Regression analysis
This is an attempt to fit a straight line to show the agreement or disagreement between two arrays of data where one is the 'predictor' (predicate) and the other is the 'response' (propositus).

$$y = a + bx$$

y = response (dependent)
x = predictor (independent)
a = intercept
b = slope

Formula 8 Correlation coefficient
Correlation coefficient (r) expresses the degree and type of correlation between two data arrays. A value of r of negative one (− 1) implies perfect inverse correlation; a value of 1.0 implies perfect correlation. Values of r near zero indicate a random relationship between the arrays.
The parameter being evaluated strongly influences the interpretation of the r value.

$$r = \frac{n\Sigma xy - (\Sigma x)(\Sigma y)}{\sqrt{(n\Sigma x^2 - (\Sigma x)^2)(n\Sigma y^2 - (\Sigma y)^2)}}$$

Formula 9 Specificity index
When comparing two devices or methods, the Specificity Index protocol requires that the predicate and propositus systems assay each specimen in duplicate. The minimum count of specimens must be 31.
Differences between the first sample result and second sample result of the test device are calculated as:

$$Difference = Sample \, Result_1 - Sample \, Result_2$$

The standard deviation (s) of the array of propositus differences represents the dispersion of these differences ($S_{propositus}$). The standard deviation of the differences for the predicate device represents the dispersion of those differences ($s_{predicate}$). The standard deviation of differences between sample$_2$ of propositus and predicate represents the dispersion of disagreement ($s_{accuracy}$). Total imprecision is calculated as:

$$s_{precision} = \sqrt{(s^2_{propositus}) + (s^2_{predicate})}$$

Specificity Index is calculated as:

$$Sp_{index} = \frac{s_{precision}}{s_{accuracy}}$$

Formula 10 Confidence limits (non-Parametric)
The interpretation of 95% Confidence is the same for parametric and non-parametric analysis (see parametric); however, the calculation process is different. For non-parametric analysis, the data array is sorted as function of the magnitude of x_i value.

$$Array_{sorted}: (x_1 < x_2 < x_3 \ldots < x_n)$$

Each individual element in this sorted array is assigned a sequence number starting at 1 and incrementing by 1. These sequential numbers are converted to percent by dividing by event sequence and multiplying by 100.
Elements with sequence percentages equal to or greater than 2.5% and less than or equal to 97.5% represent the centre 95% of the array or 95% Confidence.

References

Arnfred, T., Christensen, S. D. and Munck, V. (1982) Coulter Model S and Model S-PLUS Measurements of Mean Erythrocyte Volume (MCV) are Influenced by the Mean Erythrocyte Hemoglobin Concentration (MCHC). *Scand. J. Clin. Lab. Invest.*, **41**, 717–721.

Brown, B. W. and Hollander, M. (1977) *Statistics, a Biomedical Introduction.* New York, Wiley.

Bull, B. S., Richardson-Jones, A., Gibson, M. *et al.* (1992) A method for the independent assessment of the accuracy of hematology whole-blood calibrators. *Am. J. Clin. Pathol.*, **98**, 623–629.

Clopper, C. J. and Pearson, E. S. (1934) The use of confidence or fiducial limits illustrated in the case of the binomial. *Biometrika*, **26**, 404–413.

Code of Federal Regulations (1992) 21 CFR 809.10. Labeling for *in vitro* diagnostic products. Washington DC: US Government Printing Office.

Code of Federal Regulations (1992) 42 CFR 493.1213. Standard: Establishment and verification of method performance specifications. Washington DC: US Government Printing Office.

Dowdy, S. and Wearden, S. (1983) *Statistics for Research.* New York: Wiley.

Galen, R. S. and Gambino, S. P. (1975) *Beyond Normality:* *The Predictive Value and Efficiency of Medical Diagnosis* New York: Wiley, pp. 10–13, 30–40.

Geigy Scientific Tables (1982) Vol. 2. Basel: Ciba-Geigy.

Gosset, W. S. (1908) The probable error of a mean. *Biometrika*, **6**, 1–25.

ICSH (1988) Expert Panel on Cytometry The assignment of values to fresh blood used for calibrating automated blood cell counters. *Clin. Lab. Hematol.*, **10**, 203–212.

ICSH (1987) Recommendations for reference method for hemoglobinometry in human blood (ICSH Standard 1986) and specifications for international hemiglobincyanide reference preparation (3rd Edition). *Clin. Lab. Hematol.*, **9**, 773–779.

ICSH Expert Panel on Cytometry (1984) Protocol for evaluation of automated blood cell counters. *Clin. Lab. Hematol.*, **6**, 69–84.

International Federation of Clinical Chemistry and International Committee for Standardization in Hematology (1987) Approved recommendations on the theory of reference values. *J. Clin. Chem.*, **25**, 645–656.

Koepke, J. A. (1977) The calibration of automated instruments for accuracy in hemoglobinometry. *Am. J. Clin. Pathol.*, **68**, 180–184.

Lewis, S. M. and England, J. M. (1992) The selection of laboratory equipment. *Clin. Lab. Hematol.*, **14**, 131–136.

NCCLS C28-P (1992) How to Define, Determine, and Utilize Reference Intervals in the Clinical Laboratory: Proposed Guideline. Villanova PA: National Committee for Clinical Laboratory Standards.

NCCLS H15-A (1993) Reference and selected procedure for the quantitative determination of hemoglobin in blood. Approved Standard. Villanova PA: National Committee for Clinical Laboratory Standards.

NCCLS H20-A (1992) Reference leukocyte differential count (proportional) and evaluation of instrumental methods. Approved Standard. Villanova PA: National Committee for Clinical Laboratory Standards.

NCCLS H44-P (1993) Reticulocyte counting by flow cytometry. Proposed Standard. Villanova PA: National Committee for Clinical Laboratory Standards.

NCCLS H20-T (1984) Reference leukocyte differential count (proportional) and evaluation of instrumental methods. Tentative Standard. Villanova PA: National Committee for Clinical Laboratary Standards.

NCCLS-NRSCL8-P2 (1993) Nomenclature and definitions for use in NRSCL and other NCCLS Documents, 2nd edn. Villanova PA: National Committee for Clinical Laboratory Standards,

Richardson-Jones, A. (1990) Assignment of assay values to Coulter controls and calibrators. *Clin. Lab. Hematol.*, **21**, Suppl. 1, 23–30.

Rümke, C. L. (1977) The statistically expected variability in differential leukocyte counting. In: Koepke, J. A. (ed.), *Differential Leukocyte Counting.* Skokie, IL: College of American Pathologists,

Weisbrot, I. M. (1985) *Statistics for the Clinical Laboratory.* Philadelphia, PA: Lippincott.

17

Targeting the usage and reporting of hematological laboratory tests to help streamline patient care

George G. Klee, Kent A. Spackman and Thomas M. Habermann

17.1 Introduction

The ever increasing pressures to provide quality health care while controlling expenditures mandate a closer scrutiny of the utilization of laboratory resources. A significant proportion of laboratory test requests may not be necessary for effective patient care. Many such tests are redundantly ordered because of lack of communication among health care providers or because of distrust of the validity of the initial test. It is common practice to repeat many laboratory determinations when a patient transfers between medical centres. Sometimes tests are inappropriately requested due to a lack of understanding of test utility. On the other hand, there are definite advantages of repeating tests for reducing the risk of problems related to erroneous test results, but in the era of cost containment and potential resource rationing, the principle of 'doing it right the first time' becomes more than a catchy slogan.

Many health care organizations and medical societies have been developing 'practice guidelines' and 'disease management strategies'. The goal of these procedures generally is to manage health care expenditures while maintaining or enhancing the quality of care. The focus of these activities has been high volume, high risk and/or high variability areas of medical practice. Guidelines are written to cover generic practice settings whereas the management strategies are more specific to characteristics and resources of a specific medical centre. While these procedures reduce the freedom of practitioners, they are not intended to restrain medical practice to so-called 'protocol medicine'. Guidelines and strategies are meant to provide consistency for uncomplicated disease evaluation and management. The professional judgement of health care practitioners is required to determine the appropriateness of the procedures for any specific patient. Deviations from the recommendations are expected to occur, and the documentation of the reasons and effectiveness of the alternative approaches may serve as the basis for updating or not following the guidelines.

The appropriate utilization of the laboratory depends on the clinical problem(s) being investigated, the clinical status of the patient, and the information available on a specific patient. This requires real time interactive data retrieval, communication systems and sound medical judgement. Computers and electronic communications systems should be of major benefit for optimizing these activities. Unfortunately, communication often is limited, and the role of computers has been mainly limited to printing laboratory reports and tracking the financial accounting. Even these computer-printed reports often do not communicate the test information clearly. Seldom does the laboratory know why a test is being requested, and seldom does the report communicate relevant information about the strengths and limitations of the tests.

From the perspective of a clinician, the quality of the laboratory is directly dependent both on the quality and also the timeliness of the laboratory report (Aller, 1991). Laboratory report quality can be assessed by determining the extent to which the clinician is able to appropriately 'close the loop' in the testing process, that is, to effectively perceive and correctly interpret the results of testing (Connelly, 1989).

Laboratory reports are often judged by the extent to which certain goals are achieved, such as:

- Data presentation is well organized and consistent
- Print is legible (large enough, properly spaced)
- Trends are easy to follow
- Critical values are highlighted
- Current results are easily located
- Paper, printing and chart bulk are minimized
- Charting labour is minimized

These are all valuable goals, but the 'state of the art' in laboratory reporting does not optimally achieve these goals. Instead, the format of reports has been influenced greatly by the technology of line printers and 24-line 80-column computer displays as implemented by vendors of laboratory information systems. In spite of their limited graphical capabilities, these technologies were used in the past because of their low cost. Today, however, graphical displays and laser printers can be obtained at a very competitive cost. Thus, the challenge is the appropriate definition and integration of new display and reporting technologies for routine use in clinical laboratories and laboratory information systems. Laboratorians can play an important role in defining and encouraging the improvements in reporting that now are possible.

17.2 Principles of information display and graphical perception

There are two important aspects of interpretation of visual information - *perception* and *cognition* (Cleveland, 1985).

Perception is instinctive. People have a built-in propensity to perceive and recognize some types of visual stimuli better than others. For example, people are very good at recognizing faces in correct orientation. A picture of a familiar face presented upside-down is often not recognized.

Cognition, on the other hand, influences the interpretation we place on what we perceive or recognize. A picture that appears to be a meaningless blob can change appearance if the cognitive frame of reference changes. What we expect to see, based on our current thoughts, has an enormous influence on what is communicated by an image or even a set of numbers. The amount of cognitive effort required to correctly perceive and interpret visual information can vary greatly, depending on the amount of visual clutter, the number of familiar visual metaphors, helpful cues and so forth. A busy or preoccupied person can fail to cross the threshold of cognitive effort required to reach a correct interpretation. There are principles that can help guide the development of more effective laboratory reporting.

There are at least three fundamental principles of graphical perception that can be used to predict the influence of various graphical techniques on the speed and accuracy of perceptual performance (Cleveland, 1985):

1. Performance deteriorates as irrelevant information increases.
2. Graphs, icons and metaphors, when used appropriately, can greatly enhance perceptual performance.
3. For quantitative judgements, there are several types of perception task on which performance strongly depends.

The effect of irrelevant information is intuitively obvious and has been confirmed by experiments. Clutter and irrelevant information slow down the ability to perceive. Many laboratory reports include unnecessary clutter such as labels, arrows, hash marks, grid lines and sample numbers. Irrelevant information is typified by the report that includes too many significant digits or unnecessary zeros after the decimal point.

Graphs, icons and metaphors have been shown to increase speed and accuracy of perception. Graphs are very useful for presenting trend information. Icons, or pictures that are intended to convey meaning, have been successfully used in user interfaces for personal computers as well as in experiments testing interpretation of medical data (Elting and Bodey, 1991). Metaphor graphics have been used to incorporate several measurements into a single picture. For example, one author (Cole, 1990) depicted respiratory rate and volume as two sides of a rectangle and depicted inspired oxygen concentration as levels of grey within the rectangle.

In making quantitative judgements from graphs, there are several types of perception tasks on which performance strongly depends (Cleveland, 1985). These types of tasks, with the most accurate listed first, include estimation of:

- Position along a common scale
- Position along identical non-aligned scales
- Length
- Angle or slope
- Area
- Volume
- Colour hue, colour saturation, colour density

This ordering suggests that when it is necessary to make quantitative judgements about the magnitude of a single value or the relative magnitudes of one or more values, it is best to use position along a common scale as the main graphical display method. Colour variations should not be used to represent purely quantitative information but can be used instead to highlight or emphasize.

Psychologists have described general laws of perception that corroborate the rank ordering given above (Cleveland, 1985). One of these laws is called Weber's law. Roughly paraphrased, it states that the magnitude of change in a physical attribute necessary for the change to be perceived is a fixed fraction of the size of the attribute. For example, the difference in length between a line 10 cm and a line 11 cm long is relatively easy to see, since the difference is 10%. A difference of 1 cm between a line 100 cm and 101 cm long is more difficult, since the difference is 1%. This law predicts that judgements of length will be less accurate than judgements of position along identical, non-aligned scales.

A second law of perception is Steven's power law. It relates the perceived scale p to the actual x by an

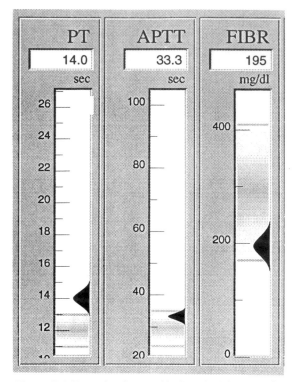

Figure 17.1 Example of a graphical method for reporting test values with their coefficient of variation (CV); PT = prothrombin time; PTT = activated partial thromboplastin time; FIBR = fibrinogen. The grey zone in the vertical bars represents the reference range

exponent β, as $p = x^\beta$. If length judgements are to be accurate, β should be equal to 1.0. Judgements of area have been found to have values of β near 0.7, and judgements of volume near 0.6. This means that in comparing two circles with different areas, the smaller circle is perceived to be larger than it really is relative to the other one, or, conversely, the area of the larger circle is underestimated. Volume comparisons are even more biased.

Laws such as these should be used to help develop guidelines for the creation of graphical displays for laboratory data. Such guidelines would indicate that whenever a quantitative judgement is to be made from a graph, the graphical technique used should be positioned along a common scale. Also, if differences in values are to be noticed, then the proportional differences should be made large. To date, there has been no development of standards for graphical display of laboratory data. Laboratorians should be creative but also careful and systematic in creating and deploying graphical displays.

17.3 Effect of presentation on outcome

The way that information is presented can have an impact on the outcome. Dramatic examples of this have been seen with altimeters for aircraft that use a dial with 2 or 3 hands of different length to represent altitude. Busy or distracted pilots have read the large hand instead of the small hand, misinterpreted their altitude, and crashed into the mountains. Similarly, data from the laboratory may be misinterpreted or overlooked with disastrous consequences.

There are four main outcomes sought by using better reporting methods. It may be possible to achieve all of these in combination with appropriately designed graphs or tables. First, we may want to decrease the perceptual effort required to interpret the report. This may extend the effectiveness of clinicians who inevitably may become less attentive because of fatigue, distractions, or monotony. Second, we may want to increase the speed of interpretation (Cole, 1990). In some cases the patient requires immediate attention and no delay is desirable. In most cases, the clinician's time for task completion needs to be conserved. Third, effective reporting can reduce errors of interpretation (Elting and Body, 1991). And fourth, properly designed reports can improve aesthetic appeal, which by itself may seem to be unimportant but can have a positive impact on the mental state of those viewing the reports.

17.4 What can be represented?

Ordinarily, we think of a laboratory report as communicating the test value and units, e.g. a serum iron of 20 μmol/l (or 1.1 mg/l). It is common also to include the reference range. However, there are numerous other aspects of testing that can also be communicated. Trends over time are very important: a fibrinogen of 100 mg/dl has an entirely different interpretation depending on whether a fibrinogen measured an hour ago was 50 or 500. A graph of the most recent values can also give a quick sense of test ordering frequency. This may be helpful in reducing unnecessary testing. For uncommon tests or those with a very wide analytic variability, it is important to communicate an answer to the question 'how high is high?' The analytic coefficient of variation (CV) can be represented graphically as a bell curve, giving information that enables quick intuitive judgements about 'borderline' or 'very high' values. In Figure 17.1, the analytic values are represented as a bell-shaped curve turned on its side. The width of the curve represents the CV of the test.

Values can sometimes be presented together to give interpretive information graphically. For example, the pH and pCO$_2$, can be plotted in two dimensions and define regions of acid–base and respiratory

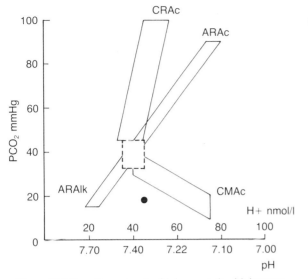

Figure 17.2 Two dimensional acid–base graph with interpretive regions. CRAc = chronic respiratory acidosis; ARAc = acute respiratory acidosis; ARAlk = acute respiratory alkalosis; CMAc = chronic metabolic acidosis. Graph derived from parameters given in R. Gilbert, Spirometry and Blood Gases, in J. B. Henry, ed., *Clinical Diagnosis and Management by Laboratory Methods*, 18th edn, p. 115

status, as in Figure 17.2, and the cross-plots of leukocyte differentials as shown later in Figures 17.5–17.9.

This type of display quickly provides interpretive information that is less cumbersome than a narrative report.

17.5 Example reporting system for coagulation assessment

Information systems and graphical reporting formats can be valuable in presenting the results of tests of hemostasis to clinicians. Two examples are given below. The first is an approach to presenting common tests of hemostasis in situations where they guide transfusion therapy; the second is an approach to presenting results of a workup of an unexplained prolonged partial thromboplastin time (PTT).

Multiple tests of hemostasis are frequently done together in situations of trauma and/or massive transfusion. The partial thromboplastin time (PTT), prothrombin time (PT), fibrinogen and D-dimer are often measured in conjunction with the hemoglobin, hematocrit and platelet count. These six values can provide valuable guidance for transfusion therapy, particularly when presented to the clinician as trend data over time along with the number of units of blood transfused. Figure 17.3 is one example of a

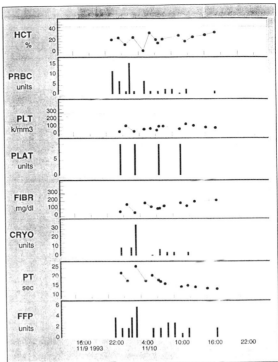

Figure 17.3 Summary of tranfusions and related hematology parameters. HCT = hematocrit; PRBC = packed red blood cells; PLT = platelet count; PLAT = transfused platelets; FIBR = fibrinogen; CRYO = cyroprecipitate; PT = prothrombin time; FFP = fresh frozen plasma

trend graph that provides a concise summary of laboratory data and transfusion status.

A common situation arises when the PTT is measured and is found to be unexpectedly prolonged. After ruling out specimen and collection errors, it is usual to perform a mixing study in which patient plasma is mixed 50:50 with a pooled normal plasma. Failure of the mixture to correct to the normal range, or prolongation after incubation and remeasurement at 60 minutes is taken as evidence for the presence of an inhibitor. Correction to the normal range is taken as evidence for a factor deficiency. Since reporting results of the mixing study often involves several numbers, there is an opportunity to apply graphical techniques to this problem. Figure 17.4 shows a graph representing the abnormal patient value at the left, the normal plasma at the right and the mixture with its 60-minute incubation value in the centre. The heavy horizontal line represents the upper limit of the normal range. This simple graph can communicate the results of the mixing study at a glance. A written interpretation of the tests can be added. This is a simple example of how graphics can be used to enhance laboratory reports.

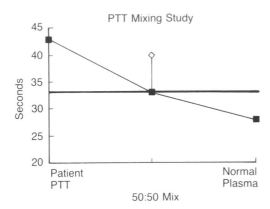

Interpretation: The abnormal PTT of the 50:50 mix at 60 minutes indicates the presence of an inhibitor

	Intermediate PTT	60 Minute PTT
Patient PTT	43	
50:50 Mix	33	40
Normal Plasma	28	

Figure 17.4 A graphical format for reporting the results of a mixing study for an abnormal partial thromboplastin time (PTT)

17.6 Clinical application of hematological laboratory tests for patients on protocols

Worldwide, most patients are not treated using institutional guidelines or national protocols. This causes wide variations in the usage patterns and expectations for laboratory services. When standardized protocols are used, it is easier to define the critical aspects of laboratory tests relative to the protocol decisions. Therefore, much of the following discussion relates to the care of patients treated on hematologic protocols.

Data from the clinical hematology laboratory are a vital part of the initial diagnostic workup in hematological disorders, an absolute requirement to the entry criteria of clinical trials, essential for the management of patients on chemotherapy, part of the toxicity evaluation, and are some of the criteria for assessing responses in certain hematological disorders.

After blood is drawn, it is forwarded to the hematology laboratory for routine as well as non-routine studies. These subsequently are recorded on the clinic chart, and the data are evaluated by physicians. In addition, these data are evaluated by data management personnel to assure that appropriate entry criteria are met before patients are entered into protocol trials. The data are utilized for entry into these studies, on a daily basis for patient management such as chemotherapy dosing, and for assessment of response. The data subsequently are abstracted and forwarded for centralized internal and external review.

Laboratory studies for clinical trials include tests to assess entry into protocols, tests to monitor the effect of therapy, tests for restaging patients, and post-treatment follow-up studies. Table 17.1 outlines specific initial diagnostic laboratory studies that are required in co-operative group trials for different hematological disorders. Further studies are essential to the initial diagnosis of these disorders but not absolutely required for entry into a protocol.

In acute leukemia, hematology data are essential to the initial diagnosis, management and evaluation of response. Leukemias are classified on the basis of the FAB classification (French–American–British classification) (Bennett *et al.*, 1976, 1980). Essential to the diagnosis of acute leukemia is bone marrow morphology and special studies on the bone marrow. After morphological determinations, further subdivisions are made based on slide-based cytochemistry, flow cytometry and cytogenetics. Histochemical stains of blast forms characteristically include peroxidase, chloracetate esterase, and non-specific esterase. These data are characteristically reported on bone marrow report forms.

Central pathology review is mandatory for quality assurance. This requires the routine submission of tissue and reports outside the institution. In acute leukemia, six unstained bone marrow films, one Romanowsky-stained film, and the cytochemical stains that have been performed at the local institution are required for review. The cytochemical-stained slides are returned to the main institution. A copy of the original pathology report with stained preparation is required. In lymphoma, representative paraffin tissue blocks or five unstained slides from a representative block upon which the diagnosis of malignant lymphoma was originally made are required.

Follow-up tests ordered vary in different diseases. In acute leukemia trials with induction and intensification therapies, a complete blood count with differential

Table 17.1 Initial diagnostic laboratory studies

Disease	Non-Hodgkin's lymphoma	Hodgkin's disease	Chronic lymphocytic leukemia	Hairy cell leukemia	Acute lymphocytic leukemia	Acute non-lymphocytic leukemia	Acute promyolocytic leukemia	Multiple myeloma	Myeloproliferative disorders
CBC									
WBC	×	×	×	×	×	×	×	×	×
Hgb	×	×	×	×	×	×	×	×	×
Platelet count	×	×	×	×	×	×	×	×	×
Differential count	×	×	×	×	×	×	×	×	×
Chemistry panel	×	×	×	×	×	×	×	×	×
BONE MARROW									
Aspirate	×	×	×	×	×	×	×	×	×
Biopsy	×	×	×	×	×	×	×	×	×
Cytogenetic study					×	×	×		×
FAB Classification					×	×	×		
OTHER STUDIES									
PTT, fibrinogen, FSP, thrombin time							×		
Serum protein electrophoresis								×	
24-hour urine electrophoresis								×	
LDH	×								
CSF for cytology	×*				×	×‡	×†		

* Strongly recommended if marrow biopsy positive for lymphoma.
† As indicated.

and platelet count is required daily during hospitalization and weekly following dismissal from the hospital after induction therapy. With each consolidation chemotherapy cycle, a complete blood count with platelet count and differential is required prior to consolidation treatment, daily and weekly. While on maintenance therapy, weekly complete blood counts are required. In Hodgkin's disease trials, a complete blood count is typically required on the day of each treatment. On follow-up visits after the completion of therapy, a complete blood count with platelet count is required at each visit.

17.7 Laboratory tests for assessing chemotherapeutic toxicity

In hematological disorders, the most common and significant complications of the diseases and toxicity of treatment are hematological. All toxicities on trials are graded according to toxicity criteria. The most common criteria incorporated into trials in the United States are the 'National Cancer Institute (NCI) common toxicity criteria'. The criteria for the complete blood count changes are outlined in Table 17.2.

Grade 4 toxicity is characterized by an absolute granulocyte count of less than $500 \times 10^6/l$. This information has different implications in the various malignancies.

The basis of treatment of acute non-lymphocytic leukemia and acute lymphocytic leukemia is cytoreduction. The treatment programmes are administered in the hospital. The peripheral white blood cell count typically is less than $200 \times 10^6/l$ at the nadir after induction and intensification therapy. Patients require intense support during this time with antibiotics and blood products. The platelet counts are characteristically less than $20 \times 10^9/l$. Daily complete blood counts are essential to the management of patients during these times.

As a measurement of effect, response rates are characterized as complete remission, partial remission and relapse. Complete remission is characterized by all of the following for at least four weeks. The peripheral neutrophil count is greater than $1 \times 10^9/l$, the platelet count is greater than or equal to $100 \times 10^9/l$, and leukemic blasts must not be present in the peripheral blood. The bone marrow aspiration and biopsy must reveal a cellularity on the bone marrow biopsy of greater than 20% with maturation of all cell lines, less than or equal to 5% blasts, and Auer rods must not be detectable. In addition, extramedullary leukemia such as central nervous system or soft tissue involvement must not be present. A partial remission requires all of the criteria of the complete remission be satisfied except that the bone marrow may contain greater than 5% blasts but less than 25% blasts. Relapse following a com-

plete remission is defined as the reappearance of blasts in the blood or the presence of greater than 5% blasts on the bone marrow on aspirate and biopsy that are not attributable to another cause such as bone marrow regeneration.

Hairy cell leukemia is an uncommon chronic leukemia with abnormal cells that resemble 'hairy projections' and demonstrate the presence of tartrate resistant acid phosphatase (Bouroncle, Wiseman and Doan, 1958; Yam, Li and Yam, 1971). Since 1984, there has been remarkable success with treatment of this disease with alpha recombinant interferon, 2'-deoxycoformycin, and 2-chlorodeoxyadenosine (Quesada et al., 1984; Spiers et al., 1987; Piro et al., 1990). In contrast to acute leukemia trials, patients on hairy cell leukemia trials have characteristically required a hemoglobin of less than 120 g/l, an absolute granulocyte count of less than $1.5 \times 10^9/l$, or circulating hairy cell count of greater than $20 \times 10^9/l$ for treatment. In addition, the toxicity profiles are different from those in acute leukemia. The treatment was entirely in outpatient setting in these trials. For a complete remission, the required hemoglobin was greater than or equal to 120 g/l, the absolute granulocyte count greater than $1.5 \times 10^9/l$, platelet count greater than $100 \times 10^9/l$, no hairy cells in the peripheral blood, no evidence of hairy cell infiltration on marrow biopsy, and absence of disease-related symptoms. For a partial response, the hemoglobin, platelet count, and white cell count were as for complete response; however, a decrease in hairy cells in the peripheral blood of greater than 50% over baseline values and a 50% reduction in the hairy cell infiltration on the bone marrow biopsy were required. The NCI common toxicity criteria were utilized for toxicity evaluations. As in acute leukemias, the doses were not adjusted as they are in other non-hematological toxicities. Typically, in grade 4 toxicities, the treatment is held or discontinued. A grade 3 toxicity requires a 50% dose reduction. However, hematological toxicities are anticipated with these drugs. A unique aspect of this trial was that if the absolute granulocyte count fell to less than $200 \times 10^6/l$ in a patient who had an initial granulocyte count of greater than $500 \times 10^6/l$, then the 2'deoxycoformycin was held until the absolute granulocyte returned to baseline.

In chronic lymphocytic leukemia, the complete blood count and differential and review of peripheral blood film provide the actual diagnosis. Since the absolute granulocyte count is markedly decreased in chronic lymphocytic leukemia, the results of the neutrophil count are less essential than in other disorders.

The different trials in lymphomas include Hodgkin's disease, low-grade non-Hodgkin's lymphoma, intermediate histology non-Hodgkin's lymphoma and high-grade lymphomas. These trials may be Phase I, Phase II or Phase III. The most significant

Table 17.2 NCI common toxicity criteria

	Toxicity grade				
	0	1	2	3	4
WBC × 10^9/l	≧ 4.0	3.0–3.9	2.0– 2.9	1.0–1.9	< 1.0
Granulocytes × 10^9/l	≧ 2.0	1.5–1.9	1.0–1.4	0.5–0.9	< 0.5
Lymphocytes × 10^9/l	≧ 2.0	1.5–1.9	1.0–1.4	0.5–0.9	< 0.5
Platelets × 10^9/l	Normal	75–normal	50–74.9	25–49	< 25
Hemoglobin, g/l	Normal	100–normal	80–100	65–79	< 65

dose-limiting toxicity of most drugs incorporated into lymphoma regimens is myelosuppression. In Phase I trials with growth factors, the reporting of complete blood counts and differentials are required three times a week. Patients may have these obtained at the laboratory of the institution at which they are being treated or in other laboratories. Electronic transfer of information is possible from the participating institution laboratory but not from other laboratories.

Table 17.3 outlines a typical dose reduction scheme that was incorporated into a PROMACE-CYTABOM protocol (cyclophosphamide, doxorubicin, etoposide, prednisone, cytarabine, bleomycin, vincristine, methotrexate, leucovorin and recombinant granulocyte macrophage colony stimulating factor) that was utilized in a dose escalation study by the Eastern Cooperative Oncology Group. These tables emphasize the need for information on the same day for the clinician so that the patient may be treated appropriately. Recent anemia protocols have evaluated erythropoietin. The dosage of this drug is not dependent on daily blood counts but may be reflected in reticulocyte counts or the reticulocyte maturation index. It is important to follow this drug over time, in weeks rather than days.

Patients undergoing bone marrow transplants are particularly dependent on accurate and timely laboratory tests. One of the primary toxicities of transplantation is again myelosuppression. This results from conditioning regimens such as high-dose cyclophosphamide and total body irradiation which are incorporated into allogeneic bone marrow transplantation for acute leukemias, aplastic anemias and non-Hodgkin's lymphomas. In addition, the multitude of drugs employed as immunosuppressive agents for patients with solid organ transplantation may be myelosuppressive or toxic to other organs such as the kidney or liver. At most centres, this data is relayed to the chart and hand-transcribed onto a flow sheet that incorporates a temperature chart, drugs, day of transplantation and other pertinent patient variables. Each of these is unique to the individual type of transplant.

All data for the patient needs to be integrated on to disease-specific, protocol-specific and cooperative group-specific reporting forms. Test information also needs to be correlated with specific drug, dose, toxicity data and dates. Data also need to be submitted for institutional review and forwarded to the operations office for central review. After the data leaves the laboratory, there are multiple ways that the data are transmitted both intra-institutionally and extra-institutionally. At this time, much data are manually transcribed. Future trends will result in more electronic communication.

17.8 Utilization and reporting of leukocyte differential counts

The complete blood count (CBC) with enumeration of the leukocyte differential is one of the most frequently requested laboratory procedures. A recent focus of instrument manufacturers has been to automate the differential counting to provide routinely enumeration of cell types with every CBC request (Hoyer, 1993). The analytic cost of this additional information is minimal; however, the cost/benefit ratio of this practice has not been formally analysed. Additional laboratory costs are incurred in purchasing the instruments and reagents along with the time and labour to achieve quality control and to re-test specimens with incomplete automated results. Additional clinical costs are incurred in interpreting the test results and follow-up of abnormalities. The laboratory benefits often are a reduction in the number of labour-intensive manual differential counts requested with a subsequent reduction in cost of personnel. These clinical benefits are a function of the abnormalities detected and the ability of the clinician to readily identify these abnormalities and carry out appropriate actions. The clinical benefits may be a function of the data presentation and reporting. These clinical benefits are not well documented, but data may become available in the future because test utilization is becoming an important focus of continuous quality improvement programmes.

The microscopic examination of the Romanowsky-stained blood film has been a fundamental part of medical practice for many years. Traditionally this had been the mechanism for enumerating

Table 17.3 Neutropenia

Granulocyte $\times$ $10^9/l$	Percent of drug to give				
	Methotrexate	Ara-C	Cyclophosphamide	Adriamycin	VP-16
$\geqslant 2.0$	100%	100%	100%	100%	100%
1.5 – 1.99	100%	100%	100%	100%	100%
1.0 – 1.49	100%	75%	50%	50%	50%
0.5 – 0.99	100%	25%	25%	25%	25%
< 0.5	50%	Hold	Hold	Hold	Hold

Thrombocytopenia

Platelet $\times$ $10^9/l$	Percent of drug to give				
	Methotrexate	Ara-C	Cyclophosphamide	Adriamycin	VP-16
$\geqslant 100$	100%	100%	100%	100%	100%
50 – 99	100%	50%	75%	75%	50%
< 50	50%	Hold	Hold	Hold	Hold

leukocyte subtypes. With modern laboratory equipment, leukocyte differential counting does not require blood films. In most moderate medical practices, attending clinicians do not review blood films on their regular patients. Therefore, it is appropriate to examine the clinical utility of the numerical leukocyte differential counts as an independent practice parameter.

17.9 Clinical utility of leukocyte differential counts

Some of the major applications for leukocyte differentials are investigation of bacterial, viral and allergic inflammations, evaluation and management of leukemias and lymphomas, investigation of leukopenia, and 'case-finding' to detect clinically unrecognized disease. In patients with unexplained fever not treated with chemotherapeutic agents, neutrophilic leukocytosis suggests pyogenic infection or tissue necrosis, whereas low neutrophil counts suggest non-pyogenic infections, diseases such as tuberculosis, brucellosis and malaria (Diggs, 1977). In patients with jaundice, a low total leukocyte count with increased lymphocytes suggests viral hepatitis. Malignancies are characterized by neutrophilic leukocytosis or normal white blood cell counts. In patients with pulmonary disease, increased eosinophils suggests PIE syndrome (pulmonary infiltrate with eosinophilia), while marked neutropenia suggests staphylococcal pneumonia. In each of these settings, most clinicians find the leukocyte differential helpful for undertaking an appropriate action; however, formal performance characteristics in terms of sensitivity, specificity and predictive value generally are not available.

Two recent studies have evaluated the utility of the leukocyte differential for managing sepsis in in-

fants. An investigation of 1009 febrile infants at The Medical College of Wisconsin showed that a subset of 81 patients with serious bacterial infections had significantly higher leukocyte counts and absolute band counts, but the percentage of polymorphonuclear cells was not significantly different (Bonadio, Smith and Carmody, 1992). The predictive value of a positive leukocyte count varied from 8% to 35%, while the sensitivity decreased from 74% to 16% as the counts increased from 8 to 20 $\times$ $10^9/l$. A second study of 176 samples from 63 babies in an intensive care unit assessed the utility of the CBC and leukocyte differential count for: (1) predicting onset of clinically unrecognized disease; (2) assessing severity of current disease and (3) following a trend during treatment (Charache et al., 1992). They concluded that neither conventional nor automated differential counts were useful for predicting the onset of clinically unrecognized disease. The leukocyte count and the absolute immature neutrophil count correlated with severity, but prediction statistics were not provided. The leukocyte count was superior to the differential count for following trends in patients' conditions.

A nine-year study of 101 patients with adult acute leukemia evaluated the utility of CBC as an early sign of relapse (Kawamura et al., 1981). Twenty-three cases (15 acute myelocytic leukemia, 8 acute lymphocytic leukemia) relapsed after complete remission. The blood counts were measured every two weeks. In 12 patients no leukemia cells were recognized in the peripheral film. Statistically, both the percentage and absolute lymphocyte counts were significantly higher at relapse compared to 6 weeks before relapse (P < 0.01); however, the ranges of values were very similar. Predictive value information was not provided, but based on the graphical data presented, the predictive value of both percentage and absolute lymphocytes as an early sign of relapse would be low.

Several studies have evaluated the CBC and leukocyte differential counts for disease detection and found the utility to be very low. A retrospective review of 799 CBCs and 475 differential counts in an ambulatory care setting found no cases of clinically inapparent disease (Rich, Crowson and Connelly, 1983). In a study of the usefulness of routine laboratory tests on preoperative patients, only 1 out of 610 (0.15%) CBCs had an unexpected increase in leukocytes and 1 out of 390 (0.3%) had an unexpected abnormality reported with the leukocyte differential (2 nucleated red cells). Neither of these findings had a direct effect on patient outcome (Kaplan *et al.*, 1985). Two studies showed routine total leukocyte counts have little utility for general medical service inpatients (Frye *et al.*, 1987; Mozes, Haimi-Cohen and Halkin, 1989). Similarly, 387 asymptomatic well children showed that 'no unsuspected illness was discovered as a result of an abnormal total and differential leukocyte count' (Moyer and Grimes, 1990).

17.10 Appropriateness of use

These recent studies cast doubt on the usefulness of leukocyte measurements in asymptomatic patients. This low utility may in part be due to the way tests are being used and how they are reported. There has been a long controversy about the reporting of percentage versus absolute leukocyte differential counts. Also, most studies on utility have used simple reference ranges rather than population-specific or individual-specific ranges. Furthermore, there has been little attention directed to defining when these tests should be requested in terms of appropriate clinical settings and appropriate times. Perhaps further refinement of these issues could improve the clinical utility of leukocyte counts and differentials.

17.11 Percentage versus absolute leukocyte counts

Traditionally, leukocyte differential counts have been reported as percentage counts because those data were directly available from the blood film. This became the tradition to which most clinicians became accustomed. However, for more critical decisions, such as in the evaluation of leukopenia, many clinicians would calculate absolute differential counts from the total leukocyte count and the differential count.

The relationships between absolute and percentage granulocyte and lymphocyte counts are graphically illustrated in Figures 17.5 and 17.6. When the absolute counts (y) are cross-plotted against the total leukocyte count (x), the percentage counts present as diagonal lines through the origin. The values from 200 healthy volunteers measured on the Coulter S + IV (Coulter Electronics) also are displayed. The central 95% healthy reference limits are shown by the dotted horizontal and vertical lines. Note that within the normal reference range for total leukocytes, the percentage limits form tighter classification limits than the absolute limits, whereas outside this range the absolute limits are more restrictive. For example, points in the triangle below the 45% line and above the $2 \times 10^9/l$ granulocyte line would be considered normal by absolute limits but low by percentage limits. On the other hand, points in the space below the 80% line and above the $7.0 \times 10^9/l$ granulocyte line would be normal by percentage limits and abnormal by absolute limits.

From a mathematical perspective, it would appear there are advantages to both absolute and percentage differential counts; however, the clinical manifestation of disease generally is not associated with values in the triangles above or below the diagonal percentage lines (Klee and O'Sullivan, 1977). Most of the triangular area above the 80% diagonal line and below the $7.0 \times 10^9/l$ granulocytes is a virtual space because it is impossible for the granulocyte count to exceed the total leukocyte count.

Figure 17.7 depicts the tracking of 5 patients with septicemia, plotted on the same axis as Figure 17.5. Note that the absolute counts generally cross into the abnormal zones (defined by dotted horizontal lines) more rapidly and consistently than the percentage counts cross into the abnormal zones (defined by dotted diagonal lines). However, some drugs (such as glucocorticoids) and certain disease states which simultaneously suppress one cell population (lymphocytes) and increase another population (granulocytes) will cause greater percentage than absolute changes (Friedman *et al.*, 1980).

A method to further improve the reference ranges for granulocytes and lymphocytes would be to develop a multivariate range for the two absolute variables. Figure 17.8 shows a cross-plot of lymphocytes (y) versus granulocytes (x) for the same 200 healthy volunteers. Formal multivariate ranges would take into account the correlation between these two variables. However, this correlation is low (r = 0.24) so univariate absolute ranges are almost as good as these multivariate statistics.

17.12 Biologic variability

The within-person variability of lymphocyte and granulocyte counts is much tighter than the between-person variability. When expressed as a coefficient of variance (CV), Fraser *et al.* (1989) found the within-subject lymphocyte CV for elderly subjects to be 9.4% compared to 24.1–27.8% for between subjects. The CVs for granulocytes were 17.3–19.3% within-

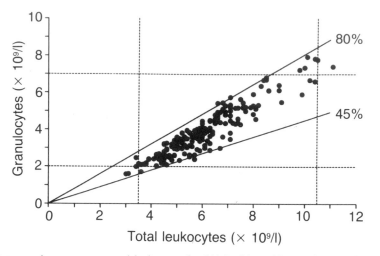

Figure 17.5 Cross-plot granulocytes versus total leukocytes for 200 healthy subjects. Diagonal lines represent percentage differential normal limits. Dotted lines represent normal limits for absolute counts.

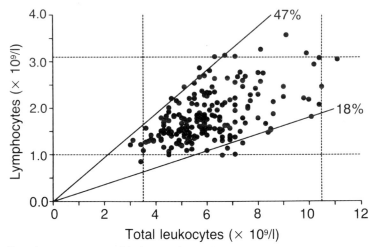

Figure 17.6 Cross-plot of lymphocytes versus total leukocytes for 200 healthy subjects. Reference line same as in Figure 17.5

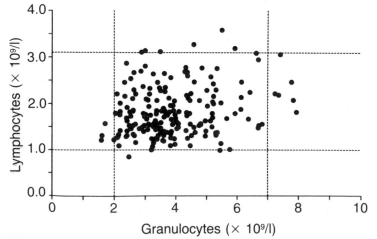

Figure 17.7 Cross-plot of lymphocytes versus granulocytes for 200 healthy subjects. Note the low correlation between these two variables.

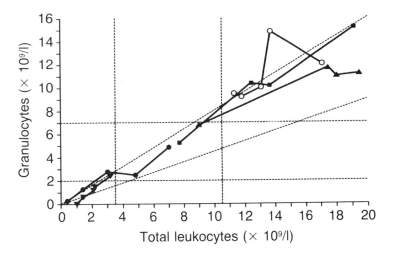

Figure 17.8 Tracking of percentage and total granulocyte changes in five patients with septicemia

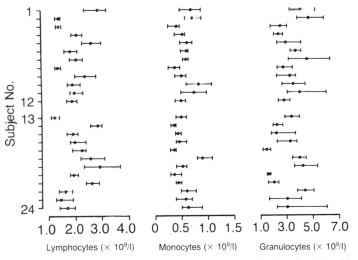

Figure 17.9 Within-person biologic changes of lymphocytes, monocytes and granulocytes for 24 healthy subjects. Reproduced with the permission of C. G. Fraser, *American Journal of Clinical Pathology*

subject and 21.2–29.7% between subjects. Other studies have shown similar differences (Statland *et al.*, 1977; Costongs *et al.*, 1985; Ross *et al.*, 1988). Figure 17.9 depicts the mean and ranges of each of the cell types of each of the 24 subjects studied by Fraser *et al.* (1989) using 9 to 10 data sets. Notice that, particularly for lymphocytes, individual ranges are much tighter than the population ranges. The individual ranges for subjects like number 2 and 3 would provide a much more sensitive index to changes with disease.

17.13 Scoring system to improve predictive value

A group from Australia developed a scoring system to

improve the predictive value of the CBC and different-ial for the early diagnosis of neonatal sepsis (Rodwell, Leslie and Tudehope, 1988). Their seven parameter scores provided a sensitivity of 96% and a positive predictive value of 31% for scores ≥3. With a score ≤2 the likelihood that sepsis was absent was 99%. Scoring systems such as this or other multivariate prediction rules (Wasson *et al.*, 1985) may help to more closely link laboratory measurements to clinical practice.

17.14 Summary

The quality revolution of industry in the 1990s has emphasized 'focusing on the needs of customers' and developing efficient systems to provide quality output with zero defects. The health care industry, in particular, is under intense pressure to change. The issues and techniques discussed in this article should provide laboratory hematologists with the background for developing a strategy to better position their laboratory for the competitive health care market. The primary users of the laboratory are the patient care physicians who, in turn, respond to the clinical needs of patients, health care regulators, and insurance companies. The timeliness and clarity of reports are critical factors for the efficient and appropriate responses of clinicians. Explicit enumeration of the critical action limits of screening laboratory tests will help to focus quality assurance programmes to optimize test performance. In addition, the monitoring of health care outcomes will help define the strengths and limitations of laboratory tests to improve the proper utilization of these procedures. The challenge for the laboratorians of the 1990s will be to develop and implement strategies to meet these health care needs efficiently while minimizing costs.

References

Aller, R. D. (1991) Information for medical decision making: Improving our laboratory reports. *Clin. Lab. Med.*, **11(1)**, 171–186.

Bennett, J. M., Catovsky, D., Daniel, M. T. *et al.* (1976) Proposals for the classification of the acute leukemias. *Br. J. Haematol.*, **33**, 451.

Bennett, J. M., Catovsky, D., Daniel, M. T. *et al.* (1980) A variant form of hypergranular promyelocytic leukemia (M3). *Ann. Intern. Med.*, **92**, 280.

Bonadio, W. A., Smith, D. and Carmody, J. (1992) Correlating CBC profile and infectious outcome. *Clin. Pediatr.*, **31(10)**, 578–582.

Bouroncle, B. A., Wiseman, B. K. and Doan, C. A. (1958) Leukemic reticuloendotheliosis. *Blood*, **13**, 609–630.

Charache, S., Nelson, L., Saw, D. *et al.* (1992) Accuracy and utility of differential white blood cell count in the neonatal intensive care unit. *Am. J. Clin. Pathol.*, **97(3)**, 338–344.

Cleveland, W. S. (1985) *The Elements of Graphing Data.* Monterey, CA: Wadsworth Advanced Books.

Cole, W. G. (1990) Quick and accurate monitoring via metaphor graphics. In: *Proceedings of the 14th Symposium on Computer Applications in Medical Care*, pp. 425–429.

Connelly, D. P. (1989) Graphical data display and medical decision making. In: Keller, H. and Trendelenburg, C. H. (eds), *Data Presentation/Interpretation.* Berlin: deGruyter, pp. 68–79.

Connelly, D. P., Lasky, L. C., Keller, R. M. *et al.* (1982) A system for graphical display of clinical laboratory data. *Am. J. Clin. Pathol.*, **78**, 729–737.

Costongs, G. M. P. J., Janson, P. C. W., Bas, B. M. *et al.* (1985) Short-term and long-term intra-individual variations and critical differences of haematological laboratory parameters. *J. Clin. Chem. Clin. Biochem.*, **23(2)**, 69–76.

Diggs, L. W. (1977) Highlights in the history of neutrophil counts. In: Koepke, J. A. (ed.), *Differential Leukocyte Counting.* College of American Pathologists, pp. 2–9.

Elting, L. S., and Body, G. P. (1991) Is a picture worth a thousand medical words? A randomized trial of reporting formats for medical research data. *Methods of Information in Medicine*, **30**, 145–150.

Fraser, C. G., Wilkinson, S. P., Neville, R. G. *et al.* (1989) Biologic variation of common hematologic laboratory quantities in the elderly. *Am. J. Clin. Pathol.*, **92(4)**, 465–470.

Friedman, R. B., Anderson, R. E., Entine, S. M. *et al.* (1980) Effects of diseases on clinical laboratory tests. *Clin. Chem.*, **26(4)**, 28D.

Frye, E. B., Hubbell, F. A., Akin, B. V. *et al.* (1987) Usefulness of routine admission complete blood cell counts on a general medical service. *J. Gen. Intern. Med.*, **2(6)**, 373–376.

Hoyer J. D. (1993) Leukocyte differential. *Mayo Clinic Proceedings*, **68(10)**, 1027–1028.

Kaplan, E. B., Sheiner, L. B., Boeckmann, A. J. *et al.* (1985) The usefulness of preoperative laboratory screening. *JAMA*, **253(24)**, 3576–3581.

Kawamura, S., Abe, I., Saitoh, A. *et al.* (1981) Changes in lymphocytes as an early sign of relapse in adult acute leukemia. *Tohoku J. Exp. Med.*, **135(3)**, 237–245.

Klee, G. G. and O'Sullivan, M. B. (1977) Screening versus diagnostic differential leukocyte counts. In: Koepke, J. A. (ed.), *Differential Leukocyte Counting.* College of American Pathologists, pp. 69–80.

Moyer, V. A. and Grimes, R. M. (1990) Total and differential leukocyte counts in clinically well children. *Am. J. Dis. Child.*, **144**, 1200–1203.

Mozes, B., Haimi-Cohen, Y. and Halkin, H. (1989) Yield of the admission complete blood count in medical inpatients. *Postgrad. Med. J.*, **65**, 525–527.

Piro, L. D., Carrera, C. M., Carson, D. A. *et al.* (1990) Lasting remissions in hairy-cell leukemia induced by a single infusion of 2-chlorodeoxyadenosine. *N England Journal of Medicine*, **322**, 1117–1121.

Quesada, J. R., Reuben, J. Z., Manning, J. T. *et al.* (1984) Alpha interferon for induction of remission in hairy cell leukemia. *N. Engl. J. Med.*, **310**, 15–18.

Rich, E. C., Crowson, T. W. and Connelly, D. P. (1983) Effectiveness of differential leukocyte count in case finding in the ambulatory care setting. *JAMA*, **249(5)**, 633–636.

Rodwell, R. L., Leslie, A. L. and Tudehope, D. I. (1988) Early diagnosis of neonatal sepsis using a hematologic scoring system. *J. Pediatr.*, **112(5)**, 761–767.

Ross, D. W., Ayscue, L. H., Watson, J. *et al.* (1988) Stability of hematologic parameters in healthy subjects. *Am. J. Clin. Pathol.*, **90(3)**, 262–267.

Spiers, A. S. D., Moore, D., Cassileth, P. A. *et al.* (1987) Remissions in hairy-cell leukemia with pentostatin (2'-deoxycoformycin). *N. Engl. J. Med.*, **316**, 825–830.

Statland, B. E., Winkel, P., Harris, S. C. *et al.* (1977) Evaluation of biologic sources of variation of leukocyte counts and other hematologic quantities using very precise automated analyzers. *Am. J. Clin. Pathol.*, **69**, 48–54.

Wasson, J. H., Sox, H. C., Neff, R. K. *et al.* (1985) Clinical prediction rules: Applications and methodological standards. *N. Engl. J. Med.*, **313**, 793–799.

Yam, L. T., Li, C. Y. and Lam, K. W. (1971) Tartrate-resistant acid phosphatase isoenzyme in the reticulum cells of leukemic reticuloendotheliosis. *N. Engl. J. Med.*, **284**, 357–360.

Part Four

Quality Assurance

18

The intralaboratory control of quality

John A. Koepke and Brian S. Bull

18.1 Introduction

For more than 30 years the College of American Pathologists (CAP) has sponsored a laboratory accreditation programme. The inspection team that visits each participating laboratory is composed of laboratory directors, supervisors and technologists. More than 4000 laboratories have participated in this programme. A series of objective questions catalogued by laboratory section ensures compliance with appropriate standards for directors and personnel, facilities, quality assurance and quality control. Biannual on-site inspections help to ensure compliance with these standards (Batjer, 1990). The Joint Commission for the Accreditation of Healthcare Organizations (JCAHO) also has a programme for hospital accreditation which also includes the laboratory service. Although JCAHO accreditation is a requirement for hospitals, many of the larger institutions present successful participation in the CAP accreditation programme in lieu of JCAHO inspection of the laboratory service. This has been satisfactory to all concerned since it avoids needless duplication of effort.

Thus, in the USA quality control and quality assurance programmes have become mandatory for laboratories wishing to be accredited by professional and/or governmental agencies. In fact, reimbursement for laboratory testing by the Health Care Financing Administration (HCFA) hinges upon such accreditation. The federal government has recently issued an updated set of standards (Table 18.1) as well as detailed regulations based upon the Clinical Laboratory Improvement Amendments of 1988 (CLIA '88) which are currently being implemented in the USA. The CAP and the JCAHO accreditation programmes were granted deemed status in 1994, thus avoiding an additional set of rules and regulations.

These requirements for quality control and quality assurance have become an increasing burden for hematology laboratories. Previously non-accredited laboratories such as found in physician offices have a particularly difficult time in implementing these requirements. It has been estimated that up to 15% of laboratory time and effort may be expended on quality assurance efforts. Some of these requirements may be misdirected in that those aspects of laboratory routine subjected to the most extensive quality control procedures (e.g. automated hematology analysers) are not the ones most likely to fail. On the other hand it may very well be that because such extensive efforts are directed toward these aspects of testing the failure rates are quite low.

There remain 'blind spots' in the overall programmes of quality control which have not been subjected to effective control procedures. Thus, for example, the erythrocyte sedimentation rate is a widely ordered test with minimal, if any, quality control of the testing. Laboratory management, if it is to be effective, should put control procedures at appropriate points but should also 'prune' those procedures which no longer generate useful information, e.g. duplicate coagulation testing (Koepke et al., 1994). Fortunately, most of the procedures mandated by CLIA '88 are those which are generally endorsed by laboratory professionals and, therefore,

Table 18.1 Federally mandated laboratory standards*

A clinical laboratory must:
Have appropriate space and environmental conditions necessary for testing
Have written procedure manuals for performance of all tests
Use test methods, equipment, instrumentation, reagents, materials and supplies that provide accurate and reliable test results and test reports
Establish and verify method performance specifications
Routinely perform control procedures to monitor method stability
Document and maintain all quality control activities
Sustantiate continued accuracy of test methods
Perform equipment maintenance and function checks
Establish remedial action policies and procedures

*Federal Register (1992).

the major impact of the regulations is in their extension to *all* laboratories doing patient testing.

Two major changes in hematology testing have dramatically changed quality assurance strategies. The first has been the widespread utilization of multichannel hematology analysers, instruments which automatically measure a dozen or more parameters on whole blood. Multichannel instrumentation has had a similar but less pervasive effect on coagulation laboratories. The second major advance has been the advent of microprocessor systems which when joined with the hematology and coagulation analysers significantly enhance the analytical, reporting and quality control aspects of hematology and coagulation testing.

In late 1989 an international symposium on quality assurance practices in hematology reviewed the state of the art of quality control/assurance practices in hematology laboratories. A number of proposals and recommendations came out of that conference (Koepke, 1990b) and since that time a number of initiatives have been pursued based upon the recommendations of the symposium. For example, the CLIA '88 requirements for the use of blood cell controls are similar to the conference's recommendations in that only two levels of controls are now required. A new reference method for the hematocrit including changes in the salt of EDTA used for blood specimen collection has helped to obtain more accurate MCV and PCV measurements (Bull and Rittenbach, 1990). More recently there has been attention focused on the blood film review and its place in the quality assurance scheme. While random error detection schemes for hematology testing have been proposed (Houwen, 1990) relatively few laboratories have implemented such methods.

Quality control procedures began many years ago in clinical laboratories primarily in the clinical chemistry section. Early on, discarded sera were pooled, mixed and aliquoted into small vials which were then frozen for storage. Every day when chemistry analyses were performed aliquots of the frozen serum was thawed, mixed and run concurrently with the patient serum samples. Acceptable limits for the serum pool were set at $\pm 2SD$ of the mean of at least 20 measurements. If the analysis of the quality control specimen failed to lie within the control limits, the analytical system was shut down until the cause of the problem had been discovered and corrected. It was, of course, understood that 5% of the runs would be 'out of control' on a statistical basis since $\pm 2SD$, by definition, covers only 95% of the results of the data.

Since those earlier days, many advances have been made in quality control procedures. For example, lots of lyophilized serum or plasma are commercially prepared with normal, low and high levels of the analyte in question. These large lots of material may be used for a year or longer in the chemistry or coagulation laboratory. This is in contrast to control materials in cellular hematology which have had a more problematic history.

Many of these practices have now become requirements for the accreditation and licensing of clinical laboratories and transfusion services. The key word now is *documentation* of the details of the quality control programmes and, quality assurance systems. Recently evidence for improvement in the quality of the testing has also been required. Together these combine into a overall system designated total quality management (TQM) or, alternatively, continuous quality improvement (CQI).

This chapter will focus on the intralaboratory practices which help to ensure accurate and precise identification and enumeration of blood cells as well as accurate measurement of coagulation factors. External quality assurance practices such as laboratory proficiency testing surveys which may have a significant effect on test accuracy are discussed in Chapter 19.

18.2 Principles

Until recently efforts at quality control have largely been focused on the individual test and the technical aspects of the testing process. But with the passage of time it has become apparent that many of the problems with laboratory testing lie beyond the testing itself but also include the entire testing process from patient preparation and specimen collection through the testing process to the final reporting of the result to the patient's physician (Boone, 1990). Therefore it is wise to study the entire process of testing from beginning to end in a systematic fashion. The critical factors are set down by a process called object-oriented programming which can help us to better understand the complexities of hematology testing. Young (1990) has developed such an approach for automated multiparameter hematology analysers (Figure 18.1). She also explains just how the various methods used for quality control in hematology analysis work together – and sometimes overlap.

18.2.1 Laboratory hematology service

Ideally one would like to use quality control materials which are indistinguishable physically and chemically from patient blood specimens, and the quality control procedure should handle the quality control materials in a manner entirely identical to that used for the handling of patient specimens. In the chemistry and coagulation laboratories this can be accomplished fairly easily, but living blood cells require more specialized procedures especially for commercial production and only within the last decade or so have these materials become reliable for quality con-

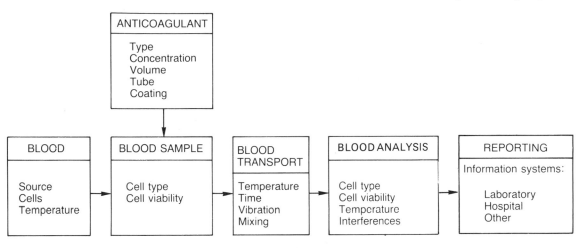

Figure 18.1 Object-orientated flow diagram for hematology testing

trol and calibration purposes. Low, normal and high concentrations of stabilized blood cells are commonly used. However it probably is as satisfactory to use just two levels of controls (as is mandated by CLIA '88). One control should be at normal levels while the other could well be a so-called 'oncology control' which has low levels of platelets and leukocytes. These levels are at or near the decision levels since it is at these concentrations that decisions regarding chemotherapy and transfusions are typically made.

Although quantitative testing in blood cell counting and coagulation testing can now be reasonably well monitored with commercial control materials, qualitative studies such as blood film reviews and bone marrow interpretation are significantly more difficult to control effectively. The skills of the expert morphologists in detecting a left shift, variant lymphocytosis or rare blast forms continue to be necessary in the hematology laboratory. Increasing amounts of effort are being put forward in this important topic with the hope that a symbiotic relationship can be fashioned between the increasingly sophisticated hematology analysers and the expert morphologists. An earlier chapter in this book discusses this aspect of laboratory hematology in greater detail (Chapter 2).

Most state-of-the-art hematology analysers are now capable of being operated in a so-called flagging mode. By that is meant that they do a panel of measurements and other studies on the blood specimens and separate out the essentially normal specimens from those which might have a significant abnormality (Koepke *et al.*, 1985b). Those potentially abnormal or so-called flagged specimens are then examined by the laboratory staff, sometimes in a hierarchical fashion as illustrated in Figure 18.2. These systems should be structured so as to have a very low incidence of false negative results – ideally this should be none whatsoever, but that may not be obtainable. As our knowledge about analysis

grows the number of false positive results should decrease thus avoiding the examination of specimens which were flagged unnecessarily. See page 191 for additional discussion.

18.2.2 Coagulation laboratory service

Although three levels of plasma controls (normal, mild and marked elevation) are frequently used for coagulation testing, control specimens at the decision level of the test would seem to be more appropriate. It is at these decision levels that the clinician may adjust the dose of warfarin, or might or might not order an infusion of cryoprecipitate (Koepke and Koepke, 1986).

It is unfortunate that the coagulation 'control' time has acquired such a following with clinicians who have been using it for years to gauge the level of anticoagulation in their patients. The ISI/INR system which standardizes the reporting of the prothrombin time is a scientifically valid solution to this problem but implementation has been slow, particularly in the USA (Chapter 3).

For the more specialized coagulation tests an increasing number of national and international reference preparations are becoming available. These include Factor VIII and fibrinogen. Chapter 13 details the preparations and materials that are now available.

18.2.3 Transfusion service

A blood bank has been defined as an establishment which collects and processes donor blood for transfusion. Blood banks recruit donors, prepare blood and blood components for transfusion including screening for antibodies and also for the agents of infectious disease transmissible by blood. A transfusion service, on the other hand, is usually located within a hospital where blood and blood products are cross-

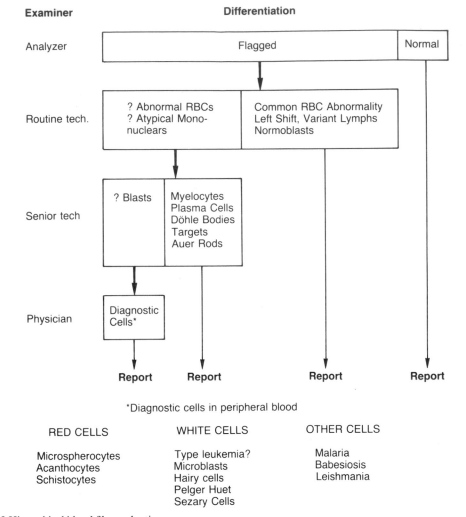

Figure 18.2 Hierarchical blood film evaluation

matched or otherwise prepared for transfusion to patients. Quality assurance practices within the transfusion service, i.e. a programme to ensure that reagents, equipment and methods function as required for the provision of safe and effective blood transfusions are described in Chapter 4. The interested reader is also referred to a previous publication on this subject by Koepke (1988).

In the USA, the production of these blood products has more and more shifted from the hospital setting into community blood banks due, in part, to the increasing complexity of production but also because of the requirements for testing for viral agents such as HBV, HIV and other infectious agents. The blood banks have therefore assumed the responsibilities of recruiting donors, processing the blood, testing the blood for infectious agents and preparing the blood components. More recently the responsibility for the development and implementa-

tion of autologous blood transfusions has also been assumed by the blood banks although they may draw some autologous blood units in the hospital outpatient setting. What this means is that hospital-based clinical pathologists and hematologists frequently no longer have the responsibility for most blood donation activities.

On the other hand, hospital-based physicians have become more involved with the transfusion practices in the hospital. This has been due to the wider array of blood components available and the increased knowledge required to use them effectively. The director of the transfusion service and his staff are in a unique position to monitor transfusion practices as well as to help educate the medical staff in such transfusion-related matters. Whole blood is now rarely transfused except perhaps to neonates. Plasma is routinely separated and more and more is being fractionated into cryoprecipitate, albumin and coagulation factor concentrates, particularly Factor VIII and Factor IX concentrates. Plasma obtained from plasmapheresis, is also being used for these purposes. Increasingly, large (600 ml) units of plasma obtained by apheresis are prepared as fresh-frozen plasma (FFP) to support long and complex operative procedures such as liver transplantation. Finally, although granulocyte transfusions are seldom used except in infant sepsis, stem cell transfusions are being used with increasing frequency in bone marrow transplantation procedures.

There should be ongoing review to determine if blood and blood components are being used appropriately. Such reviews usually validate the appropriate usage of these products. They can also help to identify areas requiring further study and possibly indicate the need for improved hemotherapy policies and procedures. In fact, such utilization review is now mandatory in many places (JCAHO, 1993). Most hospitals now have guidelines for the transfusion of blood components which have become the standard of practice. These are usually based upon published guidelines (NIH Consensus Conferences, 1985, 1987, 1988). This is a responsibility shared between the medical director of the transfusion service and the clinicians who order the blood transfusions.

To ensure the quality of blood and blood components either prepared on-site or supplied by blood banks, a system to monitor the quality of these products is necessary (Hoffman, Koepke and Widmann, 1987). Monitors or indicators can be devised for many of these products and may include monitoring of the recipients to ensure that the expected responses are obtained. Suggested monitors for blood product quality include pre- and post-transfusion measurement of the platelet count. Better still, if available, is the pre- and post-transfusion measurement of platelet functional capacity by aggregometry. Similarly, pre- and post-transfusion measurements of the partial thromboplastin time (PTT), Factor VIII levels, the activated coagulation time (ACT) and/or the fibrinogen concentration will document the affectiveness of transfusions of fresh frozen plasma or specific components such as cryoprecipitate of Factor VIII concentrates. Such studies are also useful for identifying the presence of inhibitors or antibodies to blood products.

18.3 Practices

18.3.1 Hematology laboratory

While the previous section has outlined the principles to guarantee quality, this section will give examples of the practices (Koepke and Klee, 1990). As noted earlier many practices have now become requirements for the accreditation and licensing of clinical laboratories and blood banks (Table 18.2).

Most would agree that the lack of robust blood cell and plasma preparations is responsible for most of the problems in hematological quality control. With today's hematology analysers electronic problems are uncommon whereas the mechanical and hydraulic aspects of the typical analyser are more troublesome. These potential problems as well as variability arising from ambient temperature variations necessitate that the analyser be monitored frequently in a comprehensive quality control programme. This is more of a challange than it should be since there is a lack of robust blood cell quality control preparations.

The ideal control materials should be stable indefinitely and yet respond to testing in a manner similar in all respects to fresh blood. Such a material would be sampled directly like patient specimens and should encompass without any modifications all the tests ordinarily done on fresh blood. Such materials would certainly have wide application in hematology laboratories. Since such an ideal material has not yet been manufactured, what options are available to the laboratory?

Option 1: Partially Stabilized Whole Blood. Whole blood can be partially stabilized so that assay values can be expected to remain unchanged for days up to months. Unfortunately there has often been a drift in the assigned values, particularly for leukocyte and platelet counts and the packed cell volume. If the product is 'overstabilized' the material may become insensitive to minor analytical problems and the material is no longer a satisfactory surrogate for whole blood. Finally such materials are relatively expensive as compared to chemistry control materials.

Option 2: Fresh Whole Blood. If reference measurements on fresh whole blood were performed on a daily basis, such specimens could serve as controls.

Table 18.2 Federally mandated quality control practices for moderate and/or high complexity tests*

General — Establish written quality control procedures for monitoring and evaluating the quality of the analytical testing process of each method to assure the accuracy and reliability of patient test results and reports.

— Follow manufacturer's instructions for instrument or test system operation and test performance
— Perform and document calibration at least once every six months
— Perform and document control procedures for automated hematology and coagulation testing using at least two levels of control materials every 8 hours of testing
— For manual cell counts and manual coagulation testing must be done in duplicate
— For blood typing and compatibility testing, follow reagent manufacturer's instructions, including use of appropriate controls

*Federal Register (1992).

However, the cost in technical time and effort would be considerable and the chances of erroneous assignment of values would be particularly high if the technologists performing these studies were not well trained. Periodic use of reference methods to confirm calibration of the hematology analysers has been required by the CLIA '88 regulations (Table 8.2), but the infrequent checking without good methods for ongoing quality control is not a satisfactory solution.

A variation of this concept depends upon the assumption that if a blood specimen is analysed on a properly calibrated and controlled instrument, the specimen in effect becomes a secondary 'standard' for all the parameters of the blood count. As such it can then be used to recheck the same instrument later in the day or even on the following day. Such specimens can also be used used to control analysers in satellite laboratories which may be scattered throughout the hospital. A statistical analysis of this method of quality control concluded that it offered great promise (Hackney and Cembrowski, 1990). We have used this method successfully for many years and in addition to its statistical validity, significant cost savings have been realized.

Option 3: Whole Blood Surrogates. For those hematology analyses for which stable statistical averages are not acceptable (e.g. leukocyte and/or platelet counts), whole blood surrogate materials such as latex spheres may be a feasible alternative. However, this approach does require a compromise since the surrogate material is significantly different from patient specimens since the material is both physically and chemically different from whole blood.

Whole blood control preparations have been available for many years and their quality and reliability have improved. A number of commercial suppliers of controls have also developed extensive intra- and interlaboratory comparisons which provide historical documentation of the quality control programme (Anderson, 1990). The control limits should be confirmed by comparison with contemporary controls when the new controls are first received. However, most controls now come with so-called 'assigned values' (a control/calibration oxymoron) which have been supplied by the manufacturer by running the particular lot of control on very closely controlled instruments in the manufacturer's quality control laboratory (Richardson-Jones, 1990). Although they are not truly calibrators, many laboratories have used them to calibrate and/or verify their instruments (Gilmer *et al.*, 1977), Subsequent surveys showed little evidence of any change in this undesirable practice.

Precision and accuracy

Imprecision, the antonym of precision, is the sum of all random errors that occur while a procedure is being carried out. The sum is usually expressed as a standard deviation (SD or s) or the related coefficient of variation (CV). For monitoring the precision of most cellular hematology tests excess patient samples work quite well. They are ideal because they are fresh whole blood and the handling procedures are identical to those used for the patient specimens. Thus, the two requirements for quality control programmes noted above, i.e. similarity to patient blood specimens and identity with procedures used for patient specimen analysis, are ideally satisfied. Most multichannel hematology analysers are equipped with microprocessor software for the required statistical calculations and files. Since modern analysers require such small quantities of blood for analysis, most adult blood specimens will, after the completion of the requested tests, provide ample blood for multiple (usually 10) replicate analyses needed for the determination of short term imprecision. Chapter 16 provides more details for the determination of short-term precision. Long-term precision studies are more problematic.

Accuracy, the related, but yet quite distinct characteristic of a laboratory test, is a function of the availability and adequacy of appropriate standards and calibrators – assuming the presence of a reasonably precise analyser. There is little to be gained by reducing the coefficient of variation of an analysis from 1.0 to 0.5% if the setpoint of the analysis cannot be guaranteed any closer than ± 2%.

The reason that inaccuracy degrades the usefulness of a measurement so quickly is that most clinician users of laboratory data have certain numerical thresholds outside of which they will subject a patient to additional study. A typical example would be a workup for the cause of macrocytosis on all patients in whom the mean cell volume (MCV) exceeded 102 fl. It is evident that inevitably there will be some normal patients worked up for macrocytosis along with those patients who are truly macrocytic. If an MCV analyser drifts upward 4 fl, which is close to the minimum bias that can be guaranteed with present analysers and calibrators, almost two and a half times as many patients will be investigated unnecessarily. The alternative to set action limits at 106 fl is obviously not appropriate as this will exclude many samples that are abnormal because of disease.

It is critical, therefore, for quality control programmes to ensure that the hematology analyzers are set accurately to begin with and that any drift from the setpoint can be detected promptly. These are the two most important goals for any effective quality control programme.

Standard statistical techniques are used to determine if the instrument is 'in control'. Although the application of the so-called Westgard rules for clinical chemistry control seems reasonable, in fact, such a method of analysis is rarely used in hematology laboratories (Koepke, 1990a). In Europe control data is frequently plotted on a cumulative summation (cusum) plot. This method is especially useful to detect drifts or trends in instrument performance (ECCLS, 1985). Cusum plots are much poorer in quantitating the extent of the drift so that it can be quantitatively corrected. This is because the cusum calculation transforms the bias of the analyser into the slope of the cusum plot and slopes are difficult to quantitate by inspection.

Ensuring accuracy in erythrocyte analysis

Calculation of the population average MCV, MCH and MCHC (sometimes, though incorrectly, referred to as a moving average calculation) has been used for many years as a procedure to control hematology analysers. The mean erythrocyte indices are likely to be within normal limits in the majority of anemic and polycythemic patients in an acute care hospital. Furthermore, the statistical effect of the normal values will dilute the variability caused by the relatively few macrocytic and microcytic samples (Bull and Hay, 1989). Most of the larger hematology analysers now include this method of control in their operating systems. Although it had been thought that this method of control is only useful for red cell parameters, it has been shown that the accuracy of red count counting can be transferred to leukocyte and platelet counting as well as to other parameters (Bull, 1991).

Statistical averages have more recently been explored by manufacturers as a way of ensuring the accuracy of labelled values on whole blood calibrators. Manufacturers have the ability to use an entire country as the data source for statistical averages of both the control material provided and the patient results achieved on instruments calibrated by the quality control materials that they have manufactured. Such a data base, if properly utilized (Bull et al., 1993) can document the accuracy of quality control material for the entire circuit from the time it leaves the manufacturing plant until it is used to calibrate an end-user's analyser.

One disadvantage of the use of statistical averages for control in the laboratory is the requirement for a significant number of specimens each day so that real time quality control is possible. Therefore laboratories doing less than 60 blood counts per day should not attempt to use this method as their primary quality control method. On the other hand, if a sufficient number of patient specimens are available, use of this approach can result in significant cost savings, particularly if multiple hematology analysers are being used in the laboratory. It is also useful as a cross-check on the accuracy of the two levels of control material required to be run each eight hours under present CLIA '88 regulations.

Ensuring the accuracy of the platelet count

Although it may be theoretically attractive to calibrate the hematology analyser platelet counts using platelet counts by phase contrast microscopy as the reference method, because of its low precision this approach is very demanding. The poor reproducibility of the phase counting procedure (Brecher, Schneiderman and Cronkite, 1953) requires that unmanageably large numbers of platelet counts be averaged each time recalibration is performed.

A far simpler method that has proved workable in the laboratory of one of the authors (BSB) is to note the ratio between the amplifier settings of the red cell and platelet count channels. From time to time the analyser will be recalibrated to eliminate bias in the red count by adjusting the red cell amplifier card. If, at the same time, the platelet amplifier card is adjusted appropriately to maintain the expected ratio between the two settings, it will be found that the platelet count will also retain its freedom from bias.

The reason for this behaviour is not difficult to follow. All the fluid handling and dilution steps up to and even including the transducer itself on most analysers are identical between platelets and red cells. Thus, any variation in any of these steps that must be corrected by adjusting the red cell count will affect the platelet count in an identical fashion. The only analyser breakdown that would be missed by this procedure is a partial or subtle electronic failure in the amplifier/counting circuits of red cell or platelet computation circuits. Such failures are extremely rare with mean time failure in the order of years for most modern analysers. An illustration of how stable this ratio proves to be on two analysers using commercial platelet calibrators over a period of two years is shown in Table 18.3. The majority of the variability is that induced by differences between successive lots of red cell and platelet calibrator material.

Ensuring the accuracy of the total leukocyte count

In normal patients the physiological variability of the total leukocyte count is of the order of ±35% CV. The absolute neutrophil count is the most variable. It is significantly affected by exercise, eating and other stimuli. Because of this variability, at least 100 patient samples would be required in order to reduce the confidence interval of the average leukocyte count to <5%, and more than 500 samples are needed to reduce it to <2% before such procedures would be useful for quality control purposes. Indirectly the leukocyte count is already at least under partial quality control surveillance. The sampling, dilution and even the mixing steps are identical to those used for the hemoglobin determination. Only the setpoint of the particle counting transducer is not covered.

Table 18.3 Constancy of the ratio between the red cell and the platelet amplifier circuits. The use of this ratio in quality control

		Analyser 1				Analyser 2	
A RBC Cal	B Plt Cal	B/A Ratio		A RBC Cal	B Plt Cal	B/A Ratio	
Year 1							
	1.13	0.985	0.8717	1.152	0.969	0.8411	
	1.295	1.124	0.8680	1.102	0.969	0.8793	
	1.157	1.054	0.9110	1.137	0.969	0.8522	
	1.113	0.99	0.8895	1.044	0.893	0.8554	
	1.122	0.99	0.8824	1.057	0.893	0.8448	
	1.136	0.99	0.8715	1.046	0.893	0.8537	
Year 2							
	1.175	0.99	0.8426	1.048	0.893	0.8521	
	1.122	0.99	0.8824	1.079	0.892	0.8267	
	1.157	0.99	0.8557	1.126	0.957	0.8499	
	1.127	0.99	0.8784	1.137	0.957	0.8417	
	1.152	0.99	0.8594	1.109	0.957	0.8629	
	1.152	0.99	0.8594	1.114	0.957	0.8591	
Mean:	1.153	1.006	0.873	1.096	0.933	0.852	
S.D.:	0.048	0.042	0.018	0.040	0.036	0.013	
CV%	4.191	4.128	2.057	3.613	3.860	1.522	

(Both analysers were S-Plus IVs, data collected 1985–86).

To calibrate the setpoint, a laboratory might elect to use rather tedious reference procedures on a set of three normal patient samples using the resulting counts to calibrate the multichannel analyser. A second method is to transfer the accuracy of the erythrocyte count to the leukocyte counting channel by preparing a suspension of accurately counted red cells, fixing them in glutaraldehyde and subsequently counting them to confirm the accuracy of the leukocyte count. Finally, the method used by most laboratories involves the use of commercially stabilized blood on which the manufacturer has determined the leukocyte count values as well as the flow cytometric differential count.

Ensuring the accuracy of the differential leukocyte count

While it may seem simple to develop a quality control programme using patient samples to control the manual leukocyte differential count, the inherent variability of the routine 100 cell differential count is so imprecise (Rümke, 1979) that little could be gained by such a programme. The quantitative enumeration of the four major cell types (neutrophils, lymphocytes, eosinophils and monocytes) have coefficients of variation of 5% or greater depending upon the relative proportion of cells. The qualitative findings such as left shifts, variants lymphocytes and rare blasts are even less amenable to effective quality control procedures.

The advent of multichannel analysers which are capable of performing reasonably precise quantita-

tive leukocyte differential counts seemingly provides the answers to many of the problems encountered with 100 cell manual/visual differential counts. There is little doubt that the statistical accuracy of common cell identification has been greatly improved. However, is is not clear that instrument-performed leukocyte differentials are more clinically relevant since many of the instruments cannot reliably identify band neutrophils, variant lymphocytes and other immature cells (NCCLS, 1992). However, these instruments do provide methods for the flagging of blood specimens which may contain abnormal cells. Such flagging has proven to be useful in the diagnosis as well as management of hematological disorders. The setting of the flag is determined by the way in which the analyser differentiates the various cell types. Certain characteristic patterns for cell identification are programmed into the microprocessor software. When the specimen scattergram does not fit these patterns, an electronic flag is raised and the specimen is identified as requiring further study. Typically, this requires the preparation of a stained blood film and a review of that film by a knowledgeable morphologist.

The flagging rate of an instrument is dependent upon the technology of the cell analyser, the sophistication of the software programming and probably most importantly upon the patient mix. A well designed analyser should substantially decrease the number of required blood film reviews. Usually the healthier the patient population the more effective is the screening process. Unfortunately because it is in large

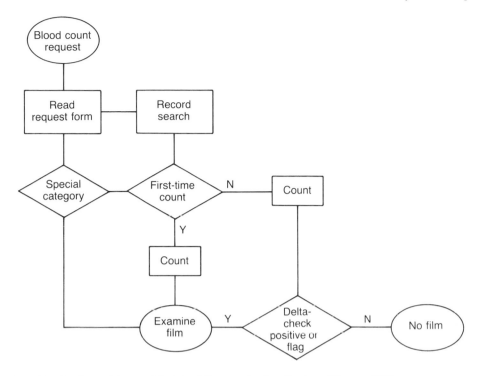

Figure 18.3 Algorithm for determining need for blood film examination (Lewis and Rowan, 1991)

acute care hospital populations where the analysers would be most cost effective in decreasing the need for tedious and demanding blood film reviews.

Blood film reviews

When a blood film is examined there must be assurance that a qualified observer has examined the blood film for a broad spectrum of abnormalities. A quality control programme should ensure that the observer is, in fact, qualified and that the blood has been examined in such a fashion that all significant abnormalities have been identified. A variety of ways of achieving this objective have been proposed. They include an ongoing statistical analysis of each individual technologist's differential counts, an analysis of each technologist's clustering of abnormalities (e.g. does one technologist report significantly more left shifts?) and/or an ongoing comparison of manual/visual and instrument generated blood counts (Bull, 1991).

In addition to the blood film reviews ordered by the clinicians, the blood film review is an integral segment of the quality control of hematology instruments as well as an important part of hematology laboratory medicine. In one of our laboratories (JAK) we have used a hierarchic system for the examination of blood films for many years. The method is illustrated in Figure 18.2. The first step is the analysis of the blood specimen on the automated

hematology analyser. Applying a set of quantitative and qualitative criteria, a proportion of the blood specimens will not have any significant abnormalities and no blood film review is necessary on such specimens. These tests can be promptly reported to the clinic or inpatient unit resulting in significant savings in time as well as money.

Specimens with questionable cells (e.g. possible blasts) are referred to the senior morphologists in the laboratory for review. At this level a variety of abnormal cell types can be confirmed and reported. However, if there are cells which might be diagnostic of leukemia, malaria or other such conditions they must be confirmed by the medical director of the laboratory before being reported (Figure 18.2).

A similar process for selecting the cases requiring inspection of blood films was described by Lewis and Rowan (1991). Using the algorithm illustrated in Fig. 18.3, they proposed the following criteria for this selection:

1. Special cases where a film is obligatory – follow-up of diagnosed blood diseases; all patients receiving chemotherapy or radiotherapy; neonates; other patients when indicated by clinical information (e.g. infectious mononucleosis, lymphadenopathy; chronic renal disease);
2. First-time blood counts when any component is outside normal reference limits;
3. Instrument flags as established for the counter;

4. A repeat count showing significant differences from earlier counts.

In this way, in two major laboratories the numbers of films to be inspected were reduced by 30–40% and it seemed likely that an even smaller proportion of films would need to be examined in any general hospital not handling the large number of unusual cases which were seen in these referral centres. A study of the validity of this concept showed that by combining automated blood counts with scrutiny of the selected films it would be unlikely for any significant error to occur in routine tests.

18.3.2 Quality control of multisite testing

In our medical centre (JAK) there are seven different locations for the hematology laboratory. Assurance of comparable results among all seven laboratories is accomplished in two ways. One is to run three patient blood samples in all seven locations every other day. The data (including the instrument differential count) are pooled, and results from each laboratory are evaluated against predetermined acceptable limits about the mean or median values of all parameters. Any laboratory data outside these limits must be evaluated and the problem remedied before any patient results are reported.

For more than a decade a weekly exchange of normal and abnormal blood films has been carried out among the various laboratory sections and shifts. In rotation each laboratory prepares enough slides for all the laboratories. Each member of the laboratory staff examines the slide and reports back the blood film review findings to the hematology quality assurance coordinator who collates the results from all laboratories. Concurrently, the director reviews the blood film and prepares a short critique of the reports from all the laboratories. In this way a certain level of standardization is achieved in the hematology laboratory service. If there are common morphological identification problems, inservice training sessions are scheduled. New employees are asked to review slides from the blood film library so that their level of expertise can be evaluated prior to assuming responsibilities for blood film reviews in the laboratory.

18.3.3 Coagulation laboratory

For routine coagulation testing a wide variety of lyophilized plasma preparations suitable for both controls as well as calibrators is available (see Chapter 13). This is a situation similar to that in clinical chemistry and has functioned quite well for many years.

However, the standardization of the reporting of the prothrombin time in patients undergoing oral anticoagulation therapy has been more problematic, especially in the USA. There has been slow but steady progress in the implementation of the ISI/INR system. Major manufacturers supply the appropriate ISI information with their thromboplastins enabling laboratories to report the prothombin time as an International Normalized Ratio. The laboratory director should take a leadership role in the implementation of this internationally recognized standard since the benefits for patient care are quite evident. A recent American study has shown the clinical usefulness of this method of reporting prothrombin times. This topic is discussed in greater detail in Chapter 3.

Although standards and controls are widely available for the common coagulation tests, this is not so for the more esoteric tests. For example, platelet aggregation studies usually require a normal control specimen. The donor for the control specimen usually turns out to be one of the laboratory staff who is not taking medications of any kind (including aspirin). Despite the advent of much improved instrumentation including whole blood aggregometers, platelet aggregometry remains very much an art which require considerable skill both in the performance and in the interpretation of the results. This is unfortunate because the only other generally available assay of platelet function is the bleeding time. This is a test subject to such frequent false-positive artefactual results as to render it nearly useless (Rogers and Levin, 1990).

18.4 Documentation of quality measurements and monitors

In order for a hospital to be accreditated in the USA the Joint Commission on Accreditation of Healthcare Organizations (JCAHO) has required the monitoring of so-called indicators or measures which reflect the quality of services provided by the hospital (JCAHO, 1993). These indicators, chosen by the hospital staff, should be objective, i.e., they must be susceptible to assessment on a continuing basis in order that trends can be monitored (hopefully to show improvement) as well as documenting compliance with pre-selected guidelines.

For years laboratories have 'counted' blood cells, molecules, workloads and other things. The laboratory service should choose useful indicators which can be counted easily and develop appropriate analyses for further discussion and debate (Koepke and Klee, 1990).

The indicator or measure should truly be a reflection of the quality of the laboratory service. Thus, for example, a cross-match to transfusion (C/T) ratio of 2.0 or less would indicate that excessive cross-matching of blood was not occurring. In hematology the proportion of instrument blood counts which

Table 18.4 Examples of quality measures

Measures of Laboratory Data Reliability
— Performance in proficiency testing trials (92–08)*
— Monitors of reporting errors (90–15A)
— Monitors of specimen acceptability (92–05)
Measures of Quality Laboratory Management
— Quality assurance programmes (90–18A)
— Monitors of testing turnaround times (89–03A, 90–13A, 91–05A)
— Critical values (92–04)
— Complications of phlebotomy (90–10A)
— Wristband identification errors (91–01A)
Measures of Appropriate Laboratory Utilization
— Differential/screening blood count ratio
— Coagulation test utilization (90–19A)
— INR and monitoring of oral anticoagulation (91–10A)
— Crossmatch/transfusion ratio (89–08A)
— Blood transfusion utilization (89–08A, 91–07A, 93–06)
— Appropriateness of autologous transfusion (90–11A, 92–01)

*Subject of CAP Q-Probe studies are indicated by their ID numbers.

also have a manual/visual differential leukocyte count may reflect the avoidance of unnecessary blood film reviews.

18.4.1 Types of quality indicators

Several of the hospital-wide measures which JCAHO requires to be monitored (e.g. blood usage, infection control and pharmacy) have close linkages with laboratory medicine. The laboratories provide a major source of information needed to monitor these activities. Several more specific laboratory quality indicators are proposed. These include:

- measures of laboratory data reliability
- measures of quality laboratory management
- measures of appropriate laboratory utilization, including blood transfusions

Each of these indicators can be used to estimate the quality of the laboratory service. Table 18.4 lists a wide variety of useful measures of laboratory quality many of which we have used. Laboratory data reliability, in addition to being monitored on a real time basis with comprehensive quality control programmes, has also been checked for many years in proficiency testing programmes (Chapter 19).

Workload recording and productivity or the assessment of test turnaround times are examples of measures of quality management. Many of these have been the subject of the College of American Pathologists Q-Probes programme (Bachner and Howanitz, 1991). This programme which was begun in 1988 has enrolled hundreds of laboratories. They submit de-

tailed data regarding the subject of the Q-Probe (Table 18.4). The data is merged and statistical evaluations including percentile ranking of the participants is done. In this way each laboratory can assess their level of compliance with developing standards of laboratory performance.

Laboratory utilization is more problematic since requests for laboratory services are initiated by the clinical staff. But laboratories are in a strategic position to monitor test utilization patterns. For example, the ratio of automated blood counts (without a manual differential count) to so-called complete blood counts (which include a complete manual/visual blood film differential and review) would be indicative of the rate of possibly inappropriate ordering of complete blood counts when only one or more of the parameters found in the automated count would be sufficient. Ideally, the monitoring of the appropriate use of laboratory testing is done conjointly with the quality assurance programmes in clinical departments such as medicine or surgery.

A recent study reviewed the indications for coagulation tests in a large group of hospitals and concluded that about 40% of prothrombin times and partial thromboplastin times were associated with inappropriate indications (Meier *et al.*, 1992). While clinicians disagreed with some of the guidelines used in the studies, it is evident that coagulation tests are ordered more often than necessary.

18.4.2 Measures of laboratory data reliability

External quality assessment

For about 30 years proficiency testing (PT) or external quality assessment (EQA) has been one of the few objective indicators of laboratory quality. Whether or not performance in these programmes can be validly used as an indicator of the quality of the performing laboratory continues to be debated (Koepke, 1992). Certainly if a laboratory consistently performs poorly in such exercises, it can reasonably be inferred that the laboratory may be unreliable. The converse is not necessarily true since a number of extraneous factors may influence the proficiency testing process. The place of such programmes in laboratory medicine is reviewed in much more detail in chapter 19.

In most larger laboratories there is an ongoing programme to monitor the performance of each section in proficiency testing surveys. Table 18.5 summarizes survey testing experience at our hospital (JAK) over a four year period of time. The left-hand side of the table categorizes the unacceptable survey results as if they were patient samples and makes a judgement as to the severity of the error using the Thompson severity scale as a model. On the right-hand side the errors are divided according to their

Table 18.5 Analysis of proficiency testing measure exceptions (1989–1992) *

Exception Severity (Thompson Scale 0–5)		Source of Exception	
0 Survey problems	12%	Methodologic inadequacies, substandard methods	36%
1 Statistically expected + 2SD⟩⟨ + 3SD	32%	Technical problems	28%
2 Defensible differences in qualitative tests, insensitive methods	25%	Clerical errors	21%
3 Clerical error or technical problems with minimal clinical risks	25%	Problems with survey materials	9%
4 Clerical error or technical problems with significant clinical risks	4%	Other problems	6%
5 Unconventional laboratory practice	2%		

*Analysis of 3% exceptions from an average of 3300 annual survey challenges.

etiology. This method of analysis has been useful in identifying problem areas and equipment and methods that need improvement.

Proficiency testing performance is now monitored by the federal governmental agencies responsible for laboratory regulation. Any failure to achieve an acceptable performance requires an explanation as well as a plan to remedy the problem if it has not already been corrected. If a continuing pattern of poor performance is found, more drastic steps are required. For the last two years, the CAP proficiency testing reports have incorporated a similar flagging programme which indicates problematic analytes and which if difficulties continue may cause a withdrawal of laboratory accreditation for that analyte (Federal Register, 1992).

Blood film reviews

As noted earlier, in our laboratories a weekly exchange of normal as well as abnormal blood films has been carried out among the various laboratory sections and shifts for more than a decade. Concurrently, the director (JAK) reviews the blood film. In this way a continuous record of the consensus of morphological evaluations of the blood films is maintained. Portions of this ongoing programme have been published and have proven to be useful measures of the state of the art of differential leukocyte counting (Koepke, Dotson and Shifman, 1985a). It has been gratifying to see the improvement in blood film review performance over the ten years this programme has been in place.

Error detection

Comprehensive programmes for error detection are becoming more common. In fact, the CLIA '88 regulations require such a programme (Federal Register, 1992). Ideally, such a programme will evaluate and promptly correct errors in laboratory testing (Houwen, 1990) A continuing monitoring of such problems should be maintained and any patterns of error generation investigated and hopefully corrected. A critical part of such programmes is the initiation and continuation of a dialogue between laboratory workers, nursing staff and clinicians so that any perceived problems can be corrected. A weekly meeting of the laboratory director with the resident staff at their working rounds has proven to be helpful in this regard.

Types of problems which we have seen over the last several years are probably similar for most other institutions. Interestingly, less than a quarter of the problems occur within the laboratory analytic process, most being either in the pre-analytic or postanalytic phases of testing (Boone, 1990).

18.4.3 Measures of appropriate laboratory utilization

With increasing emphasis on cost containment and improved efficiency, there is a concomitant emphasis on the study of appropriate utilization of laboratory services. Standards for appropriate resource utilization, so-called practice guidelines, are being developed in all segments of medicine including laboratory medicine. As might be expected there are, as yet, few universally agreed guidelines. In the case of laboratory utilization, performance standards should be established jointly by the clinical and laboratory practitioners.

Due to the inherent risks associated with blood transfusion, transfusion services have a longer history of evaluating the appropriate utilization of blood products. Audits of overall or specific blood component usage are a requirement for continuing hospital accreditation. A listing of transfusion guidelines used in one of our hospitals (BSB) is found in Table 18.6. The College of American Pathologists has developed practice parameters for the use of fresh frozen plasma, cryoprecipitate and platelets (Practice Guidelines, 1993). These guidelines are based for the most part on the several National Institutes of Health consensus conferences on the appropriate use of these blood components (NIH Consensus Conferences, 1985, 1987). Additional guidelines for perioperative red cell transfusions were also developed using this method (NIH Consensus Conference, 1988).

In some cases initial data gathering for such laboratory medicine practice guidelines has been in the special questionnaires included with proficiency testing kits. At other times the participants of the Q-Probes programme have supplied the data. Q-Probes is a programme which develops and tests various laboratory indicators among a group of several hundred participants. Some of these Q-Probes which

Table 18.6 Practice guidelines for blood component transfusion

Packed red blood cells and whole blood	1. Documented Hgb < 8.0 g/dl 2. > 10% blood volume lost in patients > 5 kg but < 30 kg 3. > 5% blood volume lost in < 5 kg patients 4. Chemotherapy or surgery with Hgb < 10 g/dl in patients < 30 kg 5. Neonatal diagnosis of hypovolemia or Hgb < 13 g/dl 6. Other
Platelets	1. Massive blood transfusion > 15 units in adults 2. Platelet count < 50 K with active bleeding/surgery 3. CPB with platelet count < 100 K with active bleeding 4. CPB times > 120 minutes with clinical bleeding 5. CPB if patient is < 15 kg 6. Platelet count < 20 K adults; < 30 K pediatrics 7. Platelet count < 100 K and > 1 blood volume lost 8. Newborn < 50 K with invasive procedure or risk of ICH 9. Other
Fresh frozen plasma	1. INR ≥ 1.5, PTT, or specific clotting abnormality with bleeding/surgery 2. Blood transfusions > 15 units, or > 1 blood volume < 5 kg 3. Coumadin or antifibrinolytic therapy with bleeding 4. TTP 5. CPB on patients < 15 kg 6. Neonatal hypovolemia/exchange transfusion 7. Fibrinogen deficiencies prior to administration of L-asparaginase 8. Other
Cryoprecipitate	1. Factor deficiency: fibrinogen, von Willebrand's, Factors VII, XIII 2. Fibronectin: sepsis, burn, shock, blunt trauma 3. DIC/fibrin glue 4. Other
Miscellaneous blood products	Product ———————— Indications ————————

CPB = Cardio-pulmonary bypass.
ICH = Intracerebral hemorrhage
K = $10^9/l$

touch on laboratory utilization are found in the last section of Table 18.4.

18.4.4 Measures of quality laboratory management

Laboratory management has a significant influence on many aspects of laboratory performance and there are a number of indicators which can be used to monitor the effectiveness of the overall management. This is the most recent focus in management practice both within the laboratory as well as throughout business and industry. This movement has been spurred on by current efforts for cost containment in health care as well as the pressures of an economy in recession. The pressures are considerable but the solutions are not evident to any great degree since the interrelationships between the various aspects are so closely intertwined. Considerable inertia exists which resists change. But in many ways the tools are already in hand but require leaders to put them together in new and useful ways which will be of benefit to all.

However, significant progress has been made in some areas. For example, the development of increasingly sophisticated laboratory instrumentation has considerably improved the quality of the data. Near-patient testing helps with turnaround times but has other drawbacks. Laboratory information systems hold a great deal of promise but the appropriate programming and implementation of these systems is difficult.

18.4.5 Monitoring of quality measurements

In laboratory medicine it has often been difficult to establish appropriate thresholds for the evaluation of quality indicators. In the case of quantitative information, however, such as the results of proficiency testing these have been judged as 'acceptable' if the results are within ± 2SD of the mean of the comparative group. The CLIA '88 regulations now have generally included in the regulations a wider (± 3SD) acceptable range. Thus only 1% of the participants would fail to report an acceptable result. To improve laboratory services and thus patient care, the results of all quality monitors should be

Table 18.7 Quality assurance office 'file cabinet'

PLANS
   Laboratory Quality Assurance Plan
   Hospital Quality Assurance Plan
   Laboratory Quality Assurance Committee Meeting
     Minutes
   Medical Staff Quality Improvement Committee Minutes
MEASURES
   Laboratory Inspection and Accreditation Files
   Proficiency Testing Reports and Responses
   Workload Statistics
   Quality Assurance Reports (Monthly/Quarterly)
   Indicator Exception Studies and Summaries (Annual)
   Laboratory 'Blunder' Reports (Internal and Risk Manage-
     ment)
ASSESSMENTS
   Quality Measure Exception Studies and Annual Sum-
     maries
   Evaluations of New Equipment
   Special Evaluations

communicated to laboratory directors, supervisors, technologists and technicians – all should be involved. Weekly or monthly staff meetings should be held with minutes of the deliberations to document the various working monitors. Any threshold violations which have exceeded the predetermined thresholds and plans for the correction of any analyte testing problems should be discussed. Subsequent re-evaluation should document the effectiveness of these actions. The monitoring should show continuing improvement in all aspects of laboratory testing – TQI or CQM in action.

For more than a decade hospital transfusion review committees in the USA have received summaries of the transfusion service quality indicators, including blood transfusion utilization and quality control data on various blood components (see Table 18.6 for typical examples of the screening criteria applied). In addition, the investigations of all transfusion reactions are summarized for committee discussion (Koepke and Klee, 1990). Any changes in transfusion policies then have a rational basis for their genesis.

A variety of records and reports should be kept in the quality assurance office. Intitial measurement studies provide baseline data to which follow-up studies can be compared, and thus significant improvement in the provision of laboratory services can be documented. As an example, Table 18.7 lists the files which might be found in the quality assurance office.

18.5 Future quality assurance initiatives

Following the 1989 conference on quality assurance for laboratory hematology a number of proposals

and recommendations were made (Koepke, 1990b). Many of them were closely associated with data gathering and the management of such data. In order to accomplish these tasks laboratory information systems are essential. The impact of laboratory information systems as well as the individual instrument microprocessors has already been significant and undoubtedly will be even more so in the future. Data handling techniques such as filing, sorting and transferring the data have been important because of their beneficial effects on the laboratory transcription errors that are unavoidable whenever data is manually transmitted.

A growing demand for quality control analysis and documentation will significantly increase the use of laboratory-based information systems. Future quality control packages should provide for more sophisticated methods for extracting quality control information from patient data in real time. As the number of simultaneous analyses increases, the potential usefulness of cross-correlating all the data in a particular patient sample increases significantly. Such systems improve the clinical value of the data and will lead to the development of methods for instrument-aided diagnosis. It naturally follows that more sensitive and specific quality control procedures will be developed as the quality of the data improves.

The microprocessors which are now an integral part of all larger hematology analysers as well as coagulation instruments can significantly augment the process of operator-instrument interaction. For instance, if a sample should be rerun, the instrument's microprocessor should simplify this task. Likewise the selection of the most appropriate patient samples to be used for quality control purposes can be considerably simplified.

A microprocessor-controlled analyser might very well be programmed for autocalibration since there is such an extraordinary stability ($< 1\%$ CV) of the mean erythrocyte indices. The relationship between the red cell indices and platelet and leukocyte counts may well allow for an expansion of the concept to include autocalibration of hematology analysers which measure blood count parameters (Bull and Korpman, 1983).

Presently such concepts seem rather remote in coagulation testing. However, the ability of coagulation instruments to perform panels of coagulation tests is already available. Instrument-generated prompts for further more specific testing may very well be developed.

In the transfusion service the implementation of computerization has been more or less confined to the patient specimen and blood unit identification as well as filing and sorting of transfusion-related events such as cross-matching and antibody identification. Despite the apparently routine nature of these tasks the computerization of transfusion service records has undoubtedly saved the lives of not a few hospitalized patients. Any patient who has been previously transfused in a particular hospital will have his/her ABO group and Rh type in the computer file. It will thus be automatically checked whenever that patient subsequently needs a transfusion. Virtually all discrepancies will be traceable to deficiences, either personal or procedural, in the process of patient identification at the time the blood specimen for type and cross-match was obtained. Since this step remains the most susceptible to human error the simple computer match will often serve to identify the most error-prone humans. This is a significant improvement and it is most welcome.

Another aspect of transfusion service operation that has been significantly improved by computerization is the array of platelet count and coagulation test results that is now available. In the future as these systems become more user-friendly and error-free it is reasonable to expect direct application of computerization to actual component use. Practice guidelines for blood component use include criteria based upon platelet counts and/or coagulation test results (see Table 18.6). The opportunity to have these data readily available should significantly improve with the use of blood components as well as shorten the turnaround time between the ordering of the blood and the issuing of the units by the transfusion service.

However, it would be a mistake to conclude that computerization is going to supplant dedicated technologists and physicians in laboratory medicine. Indeed such individuals are needed more than ever as these systems are planned and developed. The primary reason for laboratory medicine as a profession should not be forgotten. First and foremost, we are all in this fascinating profession to take care of patients.

References

Anderson, F. C. (1990) Interlaboratory quality assurance program. *Clin. Lab. Haematol.*, **12**, (Suppl.) 111–116.

Bachner, P. and Howanitz, P. J. (1991) Q-Probes: A tool for enhancing your lab's QA. *Med. Lab. Observer*. **November**, pp. 37–46.

Batjer, J. D. (1990) The College of American Pathologists Laboratory Accreditation Programme. *Clin. Lab. Haematol.*, **12**, (Suppl.) 135–141.

Boone, D. J. (1990) Comments on random errors in haematology tests. *Clin. Lab. Haematol.*, **12**, (Suppl.) 169–170.

Brecher, G., Schneiderman, M. and Cronkite, E. P. (1953) The reproducibility of the platelet count. *Am. J. Clin. Pathol.* **23**, pp. 15–26.

Bull, B. S. (1991) Quality assurance strategies. In: Koepke, J. A. (ed.), *Practical Laboratory Hematology*. New York: Churchill Livingstone, pp. 3–29.

Bull, B. S. and Hay, K. L. (1989) The blood count, its quality control and related methods: X_B calibration and control of the multichannel hematology analyzers. In: Chanarin, I. (ed.), *Laboratory Haematology: An Account of Laboratory Techniques*. Edinburgh: Churchill Livingstone. pp. 3–9.

Bull, B. S. and Korpman, R. A. (1983) Autocalibration of hematology analyzers. *J. Clin. Lab. Automation*, **3**, 111–116.

Bull, B. S., Richardson-Jones, A., Gibson M. *et al.* (1992) A method for the independent assessment of hematology whole-blood calibrators. *Amer. J. Pathol.* **98**. 623–629.

Bull, B. S. and Rittenbach, J. D. (1990) A proposed reference haematocrit derived from multiple MCHC determinations via haemoglobin measurements. *Clin. Lab. Haematol.*, **12**, (Suppl.), 43–53.

ECCLS (1985) Standard for quality assurance, part 4: Internal quality control in haematology. European Committee for Clinical Laboratory Standards Document Vol. 5 No. 3.

Federal Register (1992) *Clinical Laboratory Improvement Amendments of 1988; Final Rules and Notice*. **42** CFR Part 493.

Gilmer, P. R., Williams, L. J., Koepke, J. A. *et al.* (1977) Calibration methods for automated hematology instruments. *Am. J. Clin. Pathol.*, **68**, 185–190.

Hackney, J. R. and Cembrowski, G. S. (1990) The use of retained patient specimens for haematology quality control. *Clin. Lab. Haematol.*, **12**, (Suppl.) 83–89.

Hoffman, M., Koepke, J. A. and Widmann, F. K. (1987) Fibrinogen content of low volume cryoprecipitate. *Transfusion* **27**, 356–358.

Houwen, B. (1990) Random errors in haematology tests: a process control approach. *Clin. Lab. Haematol.*, **12**, (Suppl.) 157–168.

Joint Commission for the Accreditation of Healthcare Organizations (1993) *Accreditation Manual for Hospitals*. Chicago, ILL. pp.129–136.

Koepke, J. A. (1988) Quality assurance in the transfusion service. In: Lewis, S. M. and Verwilghen, R. L. (eds), *Quality Assurance in Haematology*. London: Baillière Tindall, pp. 100–109.

Koepke, J. A. (1990a) Current practices for quality assurance in laboratory haematology. *Clin. Lab. Haematol.*, **12**, (Suppl.) 75–81.

Koepke, J. A. (1990b) Future directions for quality assurance in laboratory haematology. *Clin. Lab. Haematol.*, **12**, (Suppl.) 171–176.

Koepke, J. A. (1992) Critical factors for the definition of a quality clinical laboratory. *Arch. Pathol. Lab. Med.*, **116**, 484–485.

Koepke, J. A., Dotson, M. A. and Shifman, M. A. (1985a) A critical evaluation of the manual/visual differential leukocyte count. *Blood Cells*, **11**, 173–186.

Koepke, J. A., Dotson, M. A., Shifman, M. A. *et al.* (1985b) A flagging system for multichannel hematology analyzers. *Blood Cells*, **11**, 113–125.

Koepke, J. A. and Klee, G. G. (1990) Quality indicators in clinical pathology. *Arch. Pathol. Lab. Med.*, **114**, 1136–1139.

Koepke, J. A. and Koepke, J. F. (1986) How hematologists use coagulation tests. (Abstract) *Blood*, **68**, 335.

Koepke, J. A., McLaren, C. E., Wijetunga, A. *et al.* (1994)

A method to examine the need for duplicate testing of common coagulation tests. *Am. J. Clin. Pathol.*, **102**, 242–247.

Lewis, S. M. and Rowan, R. M. (1991) Assessment of the need for blood film examination with blood counts by aperture-impedance systems. In: Roberts, B. (ed.), *Standard Haematology Practice*, Oxford: Blackwell Scientific Publications, pp. 34–42.

Meier, F. A., Renner, S. W., Bachner, P. *et al.* (1992) Indications for coagulation tests in 645 clinical laboratories: A Q-Probe test utilization study. (Abstract) *Am. J. Clin. Pathol.*, **97**, 456.

NIH Consensus Conference (1985) Fresh frozen plasma – indications and risks. *JAMA*, **253**, 551–553.

NIH Consensus Conference (1987) Platelet transfusions. *JAMA*, **257**, 1177–1180.

NIH Consensus Conference (1988) Perioperative red cell transfusion. *JAMA*, **260**, 2700–2703.

Practice Guidelines for the Use of Fresh Frozen Plasma, Cryoprecipitate and Platelets. (1993) Northfield, ILL. College of American Pathologists.

Reference Leukocyte Differential Count (proportional) and evaluation of instrumental methods. NCCLS (1992) Approved standard H20-A. (ISBN 1–56–238) Villanova, PA: *National Committee for Clinical Laboratory Standards.*

Richardson-Jones, A. (1990) Coulter-assigned values for controls and calibrators. *Clin. Lab. Haematol.*, **12**, (Suppl.) 23–30.

Rogers, R. P. and Levin, J. (1990) A critical reappraisal of the bleeding time. *Semin. Thromb. Hemostasis*, **16** (Vol. 1), 1–20.

Rümke, C. L. (1979) The statistically expected variability in differential leukocyte counting. In: Koepke, J. A. (ed.), *Differential Leukocyte Counting.* Skokie, ILL. College of American Pathologists, pp. 39–45.

Young, C. J. (1990) Complete system control: an object-oriented approach. *Clin. Lab. Haematol.*, **12**, (Suppl.) 93–100.

General references

Cembrowski, G. S. and Carey, R. N. (1989) *Laboratory Quality Management.* Chicago: American Society of Clinical Pathologists Press, pp. 1–264.

Cooper, E. S. (ed.) (1992) Selected topics in transfusion medicine. *Clinics in Laboratory Medicine, December 1992.* Philadelphia: Saunders, pp. 655–844.

Koepke, J. A. (1991) *Practical Laboratory Hematology.* New York: Churchill Livingstone, pp. 3–29, 43–60 and 329–345.

Koepke, J. A. and England, J. M. (eds) (1990) First International Conference on Advances in Clinical Haematology: Current Practice and Future Directions for Quality Assessment in Laboratory Haematology *Clin. Lab. Haematol.*, **12**, (Suppl. 1) 1–176.

Lewis, S. M. and Verwilghen, R. L. (eds) (1988) *Quality Assurance in Haematology.* London: Baillière Tindall, pp. 1–297.

Stewart, C. E. and Koepke, J. A. (1987) *Basic Quality Assurance Practices for Clinical Laboratories.* Philadelphia: Lippincott, pp. 1–287.

19

External quality assessment

S. M. Lewis

Total quality management in the laboratory includes both external quality assessment and internal quality control as complementary components of quality assurance. Internal quality control (IQC) is a continual procedure *pari passu* with tests which are being carried out in the laboratory, whereas external quality assessment (EQA) is a retrospective and objective comparison of results from different laboratories on one or more specimens which are provided for the purpose by an external agency. Thus, EQA is a snapshot of a single event in the function of the laboratory, and assessment is based on the assumption that this reflects its every-day performance.

The concept of EQA is well established in laboratory practice, although there is some confusion with regard to what it should be called. It has been known, variously, as proficiency testing, ring tests, interlaboratory comparisons, trials or surveys (Marten, 1975; McBride, Wood and Carstairs, 1981; Jackson, and Hughes, 1985; Koepke, 1986; Lewis, 1986; Lohmann *et al.*, 1989). The term 'external quality assessment' was proposed by the World Health Organization (1981), and this term has been adopted by ICSH (1994). The eponym 'NEQAS' is used specifically to signify a national external quality assessment scheme. The College of American Pathologists (CAP) operates the largest interlaboratory comparison programme in the world with more than 25 000 laboratories being enrolled in this programme. These laboratories receive more than 140 000 individual survey kits from a list of more than 110 separate surveys. The programme in hematology was described in some detail in a previously published monograph (Koepke, 1986). However, the overall organization has been modified somewhat as a response to the requirements of the federally-mandated Clinical Laboratory Improvement Amendments of 1988 (CLIA '88). These changes (CAP, 1993) will be included, where pertinent, in this chapter.

EQA schemes may also function at a regional level and may even be organized at a local or district level. The type of scheme may depend on how health services are organized and administered in the country, the facilities and financial support available for the scheme, numbers of participants, geographic areas involved and the ease or difficulty in preparing and sending specimens and in communication between organizer and participants.

National and regional (or district) schemes are not alternatives as each serves a different function. In order to apply statistical procedures for analysing results the number of participants in a scheme (or in any group within the scheme) should not be less than 15–20, but they may range from this minimal number to several thousand, provided that there is sufficient material available to distribute a representative aliquot to each participant. The advantages of a national scheme is that sufficient data may be obtained to provide an overview, taking account of all methods and instruments used. If a scheme is too small, separation into instrument/method groups may result in insufficient data from some of the groups for reliable statistical analysis. Furthermore, if all instruments used in one district have a similar bias, this will be recognized by a national scheme but not by a district one. This might occur, for example, if one lot of a reagent or calibrant is defective and its distribution has been confined to one area. On the other hand, the advantage of a local scheme is that results are usually available more rapidly and personal contact can be monitored more easily between the participating laboratories and the organizer.

As indicated above, the essential purpose of EQA is to provide an objective independent check of laboratory results in order to establish between-laboratory compatibility. In some countries, including the USA, satisfactory performance in surveys is a requirement for laboratory accreditation and reimbursement. EQA also has other uses. It allows different instruments and methods for the same test to be compared and their reliability to be assessed. It is also possible to study new control materials and calibrants, and by means of regular checks, to monitor batch products of reagents, control materials and kits. Performance in an EQA scheme should, if possible, be included in the evaluation of any new instrument.

From EQA data the state of the art can be judged and selected methods recommended, whilst the standard of performance by the participants will indicate whether there is need for training by way of workshops and published guidelines.

EQA results will also reveal deficiencies which are the responsibility of manufacturer. Thus, for example, a test kit which performs reliably in the hands of an expert may fail in a 'routine' laboratory if used by an inexperienced person unless it is accompanied by clear and unambiguous instructions for performing the test, reading the reaction, interpreting the results, use of controls, etc. When a few laboratories fail to obtain the correct result for a test in an EQA survey it must be assumed that the fault lies with these laboratories; when a larger proportion of participants in the survey fail to get the correct answer with the same kit it is necessary to adjudicate between the suitability of the specimen, the reliability of the kit and the competence of the users. EQA data will usually help to resolve this question.

Only a few individuals will be involved in the organization of an EQA scheme and will wish to have technical information on specimen preparation and distribution, computer programming for participant registration, data handling, statistical analysis, etc. Details of these can be found elsewhere (Lewis, 1986; Bullock and Peters, 1990; Reardon, Mack and Hutchinson, 1991; Lewis, 1993; Dacie and Lewis, 1994).

Of more general interest to all laboratory workers are the principles under which schemes should function. These are described below.

19.1 Principles of EQAS

1. In each country there should be a scheme which is recognized officially by the health authorities of that country. When more than one scheme has been established in a country for the same sets of tests every effort must be made to ensure their concordance. There must be a minimum number of participants to enable results to be analysed meaningfully, and for such analysis to take account of different methods, instruments, kits or reagents which are used in accordance with current practice. To meet this requirement it may be desirable to merge regional schemes into a National EQAS.

   If a commercial organization undertaking EQA also markets material for internal quality control and calibration of equipment, participants in this scheme may be influenced to use such materials not because they are the best available for the purpose, but because they lead to better performance in the company's EQA scheme. Accordingly no country should be de-

pendent for EQA on commercially operated schemes, although these may serve a useful purpose as supplements to official schemes.

2. The organizer should have appropriate professional qualifications relating to laboratory practice. There might also be a manager with administrative qualifications.

3. Authority for the scheme must be vested in a board or committee, the members of which should include representatives of health authorities, professional societies, and possibly health insurance agencies, participants and the end-user general public. Schemes may be legally obligatory, or they may be a requirement of accreditation or they may be voluntary.

4. The organizer should be advised by a steering (or resource) committee which is concerned with technical and professional aspects. The board should arbitrate on any controversy which might arise between scheme and participants. Where participation in a scheme is obligatory and without reasonable competition, participation fees must be agreed by the board, who shall audit expenditure and agree on methods of funding, including the acceptability or otherwise of sponsorship by industry of specific projects being undertaken by the organizer.

5. Confidentiality should be maintained through participant identification number known only to the organizer. The identity and performance of any individual participant should be revealed to a third party only by permission of the participant, or to a specified authority if this is established in the contract with the participants.

6. The organizer will be responsible for the preparation and circulation of appropriate samples which parallel tests performed in laboratories, for accurate data processing, rapid return of results, production of detailed reports on individual performance for each participant together with general reports of the survey and summary reports of the performance in general.

7. An essential function of the scheme is education. The organizer is responsible for providing unbiased advice to participants and notification of state of art problems to appropriate professional bodies and/or health authorities.

   When an individual participant persistently fails to reach the required standard of performance the board has a public responsibility to ensure appropriate action by an independent professional authority or federal agency.

8. Schemes can be used to evaluate new methods, instruments, kits or reagents. The scheme has an important function to provide a continuing check of production batches of kits and reagents. It should also have a role in development of reference methods and reference materials.

9. Participants should be encouraged to handle

EQA samples in accordance with their usual routine practice. Satellite laboratories should be registered to receive independent specimens. A laboratory using more than one method/instrument system must register their main one for EQA and any others may also be registered additionally. Where a method or system used in a particular laboratory is not registered it is the responsibility of the participant to undertake appropriate procedure to ensure intralaboratory concordance.

10. Distinction is made between surveys and trials. Surveys are regular tests in a specified programme for the purpose of assessing performance of the participants.

Trials are preliminary tests used to evaluate a new material or a new test being considered for inclusion in the survey programme before the performance by participating laboratories is assessed.

19.1.1 Timetable of surveys

It is important that surveys be performed at regular intervals, although their frequency may vary, depending on the diagnostic importance of the tests, the critical limits which distinguish between normal and abnormal results, the frequency with which the tests are requested in practice and their technical reliability. It has been argued that the least frequently performed tests require the greatest amount of assessment.

A survey may contain one or more tests, some tests (eg. blood counts) should be included in every distribution. It is important, however, to remember that the laboratory work programme is not intended to be built round EQA, so that the participants should not be over saturated with the less common tests, especially time-consuming manual procedures.

Tests in surveys may be quantitative, semi-quantitative or qualitative.

For quantitative tests two or more samples are included in each survey; these are selected so as to give maximum information that will help to identify the reason for any discordant results. Thus the paired samples might be identical in order to check on imprecision, one may have a known amount of analyte added for a recovery analysis, or the samples may be at different levels of concentration to check on linearity of response or at levels of concentration which are clinically important, e.g. at the border-line of the normal reference range. For the blood count equine blood is particularly useful as the red cells have MCV of 48 fl (horse) and 58 fl (donkey), thus providing a model for human microcytosis.

For qualitative tests the specimens should give unequivocally positive or negative reactions as assessment of performance is difficult and often arbitrary with intermediate/equivocal reactions.

19.1.2 Sample preparation

Material may be human, animal or (under special circumstances) artificial. In the CAP surveys only human materials are used.

All human material distributed should be negative on testing, at least for HBsAg and HIV I and II. All human samples must be accompanied by a biological hazard label. Each batch should also be checked for microbial contamination after dispensing by culture of a proportion of the batch.

Material should be stable at least for the period during which it is likely to be tested, and it should be verified whether any sterilizing or stabilizing processes will alter the character of the material such that it will behave differently from patient material when tested in the laboratory.

For the blood count it is not possible to use the same type of specimens of blood in EDTA as is used in practice. To ensure adequate stability of the cellular elements, the blood for surveys is usually collected into acid-citrate-dextrose (ACD) or citrate-phosphate-dextrose (CPD) solutions in which red cells can be preserved for at least 3–4 weeks; even so, the samples do not accurately mimic whole blood and there are differences, especially MCV, by various blood counting systems (Wardle, Ward and Lewis, 1985). This makes it necessary to assess results separately with different instrument groups. Animal blood is useful for simulating human abnormalities. As stated above, equine (horse or donkey) red cells are microcytic. Avian red cells may be used as surrogate leukocytes in some counters but automated leukocyte differential counts require different types of preparation for each counting system.

Stabled horses (but not field grazing) have low serum and red cell folate, whilst horses and cattle have very high levels of vitamin B_{12}. Sheep blood is deficient in glucose-6-phosphate dehydrogenase (G6PD). As leukocytes remain in good condition for counting for only a few days, it may be necessary to add glutaraldehyde-fixed blood cells in order to provide simulated leukocytes. Human blood is satisfactory for platelet counts provided that the specimens reach the participants within 48 hours and are counted without delay. The platelet count of equine blood is stable for a longer period but is less suitable than human blood for red cell counts and sizing by some counting systems. With most systems partially fixed stabilized whole blood (see page 134) is suitable for blood counts, including platelet counts.

If it is customary for vitamin B_{12}, folate, iron, transferrin and/or ferritin assays to form part of the hematology service, serum is required for appropriate surveys. This should be sterile and free from cloudiness or particles. This is often difficult to achieve when the serum is a pooled collection from a large number of donor-samples. It may thus be necessary to subject the material to micropore filtration at 0.2 μm. This has the disadvantage of being time consuming and expensive, and in addition 25–30% of the initial volume is lost by the filtration.

Attempts have been made to overcome these difficulties by preceding the 0.2 μm filtration by a series of coarse filtration, e.g. at 20, 8, 3, 1 and 0.45 μm successively. This process does not entirely resolve the problem and it is preferable, as far as possible, to obtain serum either from a single donor or from a small number of selected donors.

19.1.3 Blood coagulation surveys

In blood coagulation, determination of prothrombin time (PT) and INR and partial thromboplastin time (PTT) are the usual EQA tests, while plasma fibrinogen concentration, Factor VIII:C assay and other factor assays might be included from time to time. Although there are differences between fresh and lyophilized plasma in various tests (van den Besselaar and Bertina, 1988) lyophilized plasmas and plasmas obtained by plasmapheresis from patients with mild hemophilia or von Willebrand's disease are useful for PTT and Factor VIII assay while lyophilized plasma is suitable for fibrinogen assay.

Samples obtained by plasmapheresis of patients with other coagulation defects have also been a valuable source of large volumes of material, at least for parts of the testing procedures. However, increased incidence of HIV antibody, has made it very difficult to obtain suitable material from this source.

19.1.4 Blood group serology and blood bank surveys

Survey tests include compatibility testing, ABO/Rh blood grouping, antibody screening. Plasma is obtained from one or more selected donors by plasmapheresis, pooled if more than one donor is used, defibrinated with bovine thrombin, dialysed against saline, filtered under sterile conditions and then distributed in 1.5 ml aliquots (Holburn and England, 1982). For red cells, whole blood is collected in ACD or CPD anticoagulant from donors of selected genotypes.

19.1.5 Data processing

EQA tests in surveys may be quantitative, semi-quantitative or qualitative. Each requires an appropriate procedure for analysing results, determining their closeness to the correct result and assessing whether performance is satisfactory. This assessment may be based on: (a) statistical criteria; (b) comparison with performance by selected peer or referee laboratories;

or (c) the extent to which a discrepant result might influence clinical management to a patient's detriment.

Data processing starts when results are received by the organizer. Except for small schemes, where a simple calculator will suffice, a computer facility is essential, especially for retrieving data for cumulative assessments and for retrospective studies of equipment performance, etc.

The primary object of the assessment is to evaluate the performance of individual participants and to identify problems relating to methods, instruments, reagents, controls and calibrators which have been used by the participants. Statistical analysis is by fairly simple standard computer programmes. It is, however, necessary to define a reference or target value point which can be assumed to be the true numerical value or qualitative observation. Several methods are used to establish reference points. It is, however, important to appreciate that unless the true value is established by an accurate method all reference points are subject to biased estimates.

19.1.6 Consensus mean and median

Consensus may be biased because a particular type of instrument or reagent or calibrator is used by a large majority of participants. To obtain statistically valid data for analysing a subgroup an adequate number of participants (at least 15–20) is necessary. Thus a newly introduced method or instrument suffers a disadvantage until a sufficiently large number of participants register for that group. On the other hand comparison of mean or median values provides a measure of inter-method bias without necessarily identifying any as being the *correct* value.

When analysing the data, first any obvious blunders or bizarre values are deleted, such as a result which differs by more than 100% from the overall mean. Then, assuming a Gaussian distribution, the mean ($\bar{x}$) and the standard deviation (SD) are calculated by simple statistical procedures, and re-calculated from the residual data after excluding any outlier results falling outside ±3 SD. The outliers are recorded as unsatisfactory performance (see later).

The CAP outlier detection and exclusion techniques are for the most part similar to those described above. The method used to eliminate technical and clerical errors and other bizarre results is to calculate the mean and standard deviation of the original set of peer group results, compute the limits (usually ±3SD) and treat any lying outside these limits as outliers. Outliers are excluded from the summary statistics. In the past, the acceptable limits had been within ±2SD of the mean (rather than the median). However, the federal guidelines have now more or less superseded those limits (Federal Register, 1992).

This method of excluding outliers is valid only if

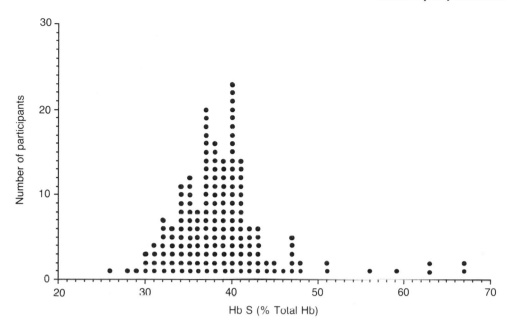

Figure 19.1 Blood count survey showing non-Gaussian distribution of results

the SD is narrow. If it is wide it is preferable to trim the data by setting the data in numerical sequence and deleting an equal number of observations from both ends (Healy, 1979). When there are less than 16 data points, one should be deleted from each end; when there are 16 or more, 10% of the total sample should be deleted. Then the trimmed mean and SD are calculated in the usual way.

In the majority of EQA surveys results tend to spread out without an obvious Gaussian distribution (Figure 19.1). In these cases the midpoint (median) is obtained instead of the mean and it is more appropriate to use non-parametric statistics; an estimate of the measure of dispersion about the *median* is obtained from the spread of the distribution of the data between the 25th and 75th percentiles (P25 and P75, respectively). This central range, which includes 50% of the results, is known as the H (or hinge) spread. It is used to estimate the standard deviation. Outliers are truncated if outside the range P25–3H to P75 +3H. SD is calculated as the 50% spread ÷ 1.349 (Tukey, 1977).

It is debatable whether it is necessary to wait for returns from the majority of participants before calculating mean or median. There is some evidence that calculation from a random 10–15% closely approximates the final result.

19.1.7 Expert laboratories

Results are obtained from a selected group of eminent laboratories of established authority who assay the specimens repeated by reference methods, thus establishing the interlaboratory and intralaboratory

precision, as well as the standard deviation of the whole set. The main disadvantage with this method is that an unnoticed bias in performance in one laboratory in a small group will disproportionately affect the reference results; enlarging the group to compensate for this effect can quickly overburden the scheme. In practice, reference results are generally consistent with the consensus median.

19.1.8 Qualitative tests

Qualitative results are obtained for tests which do not produce a numerical result, e.g. 'positive-negative'; 'low-high' or intensity of reaction (+, + +, + + +). Results may also be based on interpretation of certain features, as for example, microscopic morphology.

For qualitative procedures, correct results may be based on consensus of all participants or of a selected group of expert referees. In some instances, e.g. for sickle-cell disease and G6PD deficiency, results which are to be expected in a qualitative screening test can be confirmed by means of a quantitative estimation on the same sample. For morphological hematology the referees may have the advantage of knowing the patient's subsequent clinical course and other data from which a diagnosis may have been made; however, whilst this is important from the educational viewpoint it does not give a fair yardstick for judging performance by the ordinary participant.

In the CAP programme blood cell and bone marrow photomicrographs (see later) are reviewed by referees and by responsible committee members who define requirements for good and acceptable performance. A 90% consensus by either referees and/or survey participants is required for formal evaluation. When alternate reasonable identifications are made by a significant number of referees or participants, these may also be judged as acceptable performance.

In scoring qualitative tests account must be taken of both positive and negative misleading information in a test interpretation. Thus, for example, if the test requires identification of the presence of an abnormal feature, a correct result might be scored as $+2$, missing the feature or reaction as -1 whilst interpreting it incorrectly as -2.

In analysing blood film reports, weighted scores should be used to give higher credit for more important features, especially those which point to the specific diagnosis. Conversely, 'trivial' features such as anisocytosis should not earn a score point even if correctly identified, if there are other more important abnormalities which should have been seen, whilst a false positive identification should be penalised as -1 to -5, depending on the extent to which it might have misled the diagnosis, and the clinical importance of such an error.

19.1.9 Assessment of performance

For quantitative tests blunders will have been detected and the reason looked for in the initial stage of statistical analysis described above. Thereafter unsatisfactory performance can be identified by one of the following procedures.

19.1.10 Deviation index (DI) or standard deviation index (SDI)

This is a measure of how a test result (x) differs from the mean ($\bar{x}$) or median (m) value (Ward, Wardle and Lewis, 1982). When the mean is used it is a multiple of the truncated standard deviation (SD′), i.e. excluding results which are outside ± 3 SD in preliminary calculation. Median is recommended for most quantitative assessment in hematology as: (a) it is not dependent on the shape of distribution and (b) it is much less affected by the outlying values. The spread of the central 50% of the population between the quartiles is related to a normal Gaussian distribution to give an estimate of the standard deviation:

$$SD = 50\% \text{ spread} \div 1.349$$

Then,

$$DI = \frac{x - m}{SD'} \text{ or } \frac{x - \bar{x}}{SD'}$$

The main advantage of this method is that the index is independent of the value m or $\bar{x}$ so that it allows measurement for different samples and parameters to be readily compared. Performance is assessed in

terms of the DI as follows; DI < 0.5 = excellent; DI 0.5–1.0 = good; DI 1.0–2.0 = satisfactory but borderline; DI > 2.0 = unsatisfactory: instrument calibration and function require checking; DI > 3.0 = potentially serious problem to be investigated as a matter of urgency.

19.1.11 Variance index

Participant reference is compared with the best performance obtainable with the particular method, expressed as the chosen coefficient of variance (CCV) (Whitehead, 1977). This can refer either to the CV of the method performed under ideal conditions by expert laboratories or the CV for all results returned by participants, truncated by the exclusion of results outside the ± 2 SD. First, the variation of the individual (V) is obtained as a percentage.

$$V = \frac{x - \bar{x}}{x} \times 100$$

Then

$$Variation\ index = \frac{V}{CCV} \times 100$$

19.1.12 Ratio analysis

Most surveys include paired tests. The pairs may be random, selected to include two specific levels of analyte concentration, or they may be from the same batch either as identical samples or one with a known added amount of the analyte. By plotting the distribution of data on horizontal and vertical axes, respectively, of a graph, it is easy to see whether errors are systematic or random, whilst the actual difference found between the paired samples measures recovery of the added analyte and thus gives an indication of the reliability of the analytical method (Figure 19.2). This useful procedure, known as a Youden plot (Youden, 1960), can also be used for comparing measurements of paired samples (similar or dissimilar) by various methods.

19.1.13 Clinical relevance

To base acceptable limits of performance on statistical analysis alone is unrealistic. Thus, for example, the remarkably low CV for hemoglobin means that even a measurement at 3 SD from the mean will not result in an error of more than 10% and is unlikely to influence clinical decision, whereas platelet counts have a high CV such that 3 SD may represent an error of 50%. In the case of prothrombin time and calculation of prothrombin ratio a small difference may result in a dangerously incorrect level of therapy. In reality, therefore, poor performance is best defined as a result which might lead to inappropriate clinical

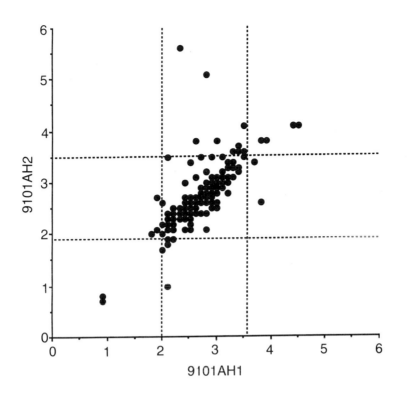

Figure 19.2 Ratio analysis: plot of results from HbA$_2$ assay on two specimens of blood. Those in the central block ($\pm$ 2SD) are satisfactory; those in bottom left and top right blocks show systematic bias; elsewhere the errors are random

action (Hartmann and Ross, 1998; CAP, 1993; Lewis, 1993).

Results are assessed by whether they fall within the limits of a given percentage deviation from the mean/median. These limits must take account of the best precision of the method/instrument. They must also take into account the normal biological variations of the measured analyte and interpretation of measurement variation in terms of clinical strategies in different clinical situations. In the USA the limits for acceptable performance have been set by government regulation (Federal Register, 1992). These limits are wider than those previously prescribed by the CAP and currently applicable in the UK (Table 19.1).

19.1.14 Interpretation

Some schemes require participants to indicate the significance of their results. This implies both technical significance (i.e. whether within normal reference values for the specified method) and clinical significance, taking account of relevant clinical information which is provided. The latter merges, perhaps, into professional audit. Incorrect interpretation of a correct quantitative result is due largely to lack of

understanding of the theory of reference values as described by IFCC and ICSH (1987) and use of inconsistent population reference ranges derived from various sources (Figure 19.3 and Table 19.2).

19.1.15 Survey reports

The aim of the report should be to present maximum information in the simplest format. Reports should be issued with a minimum of delay. Ideally each participating laboratory should receive an individualized survey report which may cover a single test or a group of tests requiring similar analysis.

The reports should contain details of statistical analysis of data from all participants by 'all methods' (if appropriate), and by group, together with the individual participant's result and assessment. This should provide each participant with a perspective of performance in relation to that of other participants.

If practical, results on paired samples should be plotted on a Youden graph. Data may also be displayed on a histogram or on a bias plot.

Examples of various types of survey reports are illustrated in Figures 19.4–19.6. Participants should also receive cumulative summaries of their per-

Table 19.1 Evaluation criteria: the limits of deviation from group mean/median value (%)

	UK NEQAS	US Federal Register
Hb	3	7
RBC	3	6
PCV	4	6
MCV	4	—
MCH	4	—
MCHC	4	—
WBC	8	15
Platelets	10	25
Vitamin B_{12}	20	—
Folate	20	—
Ferritin	20	—
HbA_2 quantitation	20	—
HbF quantitation	20	—
HbS quantitation	10	—
PTT	—	15
PT	15	15
Fibrinogen	—	20

(— = not assessed by this method).

Table 19.2 Interpretation of results in serum ferritin survey

	Specimen 1	Specimen 2
m ± SD (μg/l)	17 ± 4.4	40 ± 7.4
Method	Reported as Normal	Reported as Low
IRMA		
B–D	54%	12%
Corning	54%	0
Bio-rad	31%	0
RIA		
B–D	33%	4%
Amersham	50%	0%
ELISA	50%	4%

The numbers indicate the percentage of tests in each group.

formance, e.g. as deviation index for each test or parameter in the last six surveys (Figure 19.7). This forms the basic record for identifying persistent unsatisfactory performance (see below) and for accreditation.

19.2 Unsatisfactory performance and persistent unsatisfactory performance

In addition to the cumulative summary reports described above, participants should be encouraged to prepare their own graphic presentation of their performance. In the majority of cases an isolated incident of unsatisfactory performance will be recognized promptly and the fault rectified. If the problem is not resolved within a reasonable period official action may be required.

In some tests, especially qualitative tests such as screening for sickle cells, blood grouping and compatibility tests, even a single incorrect observation may be deemed to be potentially hazardous and to require urgent corrective action by an appropriate authority. In general, however, criteria for persistent unsatisfactory performance are results outside the set limits, deviation from the mean/median (page 202) or a DI > 2 in three or more parameters on any one sample in a survey on three occasions in a 6-month period, or similar poor results in any one of the parameters on one or both samples in three consecutive surveys (Lewis, 1988).

A variant of this procedure is to grade the extent of deviation from the median in percentiles (Woods, 1993):

Group A = ± 25 %; Group B = Next ± 10 %; Group C = Next ± 5 %; Group D = Next ± 5 %; Group E = outer ± 5 %.

Unsatisfactory performance would be indicated by a combination of DD, CE, DE or EE. Persistent unsatisfactory performance would be indicated if on the next occasion a grade of C, D or E occurs for at least one of the results.

The federal agency responsible for regulating clinical laboratories in the USA is the Health Care Financing Administration (HCFA). The final regulations were published in February 1992 (Federal Register, 1992), although some revisions have been made since then. The HCFA requires that a laboratory which performs moderate or high complexity tests on patient samples must successfully participate in a proficiency testing programme approved by HCFA. Failure to achieve an overall satisfactory performance in two consecutive testing events or in two out of three consecutive testing events is deemed unsuccessful performance. Testing event success has been defined as at least 80% satisfactory performance except for ABO group and Rhô(D) typing and compatibility testing where a 100% satisfactory score is required. Failure may result in the imposition of sanctions against the laboratory which essentially suspends laboratory testing until such time as the problems are remedied and proficiency testing again achieves a satisfactory level.

19.2.1 The blood film

The blood film has a prime role in diagnostic hematology, and thus should be an important component in EQA.

There are four aspects in blood film surveys, namely, technical skill in staining, differential count quantification, reporting on blood cell morphology and opinion of hematological diagnosis. The use of unstained blood films to assess technical aspects of staining by the participants may sometimes be unsuccessful as delay beyond 6–8 hours in staining the

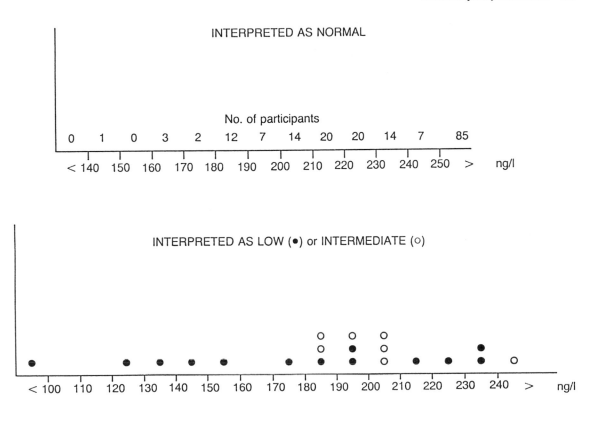

Figure 19.3 Results for vitamin B$_{12}$ on a survey specimen, showing interpretations by the participants

film, even when they are pre-fixed, may result in unsatisfactory staining. On the other hand, when films are fixed and stained in the one laboratory by a Romanowsky method, this has the possible disadvantage that participants who routinely use another staining procedure may be unaccustomed to the morphological characteristics of the stained films.

All films from a single blood specimen should be near identical but there is no absolute guarantee that the distribution of different types of cells, and especially cells which are present only in small numbers, will be similar in every film. It is desirable that each film be screened before being sent to the participants, but this is impractical in schemes with several hundred or thousands of members.

In some schemes, e.g. that of the College of American Pathologists, blood films have been replaced by 35 mm transparencies which include normal blood and bone marrow cells and various red cell and leukocyte abnormalities (CAP, 1993).

Blood film surveys are popular with participants and, at the same time, the most controversial on several counts. In some exercises the main emphasis is on quantification of the differential leukocyte count. In others identification and interpretation of

morphological features are required. UK NEQAS include both normal blood films and films from patients with blood disease. Some of these are 'bread and butter' hematological conditions, whereas others have been unusual or even rare problems, included to stimulate and provoke participants as well as to provide material for education and to give participants an opportunity to build up departmental slide libraries. In addition, the surveys also include films specifically for identifying and quantifying blood parasites. Participants report up to five morphological abnormalities and an estimate of any abnormal differential leukocyte distribution. From consensus of the total participants' results and advice from a group of referees the correct result is established. Using either an 'award' or a 'penalty' system, missed features (false negative) and incorrectly reported features (false positive) by the individual participants are noted and graded according to their significance.

The laboratory from which the material originated then provides a report of the definitive diagnosis (if this has been established) or the likely diagnosis from the retrospective information, together with an educational commentary.

There is debate whether a hematological diagnosis

U.K. National External Quality Assessment Scheme for Hematology 23/06/93

Results for Survey No. 9306   Participant Reference No. 999

System No.   2

Sample 1: Partially Fixed Human Whole Blood   Sample Quality: Satisfactory
Sample 2: Partially Fixed Human Whole Blood   Sample Quality: Satisfactory
Hemoglobin by reference method – Sample 1: 125 g/l
                                  Sample 2: 120 g/l

Instrument	Test	Result	DI	Median	SD	CV%	N	
Coulter StkS	Hb	[g/l]						
	1	127	0.45	126	2.22	1.8	916	All
			0.68	126	1.48	1.2	265	Group
	2	124	0.90	122	2.22	1.8	915	All
			1.35	122	1.48	1.2	264	Group
Coulter StkS	RCC	[×10^{12}/1]						
	1	4.18	0.14	4.17	0.074	1.8	877	All
			−0.34	4.20	0.059	1.4	264	Group
	2	3.96	0.14	3.95	0.074	1.9	875	All
			−0.15	3.97	0.067	1.7	263	Group
Coulter StkS	PCV							
	1	0.383	0.29	0.380	0.0104	2.7	883	All
			0.00	0.383	0.0067	1.7	264	Group
	2	0.370	0.36	0.366	0.0111	3.0	882	All
			0.15	0.369	0.0067	1.8	263	Group
Coulter Stks	MCV	[fl]						
	1	91.6	0.38	91.0	1.56	1.7	874	All
			0.58	91.0	1.04	1.1	264	Group
	2	93.5	0.67	92.3	1.78	1.9	873	All
			0.81	92.6	1.11	1.2	263	Group
Coulter StkS	MCH	[pg]						
	1	30.5	0.77	30.1	0.52	1.7	851	All
			1.14	30.0	0.44	1.5	262	Group
	2	31.2	0.68	30.8	0.59	1.9	849	All
			0.96	30.7	0.52	1.7	261	Group
Coulter Stks	MCHC	[%]						
	1	33.2	0.24	33.0	0.82	2.5	850	All
			0.51	32.9	0.59	1.8	263	Group
	2	33.4	0.21	33.2	0.96	2.9	848	All
			0.58	33.1	0.52	1.6	262	Group
Coulter StkS	WCC	[×10^9/1]						
	1	5.0	−0.54	5.2	0.37	7.1	887	All
			−2.00	5.3	0.15	2.8	264	Group
	2	4.7	−0.27	4.8	0.37	7.7	887	All
			−0.91	4.9	0.22	4.5	263	Group
Coulter StkS	PLT	[×10^9/1]						
	1	137	0.21	135	9.6	7.1	853	All
			−0.24	139	8.2	5.9	264	Group
	2	108	−1.53	125	11.1	8.9	849	All
			−2.68	130	8.2	6.3	261	Group

Figure 19.4 Report to participants in a blood count survey

UK NEQAS(H) : Survey 9102 : Folate (µg/l)

Sample 9102VF3 Human whole blood CPD-A1

Referee Analysis   n = 40 mean = 175   SD = 24.0

Data Analysis : All methods result n = 196   median = 183   SD = 64.1   CV% = 35

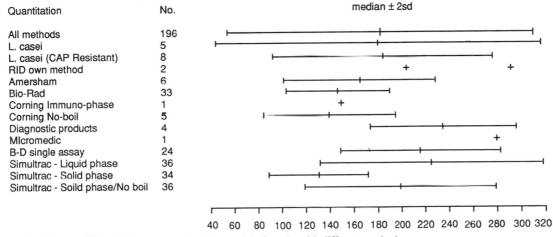

Quantitation	No.
All methods	196
L. casei	5
L. casei (CAP Resistant)	8
RID own method	2
Amersham	6
Bio-Rad	33
Corning Immuno-phase	1
Corning No-boil	5
Diagnostic products	4
MIcromedic	1
B-D single assay	24
Simultrac - Liquid phase	36
Simultrac - Solid phase	34
Simultrac - Soild phase/No boil	36

Figure 19.5 Report of blood folate survey showing spread of results with different methods

should be requested and the amount of information that should be provided to the participants. It has been argued that these exercises are intended for assessing morphological skill and thus should not be biased by providing 'leading' information whether by way of the blood count information which would usually be provided in practice with blood data or clinical comment. The contrary view is that without the film requests, the exercise becomes unrealistic and thus refutes the principles of EQA. This is linked to the question of who should report the films and whether the survey is intended for assessing technical performance or as a means for professional audit. In the UK the usual practice in the diagnostic laboratory is for blood film screening to be performed by medical technologists and for problems to be referred to the consultant hematologist. Complex problems might be subject to departmental discussion and referral to an outside expert. Undoubtedly, NEQAS is an artificial situation and NEQAS films are often subjected to an unnaturally intensive study, even the simplest abnormality being referred to several colleagues to try to ensure that a 'correct' result is submitted. It has been suggested that preliminary examination of films should be undertaken by the medical technologist without information whereas the consultant should never be expected to review a

film without relevant clinical information and the blood count parameters.

Some schemes recognize that there are different levels between the general (non-specialised) laboratories and those with access to specialised technology and expertise. The Ontario Medical Association Laboratory Proficiency Testing Programme attempted this approach for blood film surveys but it was found to be inappropriate (LPTP, Ontario Medical Review, 1980).

The essence of the problem is that in all laboratories the blood films should serve as the interface between technical performance, professional expertise and clinical judgement. This is coupled with the problem of how to establish the correct answer for each film, and whether EQA should have predominantly educational or regulatory function.

As an increasing number of laboratories install automated systems, it is necessary to assess the future role of the blood film in the diagnostic laboratory and the importance of this component of quality assessment programme; as fewer films are examined, the need for external quality assessment becomes more rather than less important. There is need to maintain a high level of competence in morphological identification of hematological abnormalities; this must include an ability to screen normal films with a

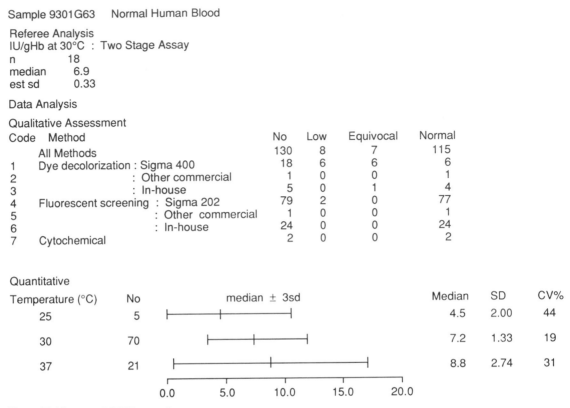

Sample 9301G63   Normal Human Blood

Referee Analysis
IU/gHb at 30°C : Two Stage Assay
n   18
median   6.9
est sd   0.33

Data Analysis

Qualitative Assessment

Code	Method		No	Low	Equivocal	Normal
	All Methods		130	8	7	115
1	Dye decolorization	: Sigma 400	18	6	6	6
2		: Other commercial	1	0	0	1
3		: In-house	5	0	1	4
4	Fluorescent screening	: Sigma 202	79	2	0	77
5		: Other commercial	1	0	0	1
6		: In-house	24	0	0	24
7	Cytochemical		2	0	0	2

Quantitative

Temperature (°C)	No	median ± 3sd	Median	SD	CV%
25	5		4.5	2.00	44
30	70		7.2	1.33	19
37	21		8.8	2.74	31

0.0   5.0   10.0   15.0   20.0

Figure 19.6 Report of G6PD screening test assay

high level of specificity and abnormal films with a high level of sensitivity.

It is, however, a sobering thought that in the Canadian experience a 32% error rate was found to be due to the use of poor microscopes which were dusty, incorrectly illuminated and inadequately maintained. Attention to these factors reduced the failure rate to 6%! (Pantalony, Wood and Jacobs, 1986)

19.2.2 Reticulocyte counts

Until the present time reticulocyte count surveys have been one of NEQAS's less successful achievements. Pre-stained films are distributed and participants carry out microscopic counts by their usual method. For over twelve years the CV has remained unchanged: 35–40% when the reticulocyte count is 1%; 25–30% at 10%; 15–20% at 15%. This is due largely to the fact that in most laboratories so few reticulocytes are included in the count especially when the reticulocyte proportion is low, that the Poisson distribution error is excessive. This could be reduced to 5%, or less, by counting greater numbers in accordance with the recommended reference method (ICSH, 1991; Dacie and Lewis, 1994). How-

ever, this is time consuming and impractical in a routine service laboratory.

The fact that reticulocyte counts are a labour-intensive test, and have such a large variance in practice has resulted in its diminishing use, albeit acknowledged in principle that it should have an important role as a measure of erythropoietic function. Unfortunately the results in NEQAS surveys do not inspire participants to use this test extensively.

The recent advent of automated methods for counting reticulocytes by flow cytometry may change this situation as many thousand cells can be rapidly counted with the high level of precision and reliability which should give this test the respect for its clinical utility which it deserves. This new development challenges ICSH to provide suitable specimens with an accurately measured and stable reticulocyte population.

Another aspect of morphology relates to cytochemistry. For some cytochemical reactions, e.g. urinary hemosiderin, participants are required to report the presence or absence of stained material, and overall results are fairly satisfactory. In quantitative tests, e.g. neutrophil alkaline phosphatase, the extent of unsatisfactory performance indicates a general prob-

UK National External Quality Assessment Scheme for Hematology *.* – Information not supplied
Performance Table for last 6 Surveys

Lab/System No	Survey No	Analysis Method	Sample	HB	RCC	PCV	MCV	MCH	MCHC	WCC	PLT	Sample quality	Results rec late	Sample post delay
999/1	9208	all	1	0.68	1.79	1.47	0.98	-0.85	-0.11	-2.73	0.85	Good	N	0
		group	1	0.17	0.59	0.48	0.17	-0.58	-0.52	-0.19	-0.76			
		all	2	0.00	2.30	1.42	0.44	-2.02	-1.35	-1.33	-1.54	Good		
		group	2	0.00	1.41	0.31	-0.79	-1.35	-0.93	0.45	0.00			
999/1	9207	all	1	0.45	0.95	1.26	0.76	-0.38	-1.06	-1.62	3.00	Good	N	0
		group	1	0.00	-0.11	-0.49	-0.38	0.23	0.68	0.00	2.54			
		all	2	0.00	0.31	0.65	0.74	-0.38	-0.67	-2.50	0.56	Good		
		group	2	-0.68	-0.58	-1.73	-0.65	0.00	0.58	-0.19	0.90			
999/1	9206	all	1	0.00	0.12	0.98	1.20	0.17	-0.76	-3.00	-1.08	Good	N	0
		group	1	-0.68	-0.07	-0.14	0.29	-0.63	-0.76	-0.49	0.73			
		all	2	*.*	*.*	*.*	*.*	.	.	*.*	*.*	Bad		
		group	2	*.*	*.*	*.*	*.*	.	.	*.*	*.*			
999/1	9205	all	1	0.00	1.46	1.15	0.45	-1.36	-0.99	-1.94	.	Good	Y	6
		group	1	-0.45	0.61	-0.42	-0.26	-1.22	-0.12	0.00	.			
		all	2	0.00	1.10	1.35	1.02	-1.02	-1.23	-3.18	.	Good		
		group	2	-1.35	0.06	-0.08	-0.27	-1.14	-0.39	-0.67	.			
999/1	9204	all	1	0.45	0.63	0.50	0.24	-0.23	-0.36	-1.35	.	Good	N	1
		group	1	0.00	-0.31	-1.34	-1.26	0.00	1.04	0.33	.			
		all	2	0.00	0.73	0.31	-0.20	0.68	-0.09	-1.08	.	Good		
		group	2	-0.68	-0.96	-1.83	-1.73	0.00	2.20	0.23	.			
999/1	9203	all	1	-0.90	0.41	1.08	0.88	-1.15	-1.63	-2.16	.	Good	N	0
		group	1	-2.03	0.56	-0.73	-0.23	-0.88	-0.14	-0.54	.			
		all	2	-2.03	0.10	0.70	0.92	-1.35	-1.23	-4.09	.	Good		
		group	2	-2.70	-0.96	-1.54	-0.35	-1.14	-0.77	-1.54	.			

UK National External Quality Assessment Scheme for Hematology
Performance Table for Last 6 Trials

Lab/System No	Trial No	Method	Sample	HB	RCC	PCV	MCV	MCH	MCHC	WCC	Sample Quality	Results rec late	Sample delay
999/1	9001	all	1	0.00	0.37	0.80	0.80	-0.94	-1.27	0.17	Good	—	1
		group	1	0.00	0.54	0.73	0.67	-1.35	-1.56	0.00			
		all	2	0.00	-0.10	-0.07	0.00	-0.60	-0.40	1.18	Good		
		group	2	0.00	0.10	-0.42	-0.39	-0.81	-0.08	0.84			
999/1	9002	all	1	0.00	0.94	1.20	0.81	-0.81	-1.14	0.00	Good	—	0
		group	1	0.00	1.18	1.23	0.45	-1.05	-1.12	-0.67			
		all	2	0.67	0.70	1.16	0.83	-0.15	-0.95	-0.22	Good		
		group	2	2.70	1.06	1.16	0.90	-0.39	-0.74	0.10			
999/1	9004	all	1	0.00	1.69	-0.45	0.34	-1.18	-1.35	-1.35	Good	—	1
		group	1	-1.35	1.93	-0.62	0.67	-1.73	-1.73	-2.25			
		all	2	0.90	-0.29	-0.13	0.00	1.50	0.37	-0.86	Good		
		group	2	1.01	0.00	-0.28	-0.41	1.20	0.63	-0.94			
999/1	9005	all	1	**	**	**	**	**		**	Bad	—	6
		group	1	**	**	**	**	**		**			
		all	2	**	**	**	**	**		**	Bad		
		group	2	**	**	**	**	**		**			
999/1	9006	all	1	-.045	1.35	0.23	0.00	-1.01	-0.45	0.00	Good	Y	0
		group	1	-0.67	1.50	-0.10	-0.90	-1.52	-0.13	-0.45			
		all	2	-0.45	1.23	0.54	-0.18	-1.46	-0.90	0.10	Good		
		group	2	-0.45	0.96	0.29	-0.90	-1.84	-0.79	0.27			
999/1	9007	all	1	0.00	0.36	0.60	0.66	0.34	0.75	4.00	Good	—	1
		group	1	0.90	0.34	0.51	1.35	0.58	0.93	1.00			
		all	2	0.90	0.40	1.14	1.42	-1.20	-1.51	3.25	Good		
		group	2	1.35	0.27	1.12	1.01	1.01	-1.20	1.56			

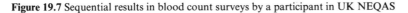

Figure 19.7 Sequential results in blood count surveys by a participant in UK NEQAS

lem of technique and lack of standardization, as illustrated by both histogram and ratio plots (Figures 19.8–19.10 and Tables 19.3 and 19.4). These surveys have also highlighted the variance in the range used for normal reference values between laboratories.

19.3 Organization of a national external quality assessment scheme (NEQAS)

The way in which an EQA scheme is organized

depends upon a number of factors. These include the role in the scheme of government health authorities and of professional bodies, whether the scheme is a commercial undertaking or run from an academic or public health institute, whether participation is obligatory or voluntary, whether it is used as the basis for licensing of laboratories and/or for recognition of laboratories for training, and what action is taken with regard to unsatisfactory performance.

In the USA and in the Ontario province of Canada there is a legal obligation to participate in an EQA

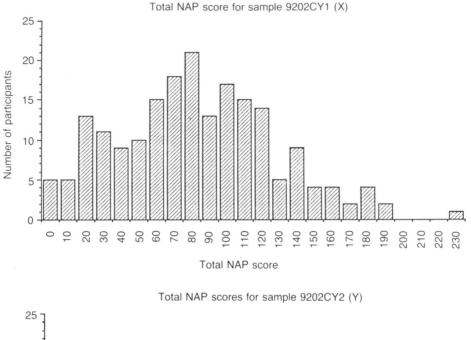

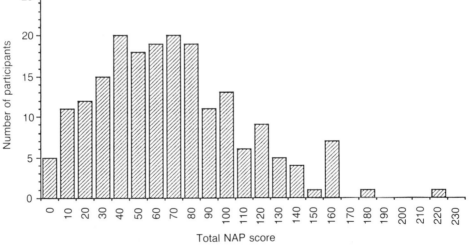

Figure 19.8 Neutrophil alkaline phosphatase survey results for paired specimens with participant assessment (see also Figure 19.9 and Table 19.3)

scheme; in some European countries also (e.g. France and Germany) participation is compulsory but in others it is voluntary. Where it is voluntary it is encouraged in different countries to varying degrees by health authorities, and by health insurance agencies who are responsible for paying the fees for the services provided. The general public do not appear to be as alert to their rights to have reliable laboratory tests as they are for other consumer services.

In a number of countries there are commercial schemes, in some cases organized by instrument

Table 19.3 Analysis of total NAP scores on samples x and y

	Sample x	Sample y
n	197	197
median	88	62
sd	43.4	40.8
CV	54	66
Reported Range	0–233	0–222

Plot of total NAP score for sample 9202CY1 (X)
vs total NAP score for sample 9202CY2 (Y)

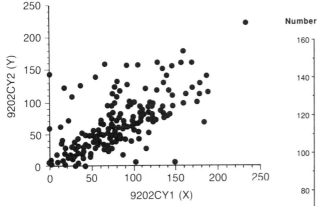

Figure 19.9 Ratio analysis of neutrophil alkaline phosphatase scores (see Figure 19.8)

Table 19.4 Participant assessment of results in NAP survey

	Low	Normal	High
x	19	138	36
y	31	143	20

Total NAP Scores

Normal Ranges reported by Participants

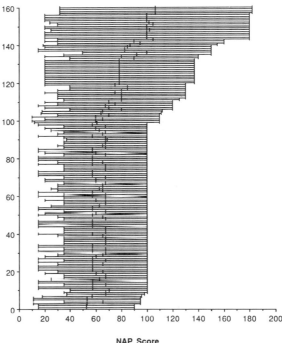

Figure 19.10 Differences in normal reference range given by participants in the survey which is illustrated in Figure 19.8 and Table 19.3

manufacturers for users of their products. Commercial schemes may complement or supplement a national scheme. As described on page 200 it is important that a national scheme be independent of any undue pressures and that the organizer of such a scheme should not have a commercial interest in any particular reagent or instrument. It is acceptable practice for materials used in surveys to be prepared under contract by a manufacturer who may also be the manufacturer of material used routinely by participating laboratories, but the specification of such survey materials must be set by the organizer and his committee.

In the UK participation in NEQAS is voluntary but strongly encouraged by the medical and technical professional bodies and participation in a recognized EQA scheme is mandatory for laboratory accreditation (Royal College of Pathologists, 1991). Virtually every National Health Service (NHS) laboratory participates, as do the majority of laboratories in the private sector. The UK NEQAS has been a good model and its organization will be described in detail. It is based on a committee structure which takes account of interrelated interests of the health authorities, professional societies and individual laboratories, and also the need to have co-ordination of different schemes concerned with various aspects of laboratory practice.

In its earlier form (Figure 19.11) co-ordination and policy decision was undertaken by a Government-appointed interdisciplinary Advisory Committee of Laboratory Standards (ACALS). Its members represent the professions and health authority, while the scheme organizers for each speciality and chairmen of the steering committees reported to the committee annually. The primary purpose of the committee was to advise the Government on the maintenance of laboratory standards. Its regular meetings ensured that the schemes in different specialties set similar standards and they provided cross-fertilization of ideas from experts involved with the various schemes.

A recent development has been the delegation of authority by the Department of Health (DoH) to a Consortium of NEQAS Organizers who constitute a Board with an Executive Committee elected from amongst its members (Figure 19.12).

The Joint Working Group on Quality Assurance (JWG) is formed by representatives of the professional bodies, Chairmen of the Advisory Panels (see below) and observers from the Department of

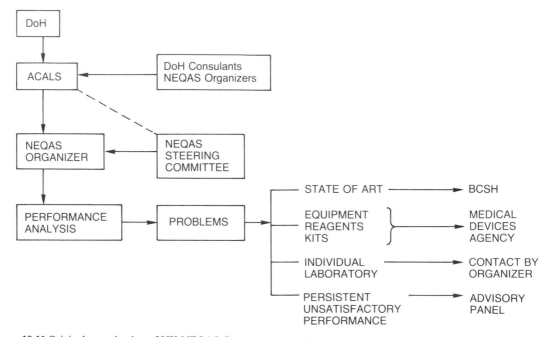

Figure 19.11 Original organization of UK NEQAS Government-appointed Advisory Committee

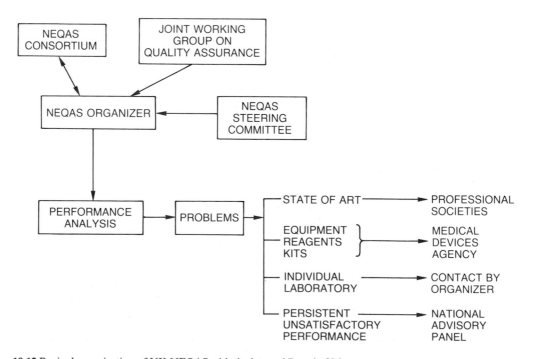

Figure 19.12 Revised organization of UK NEQAS with the internal Board of Management

Health. It has a supervisory role to ensure that each scheme is adequate for its purpose, to identify areas where a new scheme or expansion of an existing scheme is required and also to look after the interests of the participants.

Scheme Organizers are, in general, university or

public hospital consultants (specialists) within the NHS. They are not appointed directly by the DoH but facilities are provided in their institutions by contract from the DoH.

Each speciality scheme has a steering committee appointed by the DoH, chaired by an independent expert, and consisting of technical experts together with clinical advisers and representatives of the DoH who sit on each committee as observers. The role of the steering committee is to advise the organizer on the overall operations of the scheme, including such aspects as the frequency of sample distribution, type of sample, tests to be undertaken, methods of statistical analysis of results, style of data presentation. The steering committee may discuss general performance as it relates to state of the art but is not concerned with the performance of individual participating laboratories.

Review of individual participant performance is the function of an advisory panel consisting of representatives nominated by the appropriate professional bodies; in hematology these are the Royal College of Pathologists, British Society for Haematology, Association of Clinical Pathology, Institute of Medical Laboratory Sciences and the British Blood Transfusion Society. The relevant scheme organizers attend the meetings of the panel ex officio.

The scheme has been established on the basis of confidentiality between organizer and the individual participants. When there is a problem of persistent poor performance the organizer reports to the advisory panel but the identity of the laboratory is known to the panel only by a code number. Accordingly, when the chairman of the panel writes to enquire if assistance is required, this letter is passed to the coded participant by the organizer. Only if the discordance persists and no response has been received, will the identity of the participant be revealed to the panel chairman who writes directly to the head of the laboratory. In some cases members of the panel may then visit the laboratory to help resolve the problems. In the general hematology NEQAS less than ten participants a year require a chairman's letter, and only rarely has there been need for a panel visit. On the other hand, the organizer and his staff have relatively frequent direct contact by letter or telephone with participants whose problems are usually resolved by appropriate advice.

Where the problem is more general and the 'state of the art' is in question, it becomes the responsibility of the relevant professional and educational bodies to investigate the situation, to publish recommendations and guidelines in appropriate journals and to organize workshops and educational meetings. In the UK this is undertaken by the British Committee for Standards in Haematology, which is an arm of the British Society for Haematology. When the problem is traced to industry, perhaps due to an unsatis-

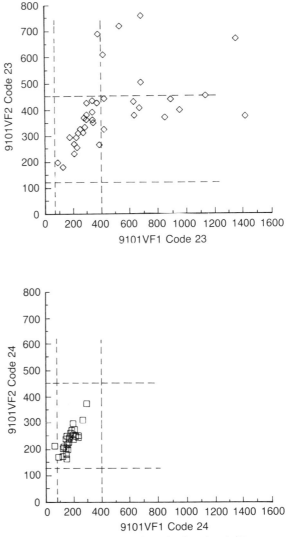

Figure 19.13 Comparison of results for vitamin B_{12} assay (ng/l) on two specimens (VF1 and VF2) by two different methods (code 23 and 24). The random imprecision by method 23 warranted referring the problem to the Medical Devices Directorate with subsequent withdrawal of the test-kit batch

factory type of instrument or a defective batch of a kit or a reagent, it is referred to the Medical Devices Directorate of the Department of Health (Figure 19.13).

Clearly NEQAS has a role beyond its basic responsibility to the individual participants. It is a valuable interface between users and manufacturers of instruments and kits. Before the need to refer formally to the Department of Health, manufacturers should be informed of problems which appear to relate to their instruments and reagents. They should be encouraged to join schemes in order to receive documenta-

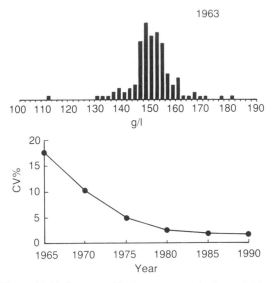

Figure 19.14 Country-wide improvement in hemoglobinometry since inception of UK NEQAS in 1963

tion even if they do not take direct part in the surveys. Harmonization of various EQA schemes could lead to pooling and strengthening of data and thus provide the facility for early recognition of failure of a new instrument, a batch of manufactured reagent or a diagnostic kit. This should be an important function in the after-manufacture control and validation of diagnostic kits and reagents.

External quality assessment must not be conceived as an isolated process. It has an important function alongside and in conjunction with internal quality control, proficiency surveillance and standardization towards the goal of reliable test performance. The value of this combination dramatically improving hemoglobinometry is illustrated in Figure 19.14. It is a model for other aspects of hematological practice.

References

Bullock, D. G. and Peters, M. (1990) A score system for external quality assessment data processing. *Endocrine EQAS in Europe*, **1**, 7.

College of American Pathologists (1993) *CAP Surveys Manual* Section II: Hematology, Coagulation, Clinical Microscopy. Northfield, ILL: College of American Pathologists.

Dacie, J. V. and Lewis, S. M. (1994) *Practical Haematology*, 8th edn. Edinburgh: Churchill Livingstone.

Federal Register (1992) *Clinical Laboratory Improvement Amendments of 1988; Final rules and notices*. February 28 1992, pp. 7188–7288.

Hartmann, A. E. and Ross, J. W. (eds) (1988) CAP Conference XIII on the evaluation of proficiency testing results

for quantitative methods in relation to clinical usefulness. *Arch. Pathol. Lab. Med.*, **112**, 327–474.

Healy, M. J. R. (1979) Outliers in clinical chemistry quality control schemes. *Clin. Chem.*, **25**, 675–677.

Holburn, A. M. and England, J. M. (1982) The UK National External Quality Assessment Scheme in blood group serology. Compatibility testing 1979–1980. *Clin. Lab. Haematol.*, **4**, 155–167.

International Council for Standardization in Haematology (1991) Guidelines for reticulocyte counting by microscopy on supravitally stained preparations. WHO/LBS/92.3. Geneva: World Health Organization.

International Council for Standardization in Haematology (1994) Rules and operating procedures. Glasgow: ICSH Secretariat.

International Federation of Clinical Chemistry/International Committee for Standardization in Haematology (1987) Approved recommendation (1986) on the Theory of Reference Values Part I. The concept of reference values. *J. Clin. Biochem.*, **25**, 337–342.

Jackson, J. M. and Hughes, W. (1985) External quality assurance in haematology. The Program of the Royal College of Pathologists of Australia. *Pathology*, **17**, 573–578.

Koepke, J. A. (1986) The College of American Pathologists Survey Programme. In: Rowan, R. M. and England, J. M. (eds), *Automation and Quality Assurance in Haematology*. Oxford: Blackwell Scientific Publications, pp. 62–83.

Lewis, S. M. (1986) External quality assessment in Europe. In: Rowan, R. M. and England, J. M. (eds) *Automation and Quality Assurance in Haematology*. Oxford: Blackwell Scientific Publications, pp. 18–61.

Lewis, S. M. (1988) External quality assessment. In: Lewis, S. M. and Verwilghen, R. L. (eds), *Quality Assurance in Haematology*. London: Baillière Tindall, pp. 151–175.

Lewis, S. M. (1992) Quality Assurance in Haematology. Document WHO/LBS/92.4. Geneva: World Health Organization.

Lewis, S. M. (1993) Quality Assurance in laboratory haematology. *Proc. R. Soc. Edinb.*, **101B**: In press.

Lohmann, R. C., Wood, D. E., Jacobs, W. I. *et al.* (1989) Reliability of white blood cell counting. *Arch. Pathol. Lab. Med.*, **113**, 989–944.

LPTP Morphological Hematology Committee (1980) Morphological hematology testing under scrutiny. Ontario Medical Review.

McBride, J. A., Wood, D. E. and Carstairs, K. C. (1981) Proficiency at haemoglobinometry in Ontario laboratories between 1975 and 1979. *Can. Med. Assoc. J.*, **125**, 180–182.

Marten, R. (1975) Instand surveys. A program for self-evaluation in the medical laboratory. Dusseldorf: Instand.

Pantalony, D., Wood, D. and Jacobs, W. (1986) Proficiency testing in hematologic morphology – a ten year experience. XXI Congress of International Society of Haematology, Sydney. (Abst.) 250.

Reardon, D. M., Mack, D. and Hutchinson, D. (1991) A whole blood control for blood count analysers, a source material for an external quality assessment scheme. *Med. Lab. Sci.*, **48**, 19–26.

Royal College of Pathologists Advisory Task Force on Standards to the Audit Steering Committee (1991): Pathology department accreditation in the United Kingdom: a synopsis. *J. Clin. Pathol.*, **44**, 798–802.

Tukey, J. W. (1977) *Exploratory Data Analysis*. Boston: Addison-Wesley.

van den Besselaar, A. M. H. P. and Bertina, R. M. (1988) Standardization and quality control in blood coagulation assays. In: Lewis, S. M. and Verwilghen, R. L. (eds). *Quality Assurance in Haematology*. London: Baillière Tindall, pp. 119–150.

Ward, P. G., Wardle, J. and Lewis, S. M. (1982) Standardization for routine blood counting – the role of interlaboratory trials. *Methods in Haematol.*, **4**, 102–120.

Wardle, J., Ward, P. G. and Lewis, S. M. (1985) Response of various blood counting systems to CPD-AI preserved whole blood. *Clin. Lab. Haematol.*, **7**, 245–250.

Whitehead, T. P. (1977) *Quality Control in Clinical Chemistry*. London: Wiley, pp. 95–105.

Woods, T. (1993) NEQAS and Haemostasis: Assessment of performance in non-INR tests. *Br. J. Biomed. Sci.*, **50**, 49–51.

World Health Organization (1981) External quality assessment of health laboratories. EURO Reports and Studies 36. Copenhagen: WHO Regional Office.

Youden, W. J. (1960) The sample, the procedure and the laboratory. *Anal. Chem.*, **32**, 23–27.

20

Regulatory and professional standards affecting clinical laboratories

Paul Bachner and William B. Hamlin

20.1 Introduction

Professional standards of performance in medicine and laboratory science traditionally have evolved from a matrix of professional education, practice and custom modified by regulatory mandate (Bachner, 1991; Derman and Dorsey, 1991). In the USA, common and accepted practice in the clinical laboratory has been influenced primarily by three sources. (1) federal government laws and regulations; (2) requirements mandated by some state governments and (3) educational, laboratory improvement and voluntary accreditation programme of organizations such as the Joint Commission on Accreditation of Healthcare Organizations (JCAHO), the College of American Pathologists (CAP), the American Association of Blood Banks (AABB), and many other organizations generally reflecting specialized areas of laboratory science.

In the federal system of government, state regulations take precedence over federal government regulations, particularly if the former are at least as stringent as those established by Congress or federal agencies. However, the history of state regulation of clinical laboratories is spotty; some states such as New York, Maryland, California, New Jersey and others have implemented systematic and rigorous statutory regulation and inspection of laboratories while others have virtually no regulations specifically designed for clinical laboratories. Over the past few years, however, an unprecedented cascade of legislative and regulatory events have emerged from Washington and have impacted on the practice of laboratory medicine. These include regulations limiting 'self-referral' to diagnostic facilities in which a physician has any financial interest; regulations limiting joint ventures and arrangements between physicians and hospitals; state and federal regulations concerning the disposal of infectious wastes; and the federal regulations pertaining to bloodborne pathogens.

The recent passage and implementation of the most widespread and comprehensive revision of regulations concerning laboratory performance, Public Law 100–578 (42 USC§263(a) section 353), popularly known as CLIA '88, has extended federal regulation of laboratories to a very large number of previously unregulated facilities and significantly increased the regulatory overhead for previously regulated facilities. Because the impact of this regulatory event has profoundly and permanently altered the way in which clinical laboratory testing is performed, this paper will examine these regulations (42 Code of Federal Regulations, 1992) in some detail.

In addition, a series of federal legislative and regulatory events of a more general nature including the Clean Air Act Amendments, the Americans with Disabilities Act, the 1991 Civil Rights Act and the Family and Medical Leave Act have contributed to the overall costs of business that impact hospitals, laboratories and all other business activities. Because of this regulatory burden, most laboratory professionals share a consensus that the balance has been shifted from a professionally-driven agenda for quality improvement to one driven by regulatory and compliance concerns.

This chapter will review widely recognized and mandated standards for laboratory practice and performance currently observed in US laboratories. Reference will be made to the situation outside the USA. Most of the standards referred to in this chapter are generic and apply to all divisions of the clinical laboratory. Although discrete standards have been established for blood banks and transfusion services by state health departments, federal agencies and the AABB (American Association of Blood Banks, 1990), standards for hematology laboratories in the USA are almost entirely a component of general laboratory standards or regulations, and will not, except for a few instances, be discussed separately.

20.2 Standards established by government regulations

20.2.1 History of clinical laboratory regulations

Historically, a myriad of federal regulatory requirements promulgated by various agencies under the auspices of existing and/or newly enacted statutes have resulted in *de facto* standards of laboratory performance.

The initial involvement of the federal government in laboratory regulation occurred in 1965 with the enactment of the Health Insurance for the Aged Act (Medicare – 42 USC§1395) which provided for the reimbursement of medical care costs to the elderly.

Responsibility for developing, implementing and enforcing the regulations was vested in the Social Security Administration (later assumed by the Health Care Financing Administration (HCFA), an agency of the Department of Health and Human Services (DHHS)). The regulations were designed to ensure that the government and its beneficiaries received the services paid for and that such services met specified minimum standards. The regulatory language defined two laboratory entities, 'hospital' and 'independent' laboratories, and provided that each must satisfy certain standards defined as 'conditions for participation' (42 CFR§405.1028 (Medicare Conditions for Participation of Hospitals) and 42CFR$ §401.1310 *et seq.* (Medicare Conditions for Coverage of Services of Independent Laboratories)).

The regulations specified that every laboratory that was to be reimbursed must be surveyed (inspected) to ensure that it satisfied the applicable 'conditions for participation'. The inspection of independent laboratories was delegated to state agencies, usually the state health department or a similar agency. The state's activities were monitored by the Social Security Administration. Hospital laboratory compliance was to be confirmed by one of two mechanisms. If the hospital was accredited by the Joint Commission for the Accreditation of Hospitals (JCAH – now the Joint Commission for Accreditation of Healthcare Organizations, or JCAHO), the Social Security Administration 'deemed' the JCAHO requirements as being 'equal to or more stringent than' the federal regulations and accepted the hospital laboratory as meeting the 'Conditions for Participation'. If the hospital was not JCAHO accredited, it would be surveyed (inspected) by the designated state agency. It is of note that the entire hospital was approved or disapproved under Part A coverage, not just the laboratory, and that JCAHO accreditation was 'deemed' to suffice only in so far as their standards were 'equal to or more stringent than' regulatory standards.

The Clinical Laboratory Improvement Act of 1967 (42 USC§263a) was passed by Congress on the premise that laboratories that accepted specimens across state borders were engaged in 'interstate commerce' and therefore subject to federal regulation. The law specified that all such facilities ('interstate laboratories') must be licensed by the federal government. The responsibility for writing, implementing and enforcing the regulations was originally assigned to the Centers for Disease Control (CDC). The CLIA '67 statute specifically provided for 'equivalency' through 'exemption from licensure' through accreditation or licensure by private sector or state programmes whose standards were 'equal to or more stringent than' those of the federal programme. Two programmes were so designated: the College of American Pathologists Laboratory Accreditation Program and the New York State Licensure Program. No other programmes were subsequently approved and both continued to be accepted until CLIA '88 was enacted. Additionally, CLIA '67 exempted from licensure any laboratory that received less than 100 specimens per year in interstate commerce; however, every laboratory that received any specimens in interstate commerce had to register and then apply for the exemption.

The regulations for all these laws included the requirement that the laboratories 'successfully' participate in proficiency testing. It is also of note that this series of statutes and their accompanying regulations did not apply to any federal government laboratories, state government laboratories or physician office laboratories (unless they were receiving specimens across state lines).

Shortly following the enactment of the Medicare statute, Title XIX of the Social Security Act (42 USC§1396 *et seq.*) established a federal-state cooperative programme for the provisions of health services to the needy (Medicaid). The programme was administered jointly by the Social Security Administration and state agencies. The laboratory regulations specified in 42 CFR§440.10 essentially paralleled Medicare requirements.

Apart from Medicare and CLIA '67 regulations which have been incorporated into or supplanted by the CLIA '88 requirements, numerous other federal regulatory mandates establish standards that prescribe and modify laboratory practice.

The Food and Drug Administration (FDA) became involved in laboratory regulatory activity when federal courts determined that human blood and blood components were 'drugs' and as such were subject to the Federal Food, Drug and Cosmetics Act (21 USC 301–360) as well as certain provisions of the Public Health Service Act (42 USC 262). These two laws require every establishment (laboratory) that processes blood or blood products to obtain both an 'establishment' licence and a 'products' licence. The FDA was the initial enforcement agency for blood banks including donor collection activities, compatibility testing and transfusion services. More recently, free standing blood banks and donor collection centres with compatibility testing remain under FDA jurisdiction while transfusion services (including associated compatibility testing) in hospital laboratories are regulated by the HCFA.

There are several federal laws and regulations that deal with laboratory safety. Initially they were not specifically directed toward the laboratory, but all apply to laboratories and are enforceable both under the primary statutes and regulations as well as CLIA '88. The Nuclear Regulatory Commission (NRC), successor to the Atomic Energy Commission (AEC), has jurisdiction over all radioactive and nuclear materials manufactured, used and disposed of in the United States. Any laboratory using radioactive isotopes, either for *in vivo* or *in vitro* testing is subject to these laws and their pertinent regulations. The NRC delegates inspection, monitoring and some enforcement responsibilities to approved state agencies and commissions.

The Occupational Safety and Health Act (29 USC 654(a) *et seq.*), enacted in 1970, directly relates to clinical laboratories. The law requires that every employer furnish each employee a place of employment that is free from recognized hazards that are causing, or are likely to cause, death or serious physical harm (29 USC 654(a) (1)). Enforcement of the law and the attendant regulations is the responsibility of the Occupational Safety and Health Administration (OSHA), an agency of the Department of Labor. OSHA may perform on site inspections to determine if an employer is in compliance with OSHA standards. Recently, there have been extensive regulatory additions relating to the use of carcinogens (Bureau of National Affairs, 1990), formaldehyde fume exposure controls (29 Code of Federal Regulations, 1992) and safety practices related to the AIDS epidemic (29 Code of Federal Regulations, 1991).

The Resource Conservation and Recovery Act (42 USC 6901 *et seq.*) directed the Environmental Protection Agency (EPA) to implement a national programme to control hazardous wastes. A clinical laboratory that generates, treats, stores, transports or disposes of materials defined as hazardous waste (essentially all laboratories) must notify the EPA of this fact, obtain an identification number, and comply with the applicable EPA regulations.

Any laboratory that ships diagnostic specimens in interstate commerce (across state lines) is subject to several additional laws and their accompanying regulations: (1) Interstate Quarantine Regulations (42 CFR 72.75) under the jurisdiction of the Public Health Service; (2) hazardous materials regulations of the Department of Transportation (42 CFR 173.386–.388) applicable to shipping by air, rail, sea or highway; (3) rules of the United States Postal Service (Postal Service Manual ($124.28) which apply to shipping diagnostic specimens in the US Mail. All of these regulations have been recently modified to further restrict the transport of human specimens as well as biologic reagents and materials.

All laboratories are subject to a variety of labour laws including the National Labor Relations Act (29 USC 151 *et seq.*), the Fair Labor Standards Act of 1938 (29 USC 20), the Equal Pay Act of 1963 (29 USC 206(d)), and the Civil Rights Act of 1964 (42 USC 20009(e)). The latter two are administered by the Equal Employment Opportunities Commission (EEOC).

Many of the requirements set forth in the aforementioned statutes and regulations have been incorporated into private, state and federal laboratory accreditation and/or licensing programmes and are, or are rapidly becoming, *de facto* 'standards' of laboratory practice.

20.2.2 The road to CLIA '88

The events leading to the enactment of the Clinical Laboratory Improvement Amendments of 1988 (CLIA '88) are of interest. In early 1988 an article appeared in the *Wall Street Journal* 'exposing' the allegedly deplorable situation relative to gynecological cytology examinations, i.e. Pap smears. This article focused on 'errors' that resulted in missed or delayed diagnoses of carcinoma of the uterine cervix. The described problems did exist to some degree but the article failed to put them in proper perspective relative to the inherent limitations of Pap testing and the significant advances in the diagnosis, treatment and cure of the disease resulting from the estimated 35 000 000 Pap smears done annually. This article, considered by many to be sensationalistic and misrepresentative, did produce a reaction in the US Congress.

Committee hearings were held in both the House of Representatives and the Senate. They were characterized by the testimony of a number of preselected, so-called 'victims' who had been misdiagnosed or not diagnosed as a result of laboratory 'error'. During the course of the hearings a television series broadcast in the Baltimore-Washington DC area further identified 'victims' of poor quality and laboratory error. Despite testimony at the public hearings, and more detailed additional information provided to committee staffs by numerous professional organizations and knowledgeable individuals that more accurately conveyed the appropriate perspective of cytology 'error' and clearly indicated the relatively minimal impact of such on patient care, Congress enacted the Clinical Laboratory Improvements of 1988. The legislation was passed despite testimony by the Department of Human and Health Services indicating that additional legislation was unnecessary since revision of the CLIA '67 regulations were in progress and all the issues could be dealt with in the context of such revisions. Proposed revisions to CLIA '67 were published by DHHS on 5 August 1988 prior to the enactment of CLIA '88 in October of 1988.

It is of note that neither the *Wall Street Journal* article nor any of the Congressional testimony revealed that the CLIA '67 regulations already applied to cytology and that all of the cited instances of unacceptable laboratory performance had been subject to enforcement under existing regulations.

The CLIA '88 statute was somewhat unique in several respects. First it applied to all clinical laboratories including physician offices, federal and state governmental facilities and research laboratories that did testing for patient care purposes. All of these had been previously either exempt or left unregulated. Secondly, the law incorporated very specific regulatory language relative to proficiency testing, particularly in cytology, certain quality control requirements, specifics of how inspections were to be done and other language that had customarily been left to the regulation writers.

Although the proposed revisions to CLIA '67 had been published and comments were being received, HCFA began the process of constructing regulations applicable to CLIA '88 while simultaneously reviewing the comments submitted relative to the 5 August, 1988 'proposed' CLIA '67 revisions. Nearly two years later on 14 March, 1990, the 'final' regulations revising CLIA '67 were published. Shortly thereafter, on 21 May 1990, most of the proposed CLIA '88 regulations were published. Subsequent publications throughout 1990–91 added segments of the regulations such as 'Approval of Accrediting Organizations', fees, sanctions, etc. The proposed CLIA '88 regulations essentially incorporated the CLIA '67 revisions and combined the Medicare, Medicaid and Interstate rules into one body of regulations.

In excess of 60 000 comments were received by HCFA relative to the CLIA '88 proposed regulations and the review of these comments with modifications of the rule ensued. On 28 February, 1992, almost two years after the proposal, the final regulations (with an additional comment period) were published.

20.2.3 Public law 100–578 (CLIA 1988)

The law and the regulations define a laboratory as any 'facility for the biological, microbiological, serological, chemical, immuno-hematological, pathological or other examination of materials derived from the human body, for the purpose of providing information for the diagnosis, prevention or treatment of any disease or impairment of, or the assessment of the health of, human beings.'

This all-encompassing definition and the final rule of February 1992 extends federal regulations from approximately 12 000 hospital and independent laboratories providing interstate services or services to

Medicare patients, to approximately 140 000 facilities, most of which have not been previously subject to any regulation.

20.2.4 The complexity model and waived tests

The complexity model constitutes the core regulatory concept and is a response to a legislative requirement that standards to ensure 'consistent performance' may vary not by site or location of testing ('site neutrality') but may reflect differences in methodology, equipment used and type of training required for test performance. The final version of the complexity model recognizes three categories: (1) waived tests; (2) moderate complexity tests and (3) high complexity tests.

Tests that are waivered require only registration with HCFA and 'good laboratory practice'. Proficiency testing, quality control or personnel standards are not required. At the time of publication of the Final Rules, waived tests included dip-stick urinalysis, visual end-point pregnancy and ovulation tests, erythrocyte sedimentation rate, stool guaiac, hemoglobin by copper sulphate method, spun hematocrit and certain capillary blood glucose monitoring devices approved by FDA for home use. Based upon the recommendations of the Clinical Laboratory Improvement Advisory Committee (CLIAC), the 'Technical Corrections' published in the Federal Register on 19 January 1993 (42 Code of Federal Regulations, 1993) added 'hemoglobin by single analyte instruments with self-contained or component features to perform specimen/reagent interaction, providing direct measurement and readout.' CLIAC has indicated an intent to review the waived list and it is probable that both additions and deletions to the list will occur. A methodology for modification and criteria for inclusion of tests into the waived category have been developed recently by the CDC and provisionally endorsed by CLIAC.

A facility may apply for waived status if it only performs 'simple' procedures that have an insignificant risk of an erroneous result. It is the belief of the authors that no test is without risk with regard to potential patient harm, that all test procedures should be subject to a documented quality control programme, and that proficiency testing should be performed if available. We also believe that performance of any laboratory test in other than a laboratory (e.g., shopping malls, drugstores, etc.) or in a physician's office laboratory (POL) without any guarantee of quality control or of access to clinical interpretation by a physician constitutes a hazard to the public health. None the less, the regulations permit tests on the waived list to be performed at any site or location without a requirement for proficiency testing, quality control, personnel standards or inspection.

All non-waived tests, including most routine

Table 20.1 Personnel – moderate complexity

February 1992 Final Rule

Director
  Pathologist
  MD, DO, and 1 year directing/supervising or 20 hours
  CME or medical residency laboratory training
  Doctorate and Board certification or 1 year directing/
  supervising
  Masters degree and 2 years experience (1 year supervising)
  Bachelors degree and 4 years experience (2 years super-
  vising)
  Qualified or could have qualified under March 1990 rule
  State qualified
Technical Consultant
  MD, DO, PhD, or MS and 1 year experience in
  speciality
  BS and 2 years experience in speciality
Clinical Consultant
  MD, DO or Doctorate and Board certification
Testing personnel
  High School graduate and appropriate training

Table 20.2 Personnel – high complexity

February 1992 Final Rule

Director
  Pathologist
  MD, DO, and 2 years directing/supervising or 1 year
  medical residency laboratory training
  Doctorate and Board certification or until 9/1/94 4 years
  experience (2 years directing/supervising)
  Serving as and qualified or could have qualified under
  March 1990 rule
  State qualified
Technical Supervisor*
  MD, DO, or PhD and 1 year experience in specialty
  Masters degree and 2 years experience in specialty
  Bachelors degree and 4 years experience in specialty
Clinical Consultant
  MD, DO or Doctorate and Board certification
General Supervisor* (must be accessible)
  MD, DO Doctorate, Masters, Bachelors and 1 year
  experience
  Associate degree and 2 years experience
  Qualified or could have qualified under March 1990 rule
Testing Personnel*
  Associate degree or until 9/1/97 high school graduate
  with appropriate training
  Qualified or could have qualified as technologist under
  March 1990 rule

*Exceptions for cytology and histopathology

hematology and chemistry procedures, require a
formal certificate of registration, quality control protocols similar to those required of hospital and independent laboratories, and successful performance of
available proficiency testing for regulated analytes.
These laboratories will be subject to HCFA inspection and will require a director (a physician may
qualify on the basis of testing experience or 20 hours

of continuing medical education credit). Testing personnel requirements for moderate complexity are
generally not onerous; however, the stringent requirements of proficiency testing may compel many POLS
and other small facilities to retain experienced consultative technical personnel.

20.2.4 Moderate and high complexity tests

All non-waived tests and laboratories performing
tests of moderate or high complexity are subject to
personnel standards, patient test management and
quality control requirements, and proficiency testing. Personnel standards are more stringent for
laboratories performing high complexity testing. Although quality control requirements for moderate
complexity tests are subject to less stringent requirements until 1994, all other requirements are essentially the same for moderate and high complexity
tests.

Tests are categorized as moderate or high complexity according to seven criteria:

1. Degree of knowledge needed to perform the test;
2. Training and experience required;
3. Complexity of reagent materials and preparations;
4. Characteristics of operational steps;
5. Characteristics of and availability of calibration,
   quality control and proficiency testing materials;
6. Trouble-shooting and maintenance required;
7. Degree of interpretation and judgement required
   in the testing process.

It has been argued that the CLIA '88 regulations
have extended the scope of federal regulations to a
large number of previously unregulated sites (POLS
in particular), and have therefore resulted in an
improvement in national standards of performance.
An alternative view is that since approximately
75% of all tests performed fall within the moderate
complexity category, the relatively lax personnel
standards for moderate complexity testing has resulted in net deregulation of the majority of tests,
previously performed under the stricter personnel
requirements of Medicare conditions of participation for hospital and independent laboratory
settings in force prior to the enactment of CLIA
1988.

20.2.5 Personnel Standards

There are no personnel requirements for laboratories
certified to perform waived tests. Laboratories certified to perform tests of moderate complexity must
meet requirements for the positions of laboratory
director, technical consultant, clinical consultant and
testing personnel. Laboratories certified to perform

tests of high complexity must meet requirements for the positions of laboratory director, technical and general supervisor, clinical consultant and testing personnel. Tables 20.1 and 20.2 summarize the education, training and experience requirements for laboratory personnel for moderate and high complexity testing. Modifications of some of the standards listed in these tables have been recommended by CLIAC and are expected to be incorporated into subsequent revisions of the regulations. These include an increase in the educational requirement for a general supervisor in a high complexity setting and a series of permanent 'grandfathering' provisions for individuals who were functioning in a position prior to the enactment of the regulations.

Laboratory director

The laboratory director, if qualified, may perform the duties of any or all of the required categories of personnel, including the technical and general supervisor, technical consultant, clinical consultant and testing personnel, but can direct no more than five laboratories. The regulations specify that the director is responsible for all activities of the laboratory including 'overall operation and administration of the laboratory including the employment of personnel who are competent to perform test procedures, and record and report test results promptly, accurately and proficiently and for assuring compliance with the applicable regulations'. Directors of clinical laboratories must be familiar with the above cited requirements which prescribe in considerable detail the spectrum of professional standards and functions that the director must directly provide, ensure or delegate. These include:

1. Responsibility for performance of delegated functions;
2. Accessibility for purposes of consultation;
3. The quality of pre-analytic, analytic and postanalytic phases of testing;
4. Physical and environmental conditions appropriate for testing and safety;
5. Methodologies appropriate for patient care;
6. Verification procedures adequate for determining accuracy, precision and other pertinent performance characteristics;
7. Performance of laboratory personnel;
8. Enrolment in and compliance with approved proficiency testing programme;
9. Quality control and assurance programmes;
10. Reporting of and provision of pertinent information required for interpretation of test results;
11. Availability of consultation to clients;
12. On site supervision by general supervisor (high complexity only);
13. Employment of sufficient number of personnel with appropriate education, training and experience;
14. Development of policies and procedures for monitoring performance of testing personnel;
15. Availability of procedure manual;
16. Specify the responsibilities and duties of all personnel.

Technical consultant (moderate complexity)

The technical consultant is responsible for the technical and scientific oversight of the laboratory. Technical consultant requirements for laboratory training or experience may be acquired concurrently in more than one of the specialties (e.g. a pathologist or medical technologist with experience can consult in each specialty). The technical consultant is not required to be on site at all times but must be available to the laboratory 'as needed'.

Clinical consultant

The clinical consultant provides consultation to the laboratory's clients concerning the diagnosis, treatment and management of patient care including appropriateness of testing ordered and interpretation of test results.

Technical supervisor (high complexity)

The laboratory must employ one or more individuals qualified by education and either training or experience to provide technical supervision for each of the specialties and subspecialties for service in which the laboratory performs high complexity testing. Requirements for laboratory training or experience in each of the specialties or subspecialties may be acquired concurrently. The technical supervisor is not required to be on site at all times but must be available to the laboratory as needed. Time in the laboratory must be adequate to supervise the technical operation.

General supervisor (high complexity)

The general supervisor is responsible for day-to-day supervision and must be accessible to testing personnel at all times that testing is performed.

Testing personnel (moderate complexity)

Testing personnel must be at least a high school graduate or equivalent with 'documented training' appropriate for the testing performed by the laboratory. Knowledge about specimen collection, proper instrument use, and the assessment of validity of patient test results is required. They must follow policies and procedures, maintain records, adhere to quality control policies, follow established corrective action policies and be capable of identifying problems and document corrective actions.

Testing personnel (high complexity)

Testing personnel are responsible for specimen processing, test performance and reporting of test results as authorized by the director. They must follow policies and procedures, maintain records, adhere to quality control policies, be capable of identifying problems and document corrective actions.

20.2.6 Proficiency testing*

The proficiency testing (PT) requirements of CLIA '88 have been perceived by the laboratory community as excessive and potentially punitive. Because proficiency testing failure is associated with severe sanctions including exclusion from testing, many believe that proficiency testing has been given status as a complete and sufficient surrogate for laboratory quality which is undeserved because of the documented limitations of proficiency testing (Boone, 1992). These include non-identity to human samples; inability of PT samples to reliably assess all instrument and reagent systems; delay in development of PT for new methods, and the influence of matrix-effects. Because of these and other factors, many believe that HCFA should incorporate safeguards to prevent the imposition of sanctions during an appeal process that is being conducted to determine if a PT failure was a true participant failure or a PT system failure. When the PT programme recognizes a system failure, those challenges that cannot be graded should be considered as 'acceptable' for determining the score.

The requirements of the regulations for proficiency testing have been summarized as follows (College of American Pathologists and American Society of Clinical Pathologists, 1992):

1. Each laboratory performing tests of moderate and/or high complexity must enrol in an approved proficiency testing programme for each specialty or subspecialty for which it seeks certification.
2. For previously regulated laboratories this requirement became effective on 1 September, 1992. Newly regulated laboratories are required to enrol in an approved PT programme by 1 January, 1994. Currently regulated laboratories are required to continue their participation in PT. Participation in PT for gynecologic cytology is required by 1994 but there appears to be no possibility that a programme will be available by that date.
3. The laboratory must notify HCFA of the approved programme(s) in which it chooses to participate, authorize the PT programme to release all data to HCFA, and for tests that are not subject to PT in these regulations, establish the accuracy and reliability of its test procedures at least twice a year. The laboratory must participate in an approved PT programme for one year and must notify HCFA before the laboratory changes PT programmes.
4. PT samples must be tested with the laboratory's regular patient workload, using routine testing methods, by personnel who routinely perform testing. The individual testing the samples and the laboratory director must attest to the routine integration of samples.
5. Laboratories that perform PT must not engage in any interlaboratory communication concerning the results until after the date the results are due to the PT programme. This includes communication between laboratories with multiple testing sites or separate locations.
6. The laboratory must not send PT samples to another laboratory and any laboratory that receives proficiency testing samples from another laboratory must notify HCFA. A laboratory's certificate will be revoked for at least one year if HCFA determines that the laboratory intentionally referred PT samples to another laboratory. The laboratory must document the handling, preparation, processing, examination and each step in the testing and reporting of PT results. The laboratory must also maintain a copy of all records, including the form used to record the PT results (including the attestation signatures), for a minimum of two years.
7. PT is required for only the test system, assays or examination used as the primary method for patient testing. The laboratory must also have a system that twice a year evaluates and defines the relationship between test results using different methodologies, reagents or instruments.
8. A laboratory must successfully participate in a PT programme approved by HCFA. 'Unsuccessful proficiency testing performance' is a 'condition level' deficiency and may result in laboratory sanctions such as suspension of the CLIA certificate and Medicare payments for the specialty, subspecialty or analyte involved. Failure to achieve an overall testing event score of satisfactory performance for two consecutive testing events or two out of three consecutive testing events is unsuccessful performance.
9. If a certificate is suspended and/or Medicare approval is terminated the laboratory must demonstrate sustained successful performance on two consecutive PT events before HFCA will consider reinstatement of the certificate for the specialty or subspecialty.
10. Failure to attain an overall testing event score of at least 80% is unsatisfactory performance for all specialties and subspecialties except ABO

---

* Also termed external quality assessment (see Chapter 19).

group and D(Rho) typing and compatibility testing (100% score required). Failure to participate in a testing event is unsatisfactory performance; however, consideration may be given to the laboratory failing to participate only if patient testing was suspended during the testing event and the laboratory notified the inspecting agency and PT programme within the time frame for submitting results that patient testing was suspended. In addition, the laboratory must have participated in the previous two testing events. Failure to return PT results for a testing event is unsatisfactory performance.

11. For any unsatisfactory testing event for reasons other than failure to participate, the laboratory must undertake appropriate training and employ the technical assistance necessary to correct the problem. All remedial action must be documented and maintained for two years.

12. For a proficiency testing programme to receive HCFA approval, it must be offered by a private nonprofit organization or a federal or state agency or entity acting as an agent for the state. The approved programme must provide technical assistance to laboratories seeking to qualify under the programme. The programme must be able to report individual laboratory performance on testing events to HCFA on a timely basis. PT report forms must include an attestation statement that PT samples were tested in the same manner as patient specimens with a signature block to be completed by the laboratory director and individual performing the test.

13. As a general rule, the PT programme must provide a minimum of five samples per testing event with at least three testing events per year. The shipments may be provided to the laboratory through mailed shipments, or, at HCFA's option, to HCFA or its agents for on site testing in the laboratory.

20.2.7 Quality control

The regulations itemize general and specific quality control (QC) standards that require each laboratory to establish and follow written quality control procedures for monitoring and evaluating the quality of the analytic process of each method to assure the accuracy and reliability of patient test results and reports. Until 1994, instruments, kits or test systems categorized as moderate complexity which have been approved by the FDA for *in vitro* diagnostic use are subject to minimal QC requirements based upon the manufacturer's instructions. For each test system, the laboratory must have a procedure manual, perform calibration procedures at least once every 6 months and perform QC with at least two levels of control each day that the test system is used. Tests of moderate complexity that have been developed 'in-house' or

FDA-approved tests that have been modified by the laboratory are subject to the full QC requirements.

The FDA will continue to evaluate products as meeting CLIA requirements for QC. The announced intent is that two years after the effective date of regulations (1 September, 1994), laboratories using tests of either moderate or high complexity which have been cleared by FDA may follow the manufacturer's instructions for much of the general QC. Laboratories using tests not cleared in this manner must follow all applicable QC requirements including standards for maintaining acceptable test methods, equipment, reagents and materials, guidelines for procedure manuals, establishment and verification of test performance specifications, calibration and control procedures, corrective actions to be taken when problems arise and QC records.

Additional specific QC requirements are listed for each specialty or subspecialty, including the subspecialties of microbiology, diagnostic immunology and chemistry, as well as hematology, cytology, histopathology, oral pathology, radiobioassay, histocompatibility, clinical cytogenetics, immunohematology and transfusion services and blood banking.

20.2.8 Patient test management

The regulations specify requirements for specimen submission and handling, test requisitions, records and reports as well as specimen referral. The laboratory may perform tests only at the written or electronic request of an individual authorized under state law to order and/or receive test results. Written authorization for oral requests must be obtained within 30 days and any test result indicating an 'imminent life-threatening condition' must be reported immediately to the individual or entity requesting the test or the individual responsible for utilizing test results. The laboratory is also required to make available a list of test methods and performance specifications.

20.2.9 Clinical laboratory improvement advisory committee (CLIAC)

The Secretary of the Department of Health and Human Services has appointed a Clinical Laboratory Improvement Advisory Committee (CLIAC) which will meet several times per year and is comprised of individuals involved in the provision or utilization of laboratory services and the development of testing. The committee reviews and makes recommendations concerning criteria for categorizing tests as moderate or high complexity, tests for inclusion in the waivered category, personnel standards, proficiency testing and quality control standards, patient test management, quality assurance standards and the applicability of the standards to new technology.

CLIAC has met on several occasions since its first meeting in October 1992 and has recommended changes pertaining to method classification (HDL-cholesterol and microbiology testing); additions to the waived test list (hemoglobin testing by 'single analyte instruments with self-contained or component features to perform specimen/reagent interaction, providing direct measurement and readout'); and recommended the creation of a physician-performed microscopy category (PPM) composed of tests most of which are of moderate complexity, are characterized by specimen lability or problems in transportation and have limited available QC. These tests (vaginal wet preps, KOH skin preparations, postcoital exam, Fern test, pinworm test, urine sediment examination, fecal leukocyte examination and wet mount examination of prostatic secretions) may be performed under the PPM category by physicians for their own patients at the time of patient visit and will be subject to inspection only under very limited circumstances. CLIAC has further recommended that Gram stains, Tzanck smears, quantitative semen analysis, histodermatology slides, polarization microscopy of synovial fluid and leukocyte differential counts not be included in PPM but agreed to include nurse practitioners, nurse midwives, pediatric nurse practitioners and physician's assistants in the personnel category for PPM. In general, most of the recommendations of CLIAC have been accepted by the DHHS or may be eventually included in the anticipated 'final' Final Rule.

Other recommendations made by CLIAC include:

1. Liberal 'grandfathering' of individuals currently performing testing or serving in supervisory positions.
2. Supported CDC recommendations for new protocols for waived status and requested CDC review of existing waived tests.
3. Endorsed modified criteria that define waived testing as 'simple laboratory examinations and procedures which have an insignificant risk of producing an erroneous laboratory testing result' and recommended deletion of previous language that related to 'risk of harm if performed incorrectly'.

20.2.10 Enforcement, inspection and sanctions

The regulations require every laboratory that is subject to CLIA regulations to undergo inspection at least once every two years. The inspection will be performed by one of 53 state or territorial agencies under contract to the Department of Health & Human Services (DHHS), unless the laboratory is located within a state that has been deemed to be exempt or has been accredited by an approved, private non-profit programme. The inspections are to be performed utilizing very specific inspection guidelines developed and recently published by HCFA (DHHS, 1993)

Failure to meet the standards of the regulations may result in sanctions applicable to all laboratories subject to CLIA. The Health Care Financing Administration (HCFA) has been given broad authority to limit or suspend CLIA certificates and impose sanctions that may include mandated and on-site supervised corrective action plans; substantial monetary penalties; suspension, limitation or revocation of the CLIA certification; criminal penalties including imprisonment for those convicted of intentional violations. For Medicare-participating laboratories, sanctions may also include suspension of payments.

Prior to CLIA '88, approximately half of the 12 000 or so hospital and independent laboratories subject to federal regulation because they provided service to Medicare patients or because they were engaged in interstate commerce, were inspected either by the College of American Pathologists (CAP) or the Joint Commission on Accreditation of Healthcare Organizations (JCAHO), the remainder by state survey agencies. Current HCFA statistics, based on a total of approximately 150 000 laboratory requests for certification applications, indicate that from the greatly expanded universe of laboratories subject to federal inspection requirements, 18% will seek accreditation via state exemption or from a private accrediting organization, 43% will request waived status, 11% will register in the category of Physician Performed Microscopy, and the remaining laboratories including a large number of physician office laboratories, will be inspected by the Federal Government, presumably by state survey agencies, organizations of widely variable but often limited resources.

DHHS or the designated organization will perform announced or unannounced, biennial inspections during which the laboratory will be expected to perform proficiency testing, provide access to records and documentation, allow employees to be interviewed, and allow inspection of all areas of the facility. The regulations provide for approval of private non-profit organizations as accrediting agencies and for extending exemption to states that maintain standards equal to or more stringent than those developed by the Secretary of DHHS. The State of Washington, the Commission on Office Laboratory Accreditation (COLA), a professional organization providing accreditation to physician office laboratories, the CAP and the JCAHO have been approved for deemed status. Applications have been received from New York State, the Commonwealth of Puerto Rico and the American Society for Histocompatibility and Immunogenetics (ASHI). The American Association of Blood Banks (AABB) and the American Osteopathic Association (AOA) have indicated their intent to apply.

Inspection by state survey agencies of previously unregulated laboratories began on 1 March 1993 and approximately 13000 facilities had been inspected by the end of January 1994. Previously regulated laboratories will not be inspected under this mechanism if they have indicated that they will maintain accreditation with an organization that has applied for deemed status or if they are located within a state that has applied for exempt status.

20.2.11 Evolution of CLIA '88

Although many of the major components of CLIA '88 have been implemented, the final form is far from complete. The evolution of the regulations has taken place within a matrix of competing political influences and professional constituencies. A 'final' Final Rule is expected to be released sometime in 1994 and will presumably reflect the commentaries received in response to the Final Rule of February 1992 and the Technical Corrections of January 1993, as well as the continuing recommendations of CLIAC. Continuing regulatory revisions are likely and many informed individuals anticipate the possibility of legislative modification. A significant group of practising physicians wishes to pursue the goal of repeal of CLIA '88 provisions that apply to physician office laboratories.

Areas of major controversy that may lead to modification of the regulations include:

1. The waived category and Physician Performed Microscopy: The physician community and organized medicine will continue to seek to increase the scope of testing available to practising physicians without a requirement for significant regulatory oversight. These efforts are likely to be opposed by many professional laboratory organizations who will stress the need for equivalent regulations, a 'level playing field', and strict construction of the site-neutral provisions of the enabling legislation.
2. In a parallel effort to facilitate the introduction of new technology with less stringent regulatory burdens, the manufacturers of laboratory equipment and tests will continue to argue persuasively about the increasing reliability and robust nature of emerging instrumentation and methods. They will support their arguments by bundling new solid-state auto-calibrated technology with robust and automatic quality controls (Burke, 1993).
3. Personnel standards will continue to be perhaps the most difficult and controversial aspect of CLIA '88. The debate concerning the need to make existing personnel requirements more or less stringent will centre around discussions of the need for quality standards versus considerations of cost and access.
4. Regulations pertaining to cytology testing and cytology proficiency testing requirements, which have not been discussed in this chapter, may prove to be the hardest to implement without imposing an inordinate burden of cost and subsequent restriction of access. It is now clear that the cytology

regulations will not be implemented as currently published but will undergo substantial revision and modification.

20.3 Standards established by professional organizations

20.3.1 Joint commission on accreditation of healthcare organizations

In recent years, the efforts of the Joint Commission on Accreditation of Healthcare Organizations (JCAHO) have been central and seminal in influencing and altering professional standards of performance in hospitals and other healthcare facilities. Through educational efforts and by virtue of the critical importance of achievement of JCAHO accreditation, a renewed emphasis on continual quality improvement (CQI) by the JCAHO coupled with an exhaustive revision of JCAHO accreditation standards have produced major changes in the application of professional standards in healthcare in general and specifically in clinical laboratories.

Prior to implementation of the 'Agenda for Change', an initiative for streamlining and refocusing assessment criteria begun seven years ago by the JCAHO, the standard-setting and monitoring process emphasized a detailed and prescriptive review of individual performance standards organized by traditional hospital and department-based categories. In recent years, a stepwise transition has taken place to a more flexible and less categorical approach to standard setting. Although the implementation of change has been characterized by varying degrees of difficulty in transferring conceptual change to the JCAHO field surveyors, the process of standard revisions that the JCAHO has undertaken has increasingly reflected the following assumptions and principles concerning quality improvement and the establishment of professional standards of performance (Bachner, 1990; JCAHO Appendix B, 1993):

1. Performance assessment is viewed in terms of structure, process and outcomes coupled with a somewhat delayed recognition (in the opinion of the authors) that an exclusive concentration on outcome is not possible because the causes of many beneficial healthcare outcomes are unknown and, if known, the practitioners and organizations do not control the causes.
2. A decreased emphasis on implicit review (peer review) usually stimulated by complications or 'errors' and based upon subjective criteria performed by different reviewers with an exclusive focus on practitioner performance, or medical audits using 'pre-defined' but not necessarily objective criteria.

3. A shift to continuous monitoring characterized by priority setting and by the use of indicators. Trends and patterns are studied, not just individual cases identified by problems.
4. An increased focus on effectiveness, appropriateness and on education that recognizes the desire of professionals to improve performance standards and skills.
5. Augmented stress on information management, utilization of human resources and a recognition that multiple causative factors determine patient outcomes.
6. A reduced emphasis on traditional departments and disciplines which, in the laboratory, will lead to more concentrated attention upon the total analytic cycle including test selection, patient and specimen preparation, test performance and interpretation, result reporting and timeliness, and the relationship of those components to patient outcomes.
7. An approach to standard setting and monitoring that is not primarily practitioner-focused, punitive or based upon unrealistic expectations, but rather emphasizes issues of appropriateness, efficiency and cost-effectiveness. These issues are of increasing importance to society but may conflict with professional principles.
8. An attempt to base performance standards on data that link local practice to processes and outcomes in other institutions.

For the past several years and as a direct result of the change in emphasis of the JCAHO, certain conflicts developed between pathologists and JCAHO surveyors (inspectors), because of a Joint Commission Standard that stated that the laboratory director was responsible for the implementation of the monitoring and evaluation process in regard to appropriateness of testing. The Standards of the JCAHO now reflect a more moderate and realistic position and state that the director of the laboratory service will monitor and evaluate the appropriate use of testing in conjunction with the medical staff, but will not be held responsible for the development and implementation of professional standards for test utilization.

Specific standards for pathology and laboratory services have been recently published as the *Accreditation Manual for Pathology and Clinical Laboratory Services* (JCAHO, 1993). These standards and scoring guidelines will be utilized in JCAHO surveys as of January 1994 and supersede laboratory standards in previous programme manuals for hospitals and other healthcare facilities. The revised laboratory standards reflect a significant elimination of redundant standards, modification of standards pertaining to decentralized testing and adaptation of standards to the requirements of CLIA '88. Specific standards and scoring guidelines for hematology and other laboratories are defined under general categories of laboratory directorship and the responsibility of the director; space, equipment, and supplies; records and reporting; communication within and outside of the laboratory; quality control and reliability of data; specific requirements for autopsy, blood transfusion and clinical pathology services.

20.3.2 College of American Pathologists

The College of American Pathologists has been involved in clinical laboratory professional standard setting in two principal areas.

Interlaboratory Comparison Programmes – The CAP began providing unknown, mailed specimens to laboratories in the early 1950s pursuant to studies (Belk and Sunderman, 1947) demonstrating significant variance between test results reported for certain analytes in patient samples by different laboratories. These initial pilot efforts ultimately resulted in the development of the CAP 'Surveys' programme which, by 1960, encompassed virtually all clinical laboratory disciplines.

The original purpose of the interlaboratory comparison programme was to stimulate laboratory improvement by allowing comparison of individual analytical results for an 'unknown' sample with those reported by all other participant laboratories. Awareness of reported values that were significantly deviant from a 'target' value or 'state of the art' capability (acceptable) would stimulate the laboratory to improve its analytical proficiency. This interlaboratory comparison process became recognized as one component of 'external' quality control. Over the ensuing years there was continual evolution of value assignment methodology and grading techniques under the continuing supervision of CAP expert 'resource' committees.

In the early 1960s the CAP Laboratory Accreditation Programme (see below) established a requirement that any laboratory wishing to be accredited must have an 'external' quality programme in place and be enrolled in 'Surveys' in all areas (specialties, subspecialties and analytes) in which it was performing analytical testing.

Interlaboratory comparisons (CAP Surveys) have since become more widely and generically referred to as proficiency testing (PT). Proficiency testing was incorporated as a regulatory requirement for Medicare and CLIA '67, and is a major component of the CLIA '88 regulations. It has become the principal means through which the government 'grades' laboratories, and can be used to deny licensure or limit testing.

Despite certain scientific limitations inherent in the use of artificially prepared, unknown analytical samples, interlaboratory comparisons, or external quality control, or proficiency testing, has become a professional 'standard of practice' for clinical laboratories.

Laboratory Accreditation – In the early 1960s the College of American Pathologists introduced the Laboratory Accreditation Programme. It was initiated as a laboratory improvement programme that encompassed several fundamental principles, and was intended to foster progressively increasing reliability and accuracy of analytical results through continuing education and on-site inspections of laboratories by knowledgeable laboratorians ('peer' review). Participation was, and continues to be, voluntary, although many laboratories have satisfied federal (Medicare and CLIA '67) requirements by virtue of CAP accreditation and a 'sub-deemed' relationship between CAP and the JCAHO.

The accreditation process was based upon broadly based 'standards' which specified a level of performance that must be attained by a laboratory if it was to attain 'accredited' status. The assessment of whether or not a laboratory satisfied the standards was accomplished through an on-site visit (or inspection) by one to several 'working' laboratorians (a team) led by a team leader who had to meet several criteria (e.g. be from an accredited laboratory, attended a training seminar or workshop, etc.). Initially, the on-site inspection was performed every three years; however when the programme was recognized as being 'equivalent to or more stringent than' the requirements set forth in CLIA '67, inspections for those laboratories using CAP accreditation for purposes of exemption from federal licensure were done annually as provided for in CLIA '67. Several years later, both the federal government and CAP modified the annual requirement and on-site inspections were done every two years (biennially). At that time, the CAP converted to a biennial cycle for all the laboratories that were participants in the Accreditation Programme. The two-year cycle (with a requirement for an interim 'self-inspection') has continued to date and has been incorporated into the CLIA '88 regulations.

The basic process for inspecting and accrediting laboratories in the context of the CAP Laboratory Accreditation Programme is an on-site visit by a team of practising laboratorians who use a series of 'checklists' as a guide to assess whether the defined standards are being met. The checklist questions are specifically designed to assist the inspector(s) in identifying activities which would ordinarily have to be carried out for a facility to satisfy the standards. Inspector observations are reported to the participant laboratory which must respond to observed problems, ('deficiencies') and areas needing improvement by submitting acceptable documentation that corrective actions have been implemented. The inspection coupled with monitoring of Survey (PT) performance is the basis of the accreditation decision, i.e. granting or denying accreditations.

This process has evolved to become a recognized professional standard. The checklists of the Commission on Laboratory Accreditation constitute a series of laboratory (discipline)-specific questions that define standards of required (phase II deficiencies) and recommended (phase I deficiencies) performance that encompass diverse and exhaustive aspects of laboratory and professional practice including directorship and supervision; space and facilities; equipment; test performance; quality control and assurance of analytic and non-analytic events; proficiency testing, safety and others. The checklists are subject to periodic review and revision by the resource committee structure of the CAP under the direction of a Checklist Commissioner and the full Commission.

The JCAHO uses a similar process for assessing laboratory performance as a component of its hospital accreditation programme. A number of states have and continue to inspect and licence (accredit) laboratories using on-site inspection and proficiency testing performance as the assessment tools. The federal government adopted this basic approach for Medicare and CLIA '67 regulations, and continues to utilize the methodology for CLIA '88.

At the present time, one of the principal differences between the various government and JCAHO programmes and the CAP accreditation programme is that the former employ inspectors on a full-time basis, thus they are not 'actively working' laboratorians. These organizations usually utilize one or two (in the case of very large facilities) inspectors for the on-site inspection. CAP inspection teams generally number 2–7 individuals all of whom are actively working in laboratories and serve in a voluntary capacity. Where specialty areas of testing are involved, individuals with experience and expertise in those areas are generally included. Rarely, if ever, is a laboratory inspected on more than one occasion by the same team.

On-site inspection, in conjunction with on-going monitoring of proficiency testing, to evaluate laboratory performance with respect to meeting professional standards has become 'state of the art' clinical laboratory practice. Professionally-driven standard setting can be expected to continue to contribute to excellence in clinical laboratory practice now that the CAP and JCAHO accreditation programme and other programmes sponsored by professional organizations are granted 'deemed status' by HCFA for purposes of CLIA 1988 inspection.

20.3.3 Practice guidelines and other standard-setting activities

In recent years, in an attempt to reduce inappropriate care and limit geographic variations in practice patterns, many national physician and medical specialty societies have issued and are actively generating systematic approaches to management and problem-solving in clinical medicine. Many of these attempts, variously referred to as practice guidelines, practice parameters, etc., incorporate recommendations concerning aspects of clinical laboratory practice. In addition, academic medical centres and independent organizations have developed guidelines. More recently, state governments, insurance companies, third-party payers and managed care organizations have implemented processes to generate guidelines for practice (Nash, 1990; Woolf, 1990).

The impetus to guideline development has been supported by the Omnibus Reconciliation Act of 1989, signed into law by President Bush in December 1989 (Public Law 101–239), that established the Agency for Health Care Policy and Research (AHCPR). In addition, other federal sources of guidelines such as the National Institutes of Health (NIH), Centers for Disease Control (CDC), Food and Drug Administration (FDA) and Office of Technology Assessment have added to this growing body of knowledge and opinion that will contribute to the process of standard setting.

Many organizations including the American Society of Clinical Pathologists and the College of American Pathologists have implemented programmes to generate practice guidelines relevant to clinical laboratories. The CAP has prepared or has in development practice guidelines pertaining to hemochromatosis; autopsy practice; fresh frozen plasma, cryoprecipitate and platelet utilization; placental pathology; testing strategies and others (College of American Pathologists, 1993).

The Q-PROBES programme of the College of American Pathologists (Bachner and Howanitz, 1991) represents an attempt to describe actual laboratory practice in peer-referenced laboratory settings with the expectation that aggregate data derived from these studies may improve individual laboratory performance and serve as a 'substrate' for guideline development. However, such descriptive 'benchmarking' programmes will need to demonstrate firm linkages to patient outcome measurements to fulfil their promise. In order to contribute to better and more efficient patient care, all forms of practice guidelines will need to be derived from experience and supported by data that describe actual practice that has been shown to be associated with desirable patient outcomes. Professional organizations with responsibilities for standard setting will need to be vigilant to guard against the inappropriate and premature use of practice guidelines in a punitive and prescriptive mode or as a 'fig leaf' for cost containment at the expense of patient care and standards of practice that have been validated by professional experience and judgement.

Many other organizations that have not been specifically mentioned in this review continue to make major contributions to professional and scientific standard setting activities in the USA and abroad. These include the National Committee for Clinical Laboratory Standards (NCCLS), the National Reference System for the Clinical Laboratory (NRSCL), the American Association for Clinical Chemistry (AACC), the American Society for Microbiology (ASM), the International Federation of Clinical Chemistry (IFCC), the European Committee for Clinical Laboratory Standards (ECCLS), the National Institute of Standards and Technology (NIST), and, of course, the sponsoring organization for this text, the International Council for Standardization in Hematology (ICSH). Their efforts, and those of others not mentioned, will continue to provide the scientific resources and professional judgement that will always constitute the bedrock of professional standard setting activities.

20.3.4 Other countries

Various countries have approached the question of accreditation in different ways. In some, participation in a national external quality assessment scheme (see Chapter 19) suffices; in others the control of laboratories is undertaken by professional associations who have the authority to issue licences which may be legally mandatory or if not, then at least virtually essential in order to comply with the requirements of health insurance schemes or other major purchasers of laboratory services, or recognition of the laboratory as being acceptable for training and certification of technical, scientific or medical staff.

In the UK an accreditation scheme was introduced in 1991 (Royal College of Pathologists, 1991). It is run as a non-profit organization, the Board of which includes representatives of the Royal College of Pathologists and other professional bodies as well as national health authorities. The requirements for accreditation are broadly similar to those in the USA, but separate departments or disciplines apply for accreditation rather than the pathology laboratory as a whole. Participation is not (as yet) mandatory; the interest which was aroused and the flow of applications to participate from laboratories, both in the public and the private sectors, suggest that there will be little need for legal compulsion for the professions themselves to ensure that a satisfactory standard is maintained.

In Germany there is a legal obligation for medical laboratories to participate in appropriate quality assurances programmes for quantitative analyses in accordance with a regulatory framework the implementation of which is assigned to a designated authority. In most other coutries in Western Europe the professions have taken responsibility for organizing and administering quality assessment and accreditation schemes.

Laboratory medicine is not unique in requiring accreditation. Quality standards have been specified by the International Standards Organization for any laboratory operating a calibration and measurement system. These specifications, which are documented as ISO 9000 series, include *Guidelines for Selection and Use of Quality Management and Quality Assurance Standards*, and models for different aspects of quality assurance. Equivalent standards have been established for the European Union (EN 29000), and they have also been adapted for use at a national level in many countries either under the ISO 9000 or EN 29000 label, or with another national identification, e.g. BS 5750 in Britain, ANSI/ASQC Q90–94 in USA, DIN ISO 9000 in Germany, AS 3900 in Australia, JIS Z 9900 in Japan. More recently, ISO has also established standards for auditing quality systems (ISO 10011 series)

In some countries authoritative bodies have been set up to certify that laboratory practice conforms to this standard. Thus, for example, in the UK, where it is known as the National Measurement Accreditation Service (NAMAS), it is directed by the Government authorized National Physical Laboratory. Similar bodies exist in Australia (NATA), Hong Kong (HOKLAS), and in most countries of Western Europe, Whilst these organizations have been set up primarily for laboratories concerned with chemical analysis and physical measurement, they might, in principle, equally be the instrument for accreditation of clinical laboratories. It is, thus, of interest to note the requirements which must be satisfied in accordance with the NAMAS Accreditation regulations (NAMAS document P5, 1992):

General
Organization and management
Quality system
Staff
Equipment
Measurement traceability and calibration
Methods and procedures for calibration and tests
Laboratory accommodation and environment
Handling of calibration and test items
Records
Calibration certificates, test reports and test certificates
Participation in inter-laboratory comparison programmes and measurement audits
Handling of complaints
Subcontracting of calibrations or tests
Outside support services and supplies
Responsibility as an accredited laboratory

When a laboratory is to be assessed there is a one-day preliminary visit by a technical officer in order to study the quality system and to advise the laboratory on any apparent non-compliance with the NAMAS requirements. This informal visitation is then followed by a full assessment by a group of independent assessors, the number of whom depending on the schedule of activities in the laboratory.

After accreditation has been granted there is an annual re-inspection to ensure continuance of compliance.

The accreditation schemes described above have agreements for mutual multilateral recognition; these agreements are especially valuable in the areas of international science and industry. By virtue of informal professional contacts the schemes which have been established for clinical laboratory show similarities in their organization and function. It might be equally useful for these schemes, too, to be harmonized in a more formal way.*

20.3.5 Conclusions

Professional autonomy and standard setting have always been the integral and related foundations of medical practice and clinical laboratory science. Within the last few decades, increasing encroachment by government regulations into standard setting – an area previously the exclusive domain of professionals – has been a source of dismay for professionals and has, in addition, redirected the efforts of professional organizations to conforming their own standard setting activities to those of government regulators. Somewhat to the surprise of professionals, the loss of professional autonomy (Mirvis, 1993) has been generally supported by a growing public demand for assessment and accountability, Relman's 'third revolution' in medical care (Relman, 1988).

The ability of professional organizations in medicine and clinical laboratory practice to respond to these trends has been hampered by the fragmentation of these organizations and their varied perceptions of the professional, social and economic impacts of regulatory events. We hope that the dual goals of limiting the role of government regulation and the restoration of professional standard setting activities to the proper source of these efforts – clinical laboratory professionals and their organizations – will serve to foster unity of action and a continuing emphasis on the care and needs of patients as well as excellence and continuing improvement in clinical laboratory practice (Berwick, 1989).

References

American Association of Blood Banks (1990) Accreditation Requirements Manual, 3rd edn, 1117 N. 19th Street, Suite 600, Arlington, VA 22209.

Bachner, P. (1990) College of American Pathologists Conference XVII on Quality Assurance in Pathology and

---

* The authors appreciate the contribution of the section on Other countries (20.3.4) by S. M. Lewis.

Laboratory Medicine: Summary. *Arch. Pathol. Lab. Med.*, **114**, 1175–1177.

Bachner, P. (1991) Quality Improvement in the modern clinical laboratory: The regulatory and accreditation perspective. *Disease Markers*, **10**, 27–35.

Bachner, P. and Howanitz, P. J. (1991) Using Q-Probes to improve the quality of laboratory medicine: A quality improvement program of the College of American Pathologists. *Quality Assurance in Health Care*, **3**, 167–177.

Belk, W. P. and Sunderman, F. W. (1947) A survey of the accuracy of chemical analyses in clinical laboratories. *Am. J. Clin. Pathol.*, **17**, 853.

Berwick, D. M. (1989) Continuous improvement as an ideal in health care. *N. Engl. J. Med.*, **320**, 53–56.

Boone, D. J. (1992) Literature review of research related to the Clinical Laboratory Improvement Amendments of 1988. *Arch. Pathol. Lab. Med.*, **116**, 681–693.

Bureau of National Affairs, Inc. (1990) Occupational exposure to hazardous chemicals in laboratories. Washington, DC., p. 96.

Burke, M. D. (1993) Turnaround time, point-of-care testing, and a future role for the clinical pathologist. *Am. J. Clin. Pathol.*, **100**, 89–90.

29 Code of Federal Regulations Part 1910.1030 (1991) *Federal Register*. December 6, 56 (No. 235): 64175–64182.

29 Code of Federal Regulations Part 1910.1048 (1992) *Federal Register*. May 27, 56 (No. 102): 22310.

42 Code of Federal Regulations Part 405, *et al.* (1992) *Federal Register*. February 28, 57 (No. 40) 7138–7243.

42 Code of Federal Regulations Part 493, *et al.* (1993) *Federal Register*. January 19, 58 (No. 11): 5215–5237.

College of American Pathologists and American Society of Clinical Pathologists (1992) A summary of major provisions of the Final Rules implementing the Clinical Laboratory Improvement Amendments of 1988. Northfield, ILL: College of American Pathologists. 60093–2750.

College of American Pathologists (1993) Glenn, G. C. CAP Practice Guidelines Status Report. Northfield, ILL: College of American Pathologists. 60093–2750.

Department of Health and Human Services (1993) Appendix C, Survey Procedures and Interpretive Guidelines for Laboratories and Laboratory Services, State Operations Manual. Publication number PB 92–146174. Available from National Technical Information Service, US Department of Commerce, 5285 Port Royal Road, Springfield, VA 22161, 703–487–4650, 800–336–4700.

Derman, H. and Dorsey, D. B. (1991) The pathology of regulation. *Clin. Lab. Med.*, **11**, 793–802.

Joint Commission on Accreditation of Healthcare Organizations (1993) Accreditation Manual for Pathology and Clinical Laboratory Services: Standards and Scoring Guidelines, Appendix A and B. JCAHO, One Renaissance Boulevard, Oakbrook Terrace, ILL. 60181.

Mirvis, D. M. (1993) Physicians' autonomy – the relation between public and professional expectations. *N. Engl. J. Med.*, **328**, 1346–1349.

Nash, D. B. (1990) Practice guidelines and outcomes: Where are we headed? *Arch. Pathol. Lab. Med.*, **114**, 1122–1125.

Relman, A. S. (1988) Assessment and accountability: the Third revolution in medical care. *N. Engl. J. Med.*, **319**, 1220–1222.

Royal College of Pathologists (1991) Pathology department accreditation in the United Kingdom: a synopsis. *J. Clin. Pathol.*, **44**, 798–802.

Woolf, S. H. (1990) Practice guidelines: A new reality in medicine. I. Recent developments. *Arch. Intern. Med.*, **150**, 1811–1818.

Index